OXFORD MEDICAL PUBLICATIONS

Oxford Handbook of
Clinical Immunology

Oxford Handbook of Clinical Immunology

GAVIN SPICKETT

Consultant and Senior Lecturer in Clinical Immunology,
Head of Regional Immunology Services,
Royal Victoria Infirmary,
Newcastle upon Tyne, UK

OXFORD
UNIVERSITY PRESS

OXFORD

UNIVERSITY PRESS

Oxford University Press, Great Clarendon Street, Oxford OX2 6DP

Oxford New York

Athens Auckland Bangkok Bogota Buenos Aires Calcutta
Cape Town Chennai Dar es Salaam Delhi Florence Hong Kong Istanbul
Karachi Kuala Lumpur Madrid Melbourne Mexico City Mumbai
Nairobi Paris São Paulo Singapore Taipei Tokyo Toronto Warsaw

and associated companies in
Berlin Ibadan

Oxford is a trade mark of Oxford University Press

Published in the United States
by Oxford University Press Inc., New York

British Library Cataloguing in Publication Data
Spickett, Gavin.
Oxford handbook of clinical immunology / Gavin Spickett.
(Oxford medical publications) Includes index.
1. Clinical immunology–Handbooks, manuals, etc. 2. Immunologic
diseases–Diagnosis–Handbooks, manuals, etc. I. Title.
II. Title: Handbook of clinical immunology. III. Series.
[DNLM: 1. Immunologic Diseases–diagnosis handbooks.
2. Immunologic Tests handbooks. WD 301 S754 1999]
RC582.S66 1999 616.07′9–dc21 98-51592
ISBN 0 19 262721 X (flexi)
Library of Congress Cataloging in Publication Data
(Data applied for)
1 3 5 7 10 8 6 4 2
ISBN 0 19 262721 X
Typeset by AMA DataSet, Preston, Lancs
Printed in Great Britain on acid free paper by
The Bath Press, Bath

Contents

Acknowledgements

Jan Klein said of the first edition of his textbook of immunology that he wrote the book for selfish reasons. I too have written this book for selfish reasons: this is the book that I wish I had had when I was starting out on my career in clinical immunology: most of the information needed to make the right decisions never seemed to be available, although now we are better served with better books and easier access to information. I hope therefore that trainees in immunology, laboratory staff carrying out immunological tests, and other interested doctors and scientists will also find it helpful. As it is written for selfish reasons, it also contains all my prejudices and reflects my own clinical and laboratory interests. Equally, the errors of commission and omission are also all mine. I would, however, welcome comments and suggestions against the possibility of further editions and for my own education.

This book is not meant to be read like a novel: it is for reference, to answer the 101 questions that land on an immunologist's desk. I hope, too, that it will increase awareness about the rational use of immunology tests and of clinical immunology problems, particularly primary immunodeficiency. This book is not a textbook of medicine: I have concentrated as far as possible only on the immunological aspects of disease, but there is no medical specialty which is not touched on somewhere. In reality clinical immunologists are probably the only true 'general' physicians, as they have to have an understanding of all other disciplines (particularly when answering obscure questions from organ-specific specialists).

I am grateful to my wife, Sally, for her patience while the manuscript took shape; as ever the whole project took longer than anticipated. I am also grateful to OUP. Many individuals have helped shape this book through their professional input to my own training and through enlightening discussions. Primacy in the list must go to Don Mason, David Webster, Helen Chapel, and John Ledingham, who taught me immunology. I am grateful to Mark Gompels and Claire Bethune for helpful discussions over various draft chapters, and to the staff of the Regional Immunology Laboratory at the RVI for their advice on technical matters on occasions too numerous to recall. I also thank my paediatric immunologist colleagues, Andrew Cant, Mario Abinun, and Terry Flood, and also my consultant colleagues, Anne Fay and Desa Lilic, again for many helpful discussions about particular points. What follows is a distillation of the experience of all of these colleagues and others too numerous to mention.

I enjoyed writing this book (well most of the time!), so I hope you will enjoy the finished version.

Abbreviations

ABPA	allergic bronchopulmonary aspergillosis
ACA	anti-cardiolipin antibody
ACE	angiotensin converting enzyme
ACh	acetylcholine
AChRAb	anti-acetylcholine-receptor antibody
ACTH	adrenocorticotrophic hormone
ADA	adenosine deaminase
ADCC	antibody-dependent cell-mediated cytotoxicity
AECA	anti-endothelial cell antibody
AGA	anti-gliadin antibodies
AIDS	acquired immune deficiency syndrome
AIHA	idiopathic autoimmune haemolytic anaemia
AIRE	autoimmune regulator
ALG	anti-lymphocyte globulin
ALL	acute lymphoblastic leukaemia
AMA	anti-mitochondrial antibody
AML	acute myeloid leukaemia
ANA	antinuclear antibody
ANCA	anti-neutrophil cytoplasmic antibody
APCED	autoimmune polyendocrinopathy candidiasis ectodermal dysplasia
APGS	autoimmune polyglandular syndrome
APP	amyloid-precursor protein
APTT	activated partial thromboplastin time
AS	ankylosing spondylitis
ASOT	antistreptolysin O titre
α-1AT	α-1-antitrypsin
AT	ataxia telangiectasia
ATG	anti-thymocyte globulin
AZT	azidothymidine (zidovudine)
BAL	bronchoalveolar lavage
BCG	bacille Calmette Guérin
BCOADC	branch-chain 2-oxo-acid dehydrogenase complex
BIS	bias index score
BM	bone marrow
BMT	bone marrow therapy
BSI	British Society for Immunology
CAH	chronic active hepatitis
CALLA	common acute lymphoblastic leukaemia antigen
cAMP	cyclic adenosine monophosphate
C-ANCA	cytoplasmic ANCA
CCV	chosen coefficient of variance
2CDA	2-chloro-deoxyadenosine
CF	cystic fibrosis
CFS	chronic fatigue syndrome
CGD	chronic granulomatous disease
CHAD	cold haemolytic disease
CHH	cartilage hair hypoplasia

CHIMP	Commission for Health Improvement
CID	combined immunodeficiency
CIDP	chronic inflammatory demyelinating polyneuropathy
CJD	Creutzfeldt Jakob disease
CK	creatine kinase
CLL	chronic lymphocytic leukaemia
CMC	chronic mucocutaneous candidiasis
CME	continuing medical education
CMI	cell-mediated immunity
CML	chronic myeloid leukaemia
CMV	cytomegalovirus
ConA	concanavalin A
COPD	chronic obstructive pulmonary disease
CPA	Clinical Pathology Accreditation
CPSM	Council for Professions Supplementary to Medicine
Cr&E	creatinine and electolytes
CREST	calcinosis, Raynaud's, oesophageal dysmotility, sclerodactyly, and telangiectasia
CRF	chronic renal failure
CRP	C-reactive protein
CSF	cerebrospinal fluid
CSF-1	colony-stimulating factor-1
CSS	Churg-Strauss syndrome
CT	computed tomography
CTD	connective tissue disease
CTLP	cytotoxic T-lymphocyte precursor
CVA	cerebrovascular accident
CVID	common variable immunodeficiency
CxR	chest X-ray
CyA	cyclosporin A
DAF	decay accelerating factor
dATP	deoxy-adenosine triphosphate
DCT	direct Coombs test
dGTP	deoxy-guanosine triphosphate
DH	dermatitis herpetiformis
DIC	disseminated intravascular coagulation
DIF	direct immunofluorescence
DM	dermatomyositis
DMARDs	disease modifying drugs anti-rheumatic drugs
DNA	deoxyribonucleic acid
DPT	diphtheria, pertussis and tetanus
dRVVT	dilute Russell's viper venom test
dsDNA	double-stranded DNA
DTH	delayed-type hypersensitivity
DV	designated value
DVT	deep vein thrombosis
EA	early antigen
EAA	extrinsic allergic alveolitis
EBNA	EBV nuclear antigen
EBV	Epstein Barr virus
ECG	electrocardiogram

ECP	eosinophil cationic protein
EDTA	ethylenediaminetetraacetic acid
EGF	epidermal growth factor
EIA	enzyme-linked immunoassay
ELISA	enzyme-linked immunosorbent assay
EM	electron microscopy
EMA	endomysial antibodies
EMG	electromyogram
ENA	extractable nuclear antigen
ENT	ear, nose, and throat
EPD	enzyme-potentiated desensitization
EPO	erythropoeitin
EQA	external quality assessment
ESR	erythrocyte sedimentation rate
Fbc	full blood count
FcR	Fc receptor
FCS	fetal calf serum
FEV_1	forced expired volume (one second)
FFA	free fatty acid
FFP	fresh frozen plasma
FITC	fluorescein isothiocyanate
FMF	familial Mediterranean fever
fMLP	N-formyl-methionyl-leucyl-phenylalanine
FSH	follicle-stimulating hormone
FT3	free triiodothyronine
FT4	free thyroxine
FVC	forced vital capacity
GABA	γ-aminobutyric acid
GAD	glutamic acid carboxylase
GBM	glomerular basement membrane
GBS	Guillain-Barré syndrome
GCA	giant-cell arteritis
G-CSF	granulocyte colony stimulating factor
GDP	guanosine diphosphate
GFD	gluten-free diet
GFR	glomerular filtration rate
GI	gastrointestinal
GLP	good laboratory practice
GM-CSF	granulocyte macrophage colony stimulating factor
GN	glomerulonephritis
GP	glycoprotein
GPC	gastric parietal cell
G6PD	glucose 6-phosphate dehydrogenase
GS-ANA	granulocyte anti-nuclear antibody
GTN	glyceryl trinitrate
GvHD	graft-versus-host disease
GvL	graft-versus-leukaemia
HAE	hereditary angioedema
H&E	haematoxylin and eosin
HANE	hereditary angioneurotic oedema

Hb	haemoglobin
HCL	hairy cell leukaemia
HCV	hepatitis C virus
HD	Hodgkin's disease
hdIVIg	high-dose intravenous immunoglobulin
HEp-2	human epithelial cell line
HGV	hepatitis G virus
HHV	human herpes virus
Hib	*Haemophilus influenzae* type b
HIGE	hyper-IgE syndrome
HIGM	hyper-IgM
HIV	human immunodeficiency virus
HLA	human leucocyte antigen
HRF	homologous restriction factor
HRT	hormone replacement therapy
Hsp	heat-shock protein
HSP	Henoch-Schönlein purpura
HSV	herpes simplex virus
5-HT	5-hydroxytryptamine (serotonin)
HTLP	helper-T lymphocyte precursor
HTLV-1	human T-cell leukaemia virus-1
ICAM	intercellular adhesion molecule
ICF	immunodeficiency, centromeric instability and abnormal facies
ID	intradermal
IDDM	insulin-dependent diabetes mellitus
IDT	intradermal test
IEF	immunoelectrophoresis
IF	intrinsic factor
IFN	interferon
Ig	immunoglobulin
IGF1-R	insulin-like growth factor-1 receptor
IIF	indirect immunofluorescence
IL	interleukin
IM	intramuscular(ly)
IMIg	intramuscular immunoglobulin
INR	international normalized ratio
IPF	idiopathic pulmonary fibrosis
ISCOMS	immunostimulatory complexes
ITP	immune thrombocytopenia
ITU	intensive care unit
IU	international units
IV	intravenous(ly)
IVIg	intravenous immunoglobulin
JCA	juvenile chronic arthritis
LAC	lupus anti-coagulant
LAD	leucocyte adhesion defect
LAK	lymphokine-activated killer cell
LC	liver cytosol
LDH	lactate dehydrogenase
LE	lupus erythematosus

LEMS	Lambert-Eaton myasthenic syndrome
LFA	lymphocyte function antigen
LFT	liver function test
LG	lymphomatoid granulomatosis
LGL	large granular lymphocyte
LIF	leukaemia inhibitory factor
LKM	liver-kidney microsomal antibodies
LM	liver microsome
LP	lumbar puncture
LPS	lipopolysaccharide
LYDMA	lymphocyte-determined membrane antigen
MAbs	monoclonal antibodies
MAG	myelin-associated glycoprotein
MAOI	monoamine-oxidase inhibitor
MBP	mannan-binding protein
MCP	macrophage chemolactic peptide
MCTD	mixed connective tissue disease
MCV	mean corpuscular volume
'ME'	'myalgic encephalomyelitis'
MFE	materno-fetal engraftment
$\beta2MG$	$\beta2$-microglobulin
MG	myasthenia gravis
MHC	major histocompatibility complex
MIS	misclassification score
MLA	medical laboratory assistant
MLR	mixed lymphocyte reaction
MLSO	medical laboratory scientific officer (Biomedical Scientist)
MMR	measles, mumps, and rubella virus
MND	multiple nuclear dots
M-PAN	microscopic polyarteritis
MPGN	membranoproliferative glomerulonephritis
MPO	myeloperoxidase
MRBIS	mean running bias index score
MRCP	Member of the Royal College of Physicians
MRCPath	Member of the Royal College of Pathologists
MRI	magnetic resonance imaging
MRVIS	mean running variance index score
MS	multiple sclerosis
MSA	mitotic spindle antigens
MUD	matched unrelated donor
NADPH	reduced nicotinamide adenine dinucleotide phosphate
NAP	neutrophil alkaline phosphatase
NAQAP	National Quality Assurance Panel
NARES	non-allergic rhinitis with eosinophilia
NB	*nota bene*
NBT	nitroblue tetrazolium test
NCAM	neuronal cell and lesion molecule
NEQAS	National External Quality Assurance Scheme
NF-AT	nuclear factor of activated T cells
NHL	non-Hodgkin's lymphoma

rbcs	red blood cells
RFLP	restriction fragment length polymorphism
RFT	respiratory function tests
RhA	rheumatoid arthritis
RhF	rheumatoid factor
RIA	radioimmunoassay
RID	radial immunodiffusion
RNA	ribonucleic acid
RNP	ribonucleoprotein
rRNP	ribosomal ribonucleoprotein
RS	Reed-Sternberg
SAA	serum amyloid A
SAC	*Staphylococcus* strain A Cowan
SAP	serum amyloid P
SBE	subacute bacterial endocarditis
SC	subcutaneous(ly)
SCAT	sheep-cell agglutination test
SCID	severe combined immunodeficiency
SCIg	subcutaneous immunoglobulin
Scl	scleroderma
SD	standard deviation
SERPIN	serine protease inhibitor
SIFTR	service increment for teaching and research
SLA	soluble liver antigens
SLE	systemic lupus erythematosus
SLVL	splenic lymphoma with circulating villous lymphocytes
Sm	Smith antibodies
SMA	smooth-muscle antibodies
SOP	standard operating procedure
SPET	single-photon emission tomography
SPT	skin-prick test
SRP	signal recognition particle
SS	Sjögren's syndrome
ssDNA	single-stranded DNA
SSP-PCR	sequence-specific primer PCR
stat.	immediately
SV40	simian virus 40
T3	triiodothyronine
T4	thyroxine
TAME	tosyl-L-arginine methyl ester
TB	tuberculosis
TC	transcobalamin
Tcr	T cell receptor
TdT	terminal deoxytransferase
TFT	thyroid function tests
TGF	T-cell growth factor
TGSI	thyroid growth stimulating antibody
Th1	T helper-1
Th2	T helper-2
THI	transient hypogammaglobulinaemia of infancy
TIA	transient ischaemic attack

TLI	total lymphoid irradiation
TNF	tumour necrosis factor
TPMT	thiopurine methyltransferase
TPN	total parenteral nutrition
TPO	thyroid peroxidase
TSH	thyroid stimulating hormone
TSH-R	thyroid stimulating hormone receptor
TSI	thyroid stimulating antibody
TTP	thrombotic thrombocytopenic purpura
UC	ulcerative colitis
UV	ultraviolet
VCA	viral capsid antigen
VCAM	vascular cell adhesion molecule
VCF	velocardiofacial syndrome
VDRL	Venereal Disease Research Laboratory
VI	variance index
VIP	vasoactive intestinal polypeptide
VIS	variance index score
VKH	Vogt-Koyanagi-Harada syndrome
VLA	very late antigen
VNTR	variable N-terminal repeat analysis
vWF	von Willebrand factor
VZV	varicella zoster virus
WAS	Wiskott-Aldrich syndrome
WASP	Wiskott-Aldrich-associated protein
WG	Wegener's granulomatosis
XLA	X-linked agammaglobulinaemia
XLPS	X-linked lymphoproliferative syndrome
ZAP	zeta-associated protein

Dedication

To the memory of the late Charles Newman, who inspired me to continue with a career in medicine, when I was assailed by doubts about my chosen path.

1 Introduction

For some obscure reason almost all books on clinical immunology seem to begin with an introductory chapter on the basic science of immunology. I have never followed the logic behind this, as the chapters are usually too brief to be of significant value, and anyway become obsolete rapidly. I intend therefore to forego the pleasure, and firmly suggest that readers find their way to a good up-to-date textbook of basic immunology (of which there are many, written by professional scientists rather than a clinician!). So all of you who hoped to read about the minutiae of the effects of interleukin-39 on CD4+ CD28- CD192+ T cells are, I am afraid, going to be sorely disappointed. However, I do promise that when such information becomes remotely relevant to managing a patient with an immunological disease it will be included.

This brings me to the purpose of this book, which is to provide a pocket reference for the diagnosis of immunological disease and, conversely, the interpretation of immunological tests. The first part of the book concentrates on the clinical diseases and detail has been provided where this is lacking in readily available textbooks. However, I have not sought simply to replicate the mass of information available in excellent reference works but to extract the important detail and give practical guidance on test selection and interpretation for both diagnosis and monitoring. Treatment is always difficult because concepts on treatment are always changing, and even well-established drugs can be used in better ways. Accordingly, although a lot of information is given on drug therapy, the reader is advised to check for up-to-date regimes and doses before embarking on treatment.

Part 2 is devoted to the individual tests used in immunological diagnosis, giving a précis of the methodology and pitfalls and advantages of each test. It is not, however, an immunological recipe book. Hopefully, it will be helpful for all those who have to sign out laboratory reports and even more for those receiving the reports and acting on them. The two parts therefore complement each other.

Clinical immunology in the UK has undergone a radical overhaul with the advent of the Calman specialist registrars. There are now two clear paths to follow, each leading to specialist accreditation: allergy or clinical immunology. Both require a broad training in general internal medicine before the specialist training commences and both training programmes place considerable emphasis on obtaining a core knowledge of basic laboratory skills, basic science, and developing clinical skills.

Laboratories are sited in major regional and sub-regional centres, although there is still a shortfall of consultant posts, with many existing consultants working single-handed. To a greater or lesser extent, these regional centres oversee the immunological testing that takes place in smaller district hospitals, often under the wing of other pathological disciplines.

Clinical immunology has developed a strong clinical base now, with most centres undertaking the direct care of patients with immunological problems and overseeing immunotherapies. Good laboratory support is essential. The major interest of most centres is in primary immunodeficiencies, which for the majority is antibody deficiency. However, it is essential that clinical immunologists can recognize the rare immunodeficiencies and ensure that they are referred to appropriate quaternary centres for treatment. In the UK there are two supra-regional referral centres for the diagnosis and management of severe combined immunodeficiency, one based at Great Ormond Street (London) and one at Newcastle General Hospital (Newcastle upon Tyne). Despite the increased number of clinical immunologists over the past 20 years (and the band is still very select), the average diagnostic delay for antibody-deficient patients has not changed much and is still around 6–8 years.

Many immunological treatments are very expensive and this has led to often heated debate about cost effectiveness. A particular example is the use of β-interferon for relapsing multiple sclerosis (MS), where both overt and covert rationing has occurred, and different health districts have developed different funding policies, so that a patient might be treated if she lived in one place but not if she moved to a different place. In a state-funded healthcare system, these debates need to become more rational and the resulting policies should be applied fairly to all.

The latest medical fad is 'evidence-based medicine': it is true that in many cases, including much immunological therapy, the evidence to support a particular approach is lacking and in some cases, such as the prophylactic use of penicillin in adult asplenic patients, will never be obtained. Although it is important to have guidelines and standards, one must never lose sight of the fact that medicine is an art not a science, and reducing one's decision making to the level of a dreary meta-analysis of half-forgotten and best-forgotten trials denies the value of experience of dealing with patients. Each patient is a learning experience far more valuable than any mountain of paper, and should form the peg on which one's personal knowledge base is hung. So my caution to those at the foot of the mountain: make sure you take every opportunity to involve yourself with your patients and learn from them. No text-book will ever teach you what they can.

Books are like friends: everyone's choice will be different. The following will be helpful in your journey through immunology:

Bradley, J. and McCluskey, J. (1997). *Clinical immunology*. Oxford University Press, Oxford.

Colvin, R. B., Khan, A. K., and McCluskey, R. T. (ed.) (1994). *Diagnostic immunopathology*, (2nd edn). Raven Press, New York.

Kay, A. B. (ed.) (1997). *Allergy and allergic disease*. Blackwell Science, Oxford.

Lawlor, G. J., Fischer, T. J., and Adelman, D. C. (1995). *Manual of allergy and immunology*, (3rd edn). Little Brown, Boston.

Maddison, P. J., Isenberg, D. A., Woo, P., and Glass, D. N. (1998). *Oxford textbook of rheumatology*, (2nd edn). Oxford University Press, Oxford.

Male, D., Cooke, A., Owen, M., Trowsdale, J., and Champion, B. (1996). *Advanced immunology*, Mosby, Philadelphia.

Paul, W. E. (ed.) (1999). *Fundamental immunology*, (4th edn). Lippincott-Raven, Philadelphia.

Peters, J. B. and Shoenfeld, Y. (ed.) (1996). *Autoantibodies*. Elsevier, Amsterdam.

Rich, R. R. (ed.) (1995). *Clinical immunology. Principles and practice*. Mosby, Philadelphia.

Stites, D. P., Terr, A. I., and Parslow, T. G. (1997). *Medical immunology*, (9th edn). Prentice-Hall International, Englewood Cliffs, New Jersey.

Weatherall, D. J., Ledingham, J. G. G., and Warrell, D. A. (1996). *Oxford textbook of medicine*, (3rd edn). Oxford University Press, Oxford.

In addition very useful information is containing in the following review periodicals:

Annual Review of Immunology
Advances in Immunology
Seminars in Immunology
Current Opinion in Immunology
Current Opinion in Rheumatology
Immunology Today
Immunological Reviews

Introduction

In general, immunodeficiencies are divided into those of the specific immune system (e.g. T cells or B cells) or those of the innate or non-specific immune system (e.g. complement and neutrophils). The age at which the patient presents gives good but not absolute clues as to the type of immune deficiency; for instance, severe combined immune deficiency (SCID) will present within the first 6 months of life. The type of infection also gives excellent clues as to the nature of the underlying immune defect. For example, recurrent meningococcal infection is a major feature of complement deficiency, while persistent respiratory syncytial virus infection in a small baby should raise the question of SCID. Other associated features also provide clues, for example ataxia (unsteadiness on the feet) together with bacterial infections suggests ataxia telangiectasia.

Immunodeficiencies may also be divided into primary (usually genetic) and secondary, where the immune defect is caused by some other non-immunological disease; for example a glycogen storage disease that causes a neutrophil defect, or a drug (for example phenytoin). Sometimes the distinction is blurred; for example, the AIDS virus (HIV-1) infects CD4+ T lymphocytes and macrophages and alters their functional capacity. This is usually referred to as a secondary immunodeficiency, despite the 'primary' effect on T cells (see Chapter 3 for a further discussion of secondary immunodeficiencies).

All patients with primary immunodeficiencies should be under the care of an immunologist, who will be familiar with the range of complications.

Causes of immunodeficiency

Genetic

- Autosomal recessive
- Autosomal dominant
- X-linked
- Gene deletions, rearrangements

Biochemical and metabolic

- Adenosine deaminase deficiency
- Purine nucleoside phosphorylase (PNP) deficiency
- Biotin-dependent multiple carboxylase deficiency
- Deficient membrane glycoproteins

Vitamin or mineral deficiency

- Zinc deficiency
- B12 deficiency
- Biotin

Undefined Primary

- Common variable immunodeficiency
- Specific antibody deficiency
- IgG subclass deficiency
- IgA deficiency

Maturational

- Transient hypogammaglobulinaemia of infancy

Secondary (see Chapter 3)

- Viral infections (HIV, CMV, EBV, rubella)
- Chronic infections (TB, leishmania)
- Malignancy
- Lymphoma/leukaemia
- Extremes of age
- Transfusion therapy
- Drugs
- Plasmapheresis
- Radiation
- Nutrition
- Chronic renal disease (including dialysis)
- Toxins (including alcohol, cigarettes)
- Splenectomy

Clinical features of immunodeficiency

Recurrent infections

There is no universally accepted definition of what constitutes 'recurrent infection' and therefore it is difficult to be categorical about who should be investigated for immunodeficiency. The following should be used as guidance:
* two major or one major and recurrent minor in 1 year;
* unusual organisms (*Aspergillus*, *Pneumocystis*);
* unusual sites (liver abscess, osteomyelitis);
* chronic infections (sinusitis);
* structural damage (e.g. bronchiectasis);
* other suspicious features.

A number of other features should raise suspicion of an underlying immunodeficiency:
* skin rash (atypical eczema): Wiskott–Aldrich syndrome, hyper-IgE syndrome, Omenn's syndrome;
* chronic diarrhoea: SCID, antibody deficiencies;
* failure to thrive: any immune deficiency in childhood;
* hepatosplenomegaly: common variable immunodeficiency (CVID), Omenn's syndrome;
* chronic osteomyelitis/deep-seated abscesses: chronic granulomatous disease;
* mouth ulceration (? cyclical): neutropenia;
* autoimmunity: CVID, hyper-IgM syndrome;
* family history.

Features associated with specific immunodeficiencies

Some features are diagnostic of particular immunodeficiencies:
* ataxia: ataxia telangiectasia, PNP deficiency;
* telangiectasia: ataxia telangiectasia;
* short-limbed dwarfism: X-linked immunodeficiency;
* skeletal abnormalities: ribs in ADA deficiency;
* cartilage–hair hypoplasia;
* ectodermal dysplasia;
* endocrinopathy (particularly with hypocalcaemia): chronic mucocutaneous candidiasis;
* partial albinism: Chediak–Higashi disease; Griscelli syndrome;
* thrombocytopenia (particularly with small platelets): X-linked thrombocytopenia, Wiskott–Aldrich syndrome;
* eczema: Wiskott–Aldrich syndrome, hyper-IgE syndrome, Omenn's syndrome;
* neonatal tetany: 22q11 deletion syndromes (DiGeorge);
* abnormal facies (leonine; fish-shaped mouth, low-set ears): hyper-IgE (leonine), 22q11 deletion syndrome (fish-shaped mouth, low-set ears), ICF syndrome (see below);
* mental retardation: 22q11 deletion syndromes, PNP deficiency, other genetic immunodeficiencies.

Investigation of immunodeficiency

History

This should include a history of all infections: site, severity, need for antibiotics, hospitalizations, operations (grommets, lobectomies, etc.); immunization history; family history, especially for serious infections, unexplained sudden deaths, diagnosed immunodeficiencies, and autoimmune diseases.

Examination

Particular features to pay attention to include:
• weight and height (failure to thrive);
• structural damage from infections (ears, sinuses, lungs);
• autoimmune features: vitiligo, alopecia, goitre;
• other suspicious/diagnostic features, as above.

Laboratory investigation

The nature of investigations undertaken should depend upon the immunodeficiency suspected and tests should be selected accordingly; there is no place for blanket screening. Equally, tests should only be done if they will affect materially either the diagnosis or the management of patients; for example, phytohaemagglutinin (PHA) proliferation is often abnormal in CVID but does not help in diagnosis (it may even confuse matters) and contributes nothing to management.

B-cell function

Full evaluation of the humoral immune system requires that all the parts are present AND functioning. The latter usually requires *in vivo* test immunization, bearing in mind the caveat that no patient with suspected immunodeficiency should receive live vaccines. The following tests comprise a full screen of humoral function:
• serum immunoglobulins (be sure to use low-level detection system for IgA to confirm absence);
• serum and urine electrophoresis (evidence for bands and urinary loss);
• IgG subclasses;
• IgE;
• antibacterial, antiviral antibodies;
• immunization responses (protein and polysaccharide antigens);
• isohaemagglutinins (IgM);
• B lymphocyte numbers;
• pokeweed mitogen (PWM) and antigen-stimulated antibody production *in vitro* (not mandatory).

T-cell function

Tests of T-cell function are less easy and less reliable than for B cells, where antibody provides a convenient read-out. 'Normal' ranges for *in vitro* proliferation assays are quite wide. It is essential that absolute T-cell counts are used, not percentages.
- T-cell numbers and surface phenotype,
  CD2, CD3, CD4, CD8, CD7, Tcr ($\alpha\beta$, $\gamma\delta$), CD40L, MHC class II
- CD40-ligand expression on activated T cells
- T-cell proliferation to antigens, mitogens (PHA, phorbol myristate acetate (PMA), ionophore, cytokines)
- T-cell cytokine production
- *In vivo* skin (delayed-type hypersensitivity, DTH) testing: the Multitest CMI is a convenient tool, but responses will depend on prior exposure

Neutrophil function

Neutrophil function tests are not widely available, so if there is suspicion of a neutrophil defect, specialist help should be sought. Interpretation is difficult and tests may be influenced by intercurrent infection and drug therapy.
- Neutrophil markers (CD11a, CD11b, CD11c, CD18, CD15)
- Up-regulation of neutrophil markers (PMA, fMLP)
- Oxidative metabolism (nitroblue tetrazolium reduction (NBT test), etc.)
- Phagocytosis
- Bacterial killing (relevant organisms should be selected)
- Chemotaxis (difficult to standardize, with wide normal range)

NK-cell function

This is of research use only at present.
- NK-cell numbers
- K562 killing assay
- Cytokine-stimulated killing (lymphokine-activated killer cell (LAK) assay)

Complement assays

- Measurement of specific components
- Functional assays (haemolytic assays)

Genetic studies

Genetic studies form an essential part of the investigation and management of primary immunodeficiencies:
- cytogenetics (deletions, translocations);
- Ig and Tcr gene rearrangements (clonality);
- X-linked gene studies;
- 22q11 microdeletions (FISH – fluorescent in situ hybridization);

- MHC studies;
- prenatal diagnosis.

Other investigations

The use of other investigative procedures depends very much on the clinical state of the patient.

- Detection of autoimmunity:
  - anti-red cell, platelet, neutrophil antibodies
  - anti-endocrine autoimmunity
- Exclusion of secondary causes:
  - renal disease, bowel disease (loss of immunoglobulins ± cells)
  - malignancy (lymph-node biopsy)
  - nutrition
  - drugs (cytotoxics, anticonvulsants)
- Detection of nodular lymphoid hyperplasia (bowel radiography)
- Lung function
- Imaging studies (lungs, sinuses)
- Direct isolation of pathogens: bacteria, fungal, and viral (serology is usually unreliable)

ANTIBODY DEFICIENCY SYNDROMES

Major B-lymphocyte disorders

- X-linked agammaglobulinaemia (Bruton's agammaglobulinaemia; XLA)
- Common variable immunodeficiency (acquired hypogammaglobulinaemia; CVID)
- Selective IgA deficiency
- IgG subclass deficiency
- Specific antibody deficiency

Rare B-lymphocyte disorders

- X-linked hyper-IgM syndrome (HIGM-1)[1]
- X-linked hypogammaglobulinaemia with growth hormone deficiency
- Selective IgM deficiency
- X-linked lymphoproliferative syndrome (Duncan's syndrome; XLPS)
- Hyper-IgE syndrome (Job's syndrome)
- Transient hypogammaglobulinaemia of infancy
- Mu-chain deficiency

---

1 As the defect in X-linked HIGM is a defect in expression of the ligand for CD40 on T cells (gp39) this disease may now be classified with T cell defects. However, the predominant abnormality is antibody deficiency.

X-linked agammaglobulinaemia (XLA)

Cause

This is a genetic disorder due to a mutation on the X chromosome affecting the *btk* gene, coding for a tyrosine kinase involved in B-cell maturation. Defects in the gene prevent B-cell maturation from pro-B cell to pre-B cell. The gene is located at Xq21.3–22. Mutations include deletions and point mutations, either conservative or leading to premature termination, with a phenotype that correlates poorly with the type of genetic abnormality. Mild phenotypes occur with some limited B-cell development. New mutations are common, so a family history may be absent. A similar defect has been described in mice, the *xid* mutation, although the features differ somewhat.

Presentation

Presentation is usually early in childhood, after 6 months of age, when maternal antibody has largely disappeared. Recurrent infections of lungs and ears (children of this age don't have sinuses) with *Haemophilus influenzae* and pneumococci are usual. Meningitis and septic arthritis (staphylococci) are also common at presentation. Milder phenotypes may present later.

Diagnosis

The history of early onset bacterial infections in a male child with a family history gives the game away; however, a family history is often absent. Neutropenia is very common at presentation but goes away with treatment and is probably due to chronic bacterial sepsis. There will often be failure to thrive and chronic diarrhoea.

The distinction of milder forms, with some B cells and low but not absent IgG, from CVID is difficult and relies on the demonstration of abnormalities of the *btk* gene. It is likely that some patients previously classified as CVID will turn out to be XLA.

XLA may rarely be associated with growth hormone deficiency (and short stature) and occasional females will be identified with the immunological features of XLA.

The differential diagnosis will include coeliac disease and cystic fibrosis, although the laboratory tests will rapidly identify antibody deficiency.

Immunology

In the complete forms the immunology is fairly distinctive:
- all immunoglobulins are absent or very low;
- B cells are low or absent;
- lymph nodes show no germinal centres; no tonsils; pre-B cells in bone marrow (BM);
- T-cell numbers and function are normal;
- NK-cell numbers and function are normal.

Mild or incomplete variants may be difficult to distinguish from CVID and may have some B cells and some residual antibody production.

Complications

The major complications relate to delay in diagnosis, leading to structural lung damage (bronchiectasis). Inadequate therapy will lead to progression of lung damage and the development of chronic sinus damage.

A chronic meningoencephalitis due to echoviruses and cox-sackieviruses may cause a progressive and fatal dementing illness; there is often muscle involvement, with a myositis and contractures. Diagnosis is by viral culture of CSF or by PCR-based techniques. No treatment appears to be helpful, although a new anti-viral is undergoing trials. This disease appears less often since the intro-duction of intravenous immunoglobulin (IVIg) therapy as standard, but it has not disappeared completely.

Ureaplasma/Mycoplasma septic arthritis may occur. This is difficult to diagnose without special culture facilities. It is a highly destructive chronic infection and requires prolonged treatment (6 months) with tetracyclines ± erythromycin.

It has been suggested that there may be an increased risk of colonic cancer.

Treatment

IVIg should be started at the earliest opportunity (Chapter 10), using a dose of 200–600 mg/kg/month given at intervals of 2–3 weeks. Longer intervals do not give satisfactory replacement. Trough IgG levels should be monitored regularly, with the aim of maintaining a level well within the normal range. Early institution of IVIg precludes the development of bronchiectasis.

Great care should be taken of the chest, with prompt antibiotic therapy (course of 10–14 days) together with physiotherapy and postural drainage if lung damage has already occurred. Ciprofloxacin is a valuable antibiotic (though not licensed for small children).

As children get older, regular lung function testing should be carried out; CT scanning is useful for identifying subclinical bronchiectasis, but imposes a significant radiation burden and should not be overused. Limited (three-cut) scanning may be better.

No oral poliovaccine should be given to these patients as they often fail to clear it, which increases the risk of reversion to wild type, with consequent paralytic disease.

Genetic studies of the patient and family will allow genetic coun-selling for carriers.

Common variable immunodeficiency (CVID)

Cause

The cause of CVID is unknown: one hypothesis suggests that an environmental insult (virus infection?) in a genetically susceptible individual triggers the disease. No conclusive viral trigger has been identified. There is some evidence for a genetic background (linked to MHC A1B8DR3C4Q0) and there may be a family history of other antibody deficiencies (especially IgA deficiency and IgG subclass deficiency) in up to 50 per cent of cases, although other family members may be entirely asymptomatic. The disease is heterogeneous.

Presentation

CVID may present at any age from childhood through to old age, although the peak of presentation is in early childhood and early adulthood.

The usual presentation is with recurrent bacterial infections, as for XLA. However, autoimmune problems, especially thrombocytopenia, haemolytic anaemia, and organ-specific autoimmunity (e.g. thyroid, diabetes, vitiligo, and alopecia), are common and may precede the development of recurrent infections.

Nodular lymphoid hyperplasia of bowel (polyclonal hyperplasia of Peyer's patches) is unique to CVID. The cause is unknown, but it is possibly premalignant. This has characteristic features on small-bowel radiology.

Granulomatous disease with lymphadenopathy and (hepato-) splenomegaly, and often involving the lung, is common in the severe form of CVID (about 25 per cent of cases). This disease resembles sarcoidosis, but is Kveim-test negative (although this test is now rarely used).

Diagnosis

The history gives the clues. Unfortunately the clues are usually missed by general physicians and an average diagnostic delay of over 7 years is typical, by which time structural lung and sinus damage is severe and irretrievable.

Immunoglobulin levels are variably low: test immunization and exclusion of secondary loss may be required.

There is frequently a lymphopenia affecting predominately the CD4+ T cells (CD45RA+ naïve cells in particular) and B cells.

When splenomegaly is present it may be difficult to exclude lymphoma, without CT scanning, lymph node biopsy, and bone marrow examination.

Immunology

Immunoglobulin levels are highly variable, and IgG may be only marginally reduced; specific antibodies are invariably low with poor/absent immunization responses. The IgM may be normal, which contrasts with lymphoma, when the IgM is the first immunoglobulin to drop (Chapter 3).

B cells may be normal or low but some cases may be late-presenting XLA in males.

There are low levels of CD4+ T cells, with specific depletion of CD45RA+ T cells. T-cell function *in vivo* and *in vitro* to antigens and mitogens is poor and there is poor NK-cell function, with reduced NK-cell numbers.

Abnormalities of 5'-nucleotidase activity on the lymphocyte surface have been described but this is not a separate syndrome as is sometimes stated. The significance of the abnormality is not known.

Classification

Three groups are identified on the basis of B-cell responses to IL-2 + anti-IgM *in vitro*:
- group A: severe disease, with granulomata (hepatosplenomegaly); no IgG or IgM production *in vitro*;
- group B: rare; IgM production only *in vitro* (?cryptic hyper-IgM);
- group C: mild disease; IgG and IgM production *in vitro*.

Complications

The major complications of CVID relate to the delay in diagnosis, with bronchiectasis and chronic sinusitis major features. Patients may also have unusual infections, such as *Campylobacter* cholangitis, and *Mycoplasma/Ureaplasma* arthritis (see XLA). Rarely, opportunist infections such as *Pneumocystis* occur.

Malabsorption may occur due to a coeliac-like enteropathy, with villous atrophy. Inflammatory bowel disease may occur with strictures.

In group A patients with splenomegaly, hypersplenism may occur with marked thrombocytopenia: splenectomy may be required.

There is a 40-fold increase in the risk of lymphoma, including intestinal lymphoma, and also a large increase in gastric carcinoma, not related to *Helicobacter pylori* colonization. Any patient with lymphadenopathy should have a lymph node biopsy and bone marrow examination to exclude the diagnosis. Lymphomas are often high grade and respond poorly to treatment.

Autoimmune disease is common and patients should be monitored for the development of overt disease (hypothyroidism, pernicious anaemia, diabetes).

Thymomas (benign or malignant) are also associated with CVID. These frequently give rise to myasthenia gravis and with haematological problems such as aplastic anaemia and immune thrombocytopenia (ITP).

Treatment

The earlier the diagnosis is made, the better the prognosis. The treatment is identical to that of XLA, with IVIg, antibiotics, and physiotherapy for chest disease. However, patients with complete IgA deficiency have a higher risk of developing anti-IgA antibodies to IVIg therapy, and a product low in IgA should be selected for them; anti-IgA antibodies should be checked at regular intervals. Patients with splenomegaly may catabolize IgG faster and may require larger doses or more frequent doses (weekly)

Regular lung function tests and limited chest CT scanning is advisable. Chronic sinus disease requires ENT review, with endoscopic inspection.

The granulomatous disease responds well to steroids (alkaline phosphatase is a good marker); these are essential if there is interstitial lung disease (reduced transfer factor). They are not necessary for asymptomatic splenomegaly. Splenectomy may be necessary for hypersplenism: such patients must have prophylactic penicillin, but immunizations are of little value. There is, however, an additional risk of infection splenectomy in CVID patients and caution is required.

A close watch must be kept for the development of malignant disease.

Selective IgA deficiency

Selective IgA deficiency is the most common primary immuno-deficiency, but mostly passes unnoticed. Depending on the racial group, between 1 in 400–800 individuals will be affected.

Cause

The cause is unknown, although it forms part of the spectrum of disease with CVID and shares the MHC type (A1, B8, DR3, C4Q0). It occurs in relatives of patients with CVID in 50 per cent of cases. Rarely it is due to a gene deletion, often including IgG2/IgG4. It has also been associated with other chromosomal abnormalities, usually involving chromosome 18 (18q syndrome and ring chromosome 18).

It is associated with drug therapy, particularly with phenytoin and penicillamine, although in many reports it is not clear whether the defect was present before drug therapy was introduced.

IgA-bearing B cells are present. IgA is synthesized but not secreted. In terms of mucosal protection, there is evidence that IgG and IgM may substitute as secretory Igs.

Presentation

- Most cases are asymptomatic. There is an increased incidence of allergic disease, connective tissue diseases (SLE, rheumatoid arthritis, and juvenile chronic arthritis), coeliac disease, and pernicious anaemia.
- Infections are rarely a problem unless there are additional humoral defects present.
- Occasional cases will come to light as a result of adverse reactions to blood products.

Diagnosis

- This requires the demonstration of undetectable IgA, NOT just a low IgA. Automated analysers do not read low enough to ascertain this beyond doubt.
- Patients should be screened for evidence of other humoral defects: IgG subclasses and specific antibodies. If there is doubt, then test immunization should be undertaken.
- Patients should be screened for anti-IgA antibodies.

Immunology

- The IgA will be undetectable (<0.05 g/l), but total IgG and IgM will be normal. IgG subclasses may be reduced (G2 and G4). Secreted IgA will be absent (secretory piece deficiency is vanishingly rare), but this is of little clinical value.
- T-cell function is normal (PHA and antigens).
- Autoantibodies may be present (NB anti-IgA antibodies). There will be an increased IgE in the presence of atopic disease.
- In the absence of IgA, IgM and IgG appear on mucosal surfaces

Complications

- The major problem with IgA deficiency is the possibility of transfusion reactions due to anti-IgA antibodies.
- Malignancy may be increased, although this may depend on other diseases present in association with IgA deficiency.
- It is possible that there may be progression to more significant humoral immunodeficiency with time.

Treatment

- Treatment is directed at the presenting disease.
- Avoid IgA-containing products: if blood transfusions are required, most transfusions centres are able to supply blood products from IgA-deficient donors. Use an IVIg (if required) with a low IgA content.
- Patients should be issued with a warning card (through some blood transfusion centres in the UK), or be encouraged to wear a Medic-Alert bracelet.

IgG subclass deficiency

Cause

The cause of IgG subclass deficiency is unknown, but it too forms part of the spectrum with CVID and IgA deficiency. It is possible that some cases represent CVID in evolution. Rarely, cases may be due to gene deletions, but these individuals may be entirely healthy.

IgG subclass levels are related to allotypes of IgG (Gm allotypes); different racial groups may therefore have different 'normal' ranges, depending on the prevalence of different allotypes. This should be taken into account when diagnosing IgG subclass deficiency.

Presentation

Presentation, like CVID, can be at any age. Recurrent infections may be a feature, particularly for IgG2 ± IgG4 deficiency. IgG4 deficiency occurring alone has also been associated with bronchiectasis.

Other conditions associated with subclass deficiency include: asthma (IgG3 deficiency), sinusitis (IgG3 deficiency), intractable epilepsy of childhood (though this may be due to anticonvulsants), and autoimmune disease (SLE).

Diagnosis

Measurement of IgG subclasses on more than one occasion is required and it is important to check that appropriate age-specific normal ranges are used (preferably related to the racial background).

Detection of low levels of IgG4 may require more sensitive assays to detect true absence: earlier normal ranges using less-sensitive assays found a significant number of individuals with undetectable IgG4. Most of these have detectable IgG4 on sensitive assays.

There is a poor correlation of specific anti-pathogen responses and IgG subclass levels. All patients should have specific antibodies measured and be test immunized.

Immunology

- A normal total IgG is entirely compatible with subclass deficiency, although low IgG1 usually reduces the total IgG (this also behaves like CVID for practical purposes). The IgA is normal or low; IgM is normal.
- B-cell and T-cell numbers are usually normal.
- Poor specific antibody responses may be present in some patients.

Complications

Long-term progression to CVID is a possibility. Bronchiectasis may occur in IgG4 deficiency.

Treatment

The treatment is controversial: only symptomatic patients should be treated. If recurrent infections are a problem, then the first step might be to use continuous antibiotics, followed by IVIg if infections are not controlled.

IVIg has been shown to be of benefit in asthma due to IgG3 deficiency (and, interestingly, a low IgG3 preparation worked), and in chronic sinusitis.

It is theoretically possible to bypass IgG2 deficiency using protein-conjugated polysaccharide vaccines to generate a protective IgG1 response.

Specific antibody deficiency with normal immunoglobulins

This syndrome is probably much more common than hitherto realized.

Cause

The cause is unknown. It is unrelated to IgG subclass deficiencies. There is usually a failure to respond to polysaccharide antigens (T-independent) and possibly other protein antigens (HBsAg?).

In small children, it may be due to a maturational delay that resolves spontaneously.

Presentation

Recurrent bacterial infection of upper and lower respiratory tract (*Haemophilus*, *Pneumococcus*, *Moraxella*) is the usual presentation.

In immunization programmes for hepatitis B, about 5 per cent of individuals fail to respond to the standard three-dose schedule; a fourth dose still leaves 1–2 per cent who fail to make a serological response.

Diagnosis

There is a history of recurrent typical infections with normal immunoglobulins and IgG subclasses. Proof requires demonstration of failure to respond to specific antigens (test immunization).

Immunology

Immunoglobulins and IgG subclasses are normal, but there are low specific antibodies, especially to capsulated organisms, and poor responses to test immunization, especially to polysaccharide antigens (Pneumovax®). Remember, children under the age of 2 years do not respond to Pneumovax®.

T and B lymphocyte numbers and T-cell function are normal.

Complications

The inevitable long delay in diagnosis leads to structural lung damage. The delay for such patients may be in the order of 15–20 years because clinicians fail to recognize immunodeficiency in the presence of normal total immunoglobulins.

Treatment

Treatment is still controversial. Continuous antibiotics are inadequate for patients with established lung disease: these should be managed on IVIg as for XLA. In small children, spontaneous improvement may occur.

Hyper-IgM syndrome (X-linked and autosomal)

Cause

Originally this was thought to be a B-cell disorder, but the demonstration in the X-linked form of a primary T-cell defect means that this form should be reclassified as a T-cell defect. X-linked and autosomal recessive forms have been documented. The X-linked form has now been shown to be due to a deficiency of the CD40-ligand on T cells (gene located at Xq26–27), required for B-cell immunoglobulin class switch. Some cases have been shown to have normal levels of CD40L but abnormal signalling through the CD40 on B cells.

The cause of the recessive and sporadic forms is currently unknown.

Presentation

- The presentation is with recurrent bacterial infections; this may include *Pneumocystis carinii* pneumonia.
- There is often neutropenia and thrombocytopenia. Autoimmune disease of all types is common.

Diagnosis

- There is usually an early onset; the diagnosis should always be considered when *Pneumocystis* pneumonia is the presenting illness. The differential diagnosis includes SCID and HIV infection.
- There will be a normal or high IgM, with low IgG and IgA.
- Genetic identification may be possible.

Immunology

There will be a raised IgM (and IgD) with a low IgG and IgA. However, the IgM may be normal in the absence of infection. There will be high isohaemagglutinins. Specific IgM responses are present but may be short-lived. IgM+ and IgD+ B cells are present

T-cell function may be normal or poor. Some patients have reduced cell-mediated immunity, as evidenced by the occurrence of *Pneumocystis* infection. The expression of CD40-ligand on activated T cells may be defective (use PMA + ionophore).

Mild variants exist, compatible with minimal disease and survival into adult life.

Complications

The complications include IgM+ lymphomas (due to chronic overstimulation), opportunist pneumonias, autoimmune disease, and aplastic anaemia. There appears to be a particular risk of cryptosporidial infection of the biliary tree, leading to a severe cholangitis and liver failure.

Treatment

IVIg should be started at the earliest opportunity: the IgM returns to normal range with adequate therapy. Prompt antibiotics are required for infections, as for other antibody deficiencies. All water should be boiled as domestic supplies cannot be guaranteed to be free of *Cryptosporidium*.

The involvement of T cells suggests that severe cases might benefit from bone marrow transplantation and some successful transplants have now been carried out. Liver transplantation may be required for liver disease secondary to *Cryptosporidium* infection.

X-linked lymphoproliferative disease (Duncan's syndrome)

This is a very rare genetic disorder, leading to failure to handle EBV correctly.

Cause

The genetic defect has been localized to Xq26, and the gene has now been cloned. The gene product (SLAM-associated protein) controls the activation of T and B cells via SLAM (signalling lymphocyte activation molecule), a surface protein. SLAM is involved in γ-IFN production and the switch from Th2 to Th1. The reason for the failure to handle EBV appropriately is not known.

Presentation

Patients are fit and well until EBV is encountered. Upon infection with EBV, three outcomes are possible:
- fulminant EBV (63 per cent);
- EBV+ lymphoma (24 per cent);
- immunodeficiency, usually profound hypogammaglobulinaemia (29%).

The mortality is 85 per cent by the age of 10 years.

Diagnosis

The diagnosis is difficult, especially if there is fulminant EBV infection. There are no diagnostic immunological findings. Genetics may help.

Immunology

The immunology is usually normal before infection, but it is rarely checked unless there is a family history.

After infection, in those that survive, there are reduced immunoglobulins (all three classes). T-cell proliferation to mitogens and antigens is poor, and there is reduced γ-IFN production. NK-cell function is also poor.

Treatment

Intravenous immunoglobulin should be used for the hypogammaglobulinaemia. Bone marrow transplantation may be an option, as part of the treatment of lymphoma.

Transient hypogammaglobulinaemia of infancy (THI)

Cause

THI is thought to be due to a delay in immune development, leading to a prolongation of the physiological trough of antibody after the age of 6 months, when maternal antibody has largely disappeared.

It is common in the families of patients with other antibody deficiencies.

Presentation

The usual presentation is with bacterial infections occurring after 6 months of age. It may last up to 36 months before spontaneous recovery takes place.

Diagnosis

There will be an early onset. The presence of normal B-cell numbers differentiates THI from XLA. IgM is frequently normal, and there may be evidence of specific antibody responsiveness.

However, there are no specific diagnostic features and the diagnosis can only be made for certain after full recovery of immune function has taken place.

Immunology

IgG and IgA are low for age; IgM is usually normal. B cells are present; T-cell numbers and function are normal. Vaccine responses may be normal or reduced.

Treatment

IVIg treatment may be required and should always be used for a fixed period and be withdrawn at intervals to check for spontaneous recovery.

By definition all recover! If there is no recovery, then the patient has CVID.

Hyper-IgE syndrome (HIGE, Job's syndrome; Buckley's syndrome)

Cause

The underlying cause for this curious illness is unknown. It is frequently classified with neutrophil defects, but the netrophil defects are secondary to the dysregulation of T- and B-cell function.

Presentation

Patients present with atypical eczema and recurrent invasive infections. Pneumatocoeles due to staphylococcal infection are a diagnostic feature. Osteopenia, probably due to abnormal osteoclast function, is a feature and may lead to recurrent fractures. Patients are described as having 'leonine' facies but not all patients have red hair as originally described.

Diagnosis

The clinical history is typical, especially the occurrence of pneumatocoeles. IgE levels are massively elevated and are usually much higher than in atopic eczema.

The occurrence of invasive as opposed to cutaneous infections distinguish HIGE from atopic eczema.

Immunology

The IgE is massively elevated (>50 000 kU/l) and there may be IgG subclass and specific antibody deficiencies, with poor/absent immunization responses.

Variable abnormalities of neutrophil function, affecting chemotaxis, phagocytosis, and microbicidal activity have been reported, but are likely to be due to inhibition by the high IgE.

The underlying defect seems to involve an imbalance of cytokine production due to a Th2 predominance (IL-4, IL-5).

Treatment

IVIg should be used for the antibody deficiency.

Cimetidine (as an immunoregulatory agent) has been recommend, although the value appears to be limited. γ-IFN is a theoretical treatment in the light of proposed Th2 predominance, but has not yet been shown to be effective in small open trials. Cyclosporin A may be very helpful. Bone marrow transplantation has been tried, although with no clear benefit.

SEVERE COMBINED IMMUNODEFICIENCY

Severe combined immunodeficiency involves both the T-cell arm and the B-cell arm. Often the major defect is on the T-cell side: B cells may be present, but in the absence of T cells fail to respond or develop appropriately. The diagnosis is frequently missed at first, which reduces the chance of a successful outcome from treatment. It is estimated that the incidence is 1 per 50 000 births.

Severe combined immunodeficiency: causes

Autosomal recessive T–B– SCID

This form has low serum immunoglobulins, low/absent B cells and low/absent T cells. NK cells are present. The disease is similar to murine SCID in which the defect is on chromosome 16 close to the genes for the surrogate λ light chains (V pre-B and λ5), leading to abnormal V(D)J recombination. RAG-1 or RAG-2 recombinase deficiency account for some cases. This form accounts for about 20 per cent of SCID.

Autosomal recessive T–B+ SCID

This form, in which T cells are absent but B cells are present in normal numbers, accounts for about 10 per cent of cases. The gene is not known for certain but in some cases is due to an abnormality in the Jak3 kinase, which is linked to the common cytokine γ-chain. B-cell and NK-cell function are normal.

X-linked T–B+ SCID

The features are low serum immunoglobulins, normal or increased B cells, low/absent T cells. B cells may be mildly affected as may NK-cell function. It is due to a mutation in cytokine receptor common γ-chain, affecting IL-2, IL-4, IL-7, IL-9, IL-15. The gene is located at Xq13.1–13.3. It accounts for 50–60 per cent of SCID.

Omenn's syndrome

This appears to be a 'leaky' form of SCID; some T cells develop, with a restricted repertoire of T-cell receptors. It may occur in families where there have been other cases of full-blown T–B-SCID. There is often eczema, lymphadenopathy, hepato-splenomegaly, and eosinophilia. It too may be due to RAG-1/RAG-2 deficiency.

A similar pattern may be seen in SCID with engraftment of maternal lymphocytes (materno-fetal engraftment, MFE) that have crossed placenta. The distinction may be difficult clinically, but cytogenetics will usually be able to distinguish maternal cells in MFE.

Adenosine deaminase (ADA) deficiency

This is a metabolic defect due to deficiency of the enzyme ADA. There are low serum immunoglobulins and a progressive reduction of T and B cells due to toxic effects of dATP and S-adenosyl homo-cysteine, which accumulate in the absence of ADA. It is an auto-somal recessive disease; the gene is located at 20q13-ter and has been cloned. ADA deficiency accounts for 20 per cent of cases of SCID. In addition to the immunodeficiency, there is abnormal flaring of the rib ends and neurological features, including cortical blindness.

Clinical features of SCID: presentation

Infections

There is onset of infections soon after birth. These include: recurrent bacterial infections (pneumonia, otitis media, sepsis); persistent thrush; persistent viral infections (RSV, enterovirus, parainfluenza, CMV); opportunist infections (*Pneumocystis carinii* pneumonia, other fungal infections).

There are very significant risks from the administration of live vaccines especially BCG and polio.

BCG SHOULD NOT BE GIVEN TO BABIES WHERE THERE IS A FAMILY HISTORY OF SCID.

Other features

These include:
- failure to thrive;
- diarrhoea (consider chronic enteroviral infection, rotavirus);
- skin rash (Omenn's syndrome, materno-fetal engraftment);
- bone abnormalities (flared ribs—ADA deficiency; malabsorption—rickets);
- short-limbed skeletal dysplasia;
- hepatosplenomegaly (BCGosis, graft-versus-host disease (GvHD) from MFE or blood transfusions; Omenn's syndrome).

Investigation of SCID

If a diagnosis of SCID is suspected, urgent investigation is required.

Plan of initial investigation

The full blood count will identify most cases—lymphopenia $<2\times10^9/l$ occurs in most cases of SCID.

THIS IS THE MOST IMPORTANT TEST AND IS USUALLY IGNORED. ANY BABY WITH LYMPHOPENIA HAS SCID UNTIL PROVEN OTHERWISE.

On suspicion, proceed to the first line investigations:
• lymphocyte subpopulations (T-, B-, NK- and T-cell subpopulations, with absolute numbers);
• immunoglobulins.

If the results are suspicious, then baby should be referred at the earliest opportunity to a specialist centre with facilities for managing SCID.

Further investigations may then be required if the first-line tests are abnormal—these are best done in the specialist referral centre:
• T-cell proliferation;
• cytokine assays;
• NK-cell function;
• specific antibodies;
• biochemical (exclusion of ADA deficiency) and genetic studies;
• HLA typing as part of work up for bone marrow transplantation.

The aims of the initial investigations are:
• to confirm the diagnosis of SCID;
• to identify unusual variants, as this may affect the conditioning protocol used prior to bone marrow transplantation;
• to provide evidence for subsequent genetic counselling of the family;
• to provide a baseline against which success of bone marrow therapy (BMT) can be measured.

Patterns of lymphocyte subpopulations in SCID and variants

• It cannot be stressed too often how important is a low total lymphocyte count as marker of SCID: low lymphocyte counts should never be ignored.
• The typical pattern is of very low/absent T cells with normal or absent B cells; immature T cells may be present in low numbers (CD3+, CD2+ CD4- CD8-).
• SCID with materno-fetal engraftment (MFE): T cells are present but are usually CD8+ and activated (CD25+, DR+); B cells are usually low or absent. Maternal origin of the cells may be confirmed by genetic studies.
• Omenn's syndrome (leaky SCID): T cells may be present, including CD4+ T cells; clonal restriction with limited Tcr β-chain repertoire (this requires genetic analysis).

• Bare lymphocyte syndrome (see below): absence or marked reduction of MHC class II antigen expression with variable MHC class I antigen expression; T cells are normal or low.
• ZAP-70 kinase deficiency and ζ-chain deficiency (see below): marked reduction/absence of CD8+ T cells; low normal CD4+ T cells.
• Absence of CD3/Tcr complexes (CD3 γ- or ε-chains) variable expression of CD3: T-cell numbers are usually normal.

Proliferation assays

• Functional studies are useful in cases when T cells are present.
• PHA response: invariably absent in all major forms of SCID, including Omenn's and SCID with MFE; may be low-normal in ZAP-70 kinase deficiency.
• Phorbol esters (PMA) ± calcium ionophore: will be normal where there is a membrane defect (e.g. ZAP-70 kinase or CD3 complex) that can be bypassed (PMA acts intracellularly on protein kinase C).
• Anti-CD3 ± IL-2: abnormal when the defect involves the CD3/Tcr complex (e.g. CD3 deficiency, ZAP-70 kinase deficiency). The normal newborn anti-CD3 response is lower than in adults.
• The reconstitution of proliferation to mitogens with IL-2 may suggest a failure to produce this cytokine.
• Other stimuli may include antigens, anti-CD2, anti-CD43 (Wiskott–Aldrich syndrome; WAS).

Cytokine assays

These are rarely used: IL-2 deficiency has been reported but is exceptionally rare.

NK-cell assays

The role of these assays in the management of SCID is experimental. It may be useful as a baseline marker for monitoring against graft failure.

Immunoglobulins

If the diagnosis is made within the first few weeks of life, maternal antibody will still be present. Even if the child has B+ SCID, immunoglobulins and specific antibody are not produced. It may be worth checking for specific antibodies if there is late presentation and the child has been immunized.

Biochemistry and genetics

Check for ADA deficiency: abnormal metabolites (dATP, S-adenosyl homocysteine) will be present.

Investigation of SCID (cont.)

It may be possible to test genetically for specific genetic abnormalities, e.g. X-linked SCID (common cytokine receptor γ-chain gene affecting IL-2, IL-4, IL-7, IL-9, IL-15), MHC class II deficiency (CIITA or RFX-5 genes), ZAP-70 kinase deficiency, γ-, ζ-chain deficiency RAG-1/RAG-2, Jak-3.

The genetics department will be able to assist in the distinction of Omenn's syndrome from SCID with MFE: skin biopsies are helpful; cytogenetics can be used if it is a male baby, otherwise molecular genetics are required.

Management of SCID

Successful management of SCID requires a multidisciplinary team used to dealing with very sick small infants. Management should be restricted to centres experienced in the diagnosis and care of SCID. It should not be undertaken in haematology–oncology bone marrow transplant units as the requirements are very different from those of leukaemic patients.

Management

The following form essential components of the management of SCID:

- aggressive treatment of infections with antibacterials, antifungals, and antivirals (good microbiology/virology support is a *sine qua non*).;
- laminar flow isolation at the earliest opportunity;
- nutritional support (total parenteral nutrition; TPN): babies are often failing to thrive;
- irradiate all blood products to prevent transfer of viable lymphocytes (causing graft-versus-host disease; use CMV-negative blood);
- intravenous immunoglobulin prophylaxis;
- PEG-ADA therapy (for ADA-deficient SCID): this may improve lymphocyte function temporarily while bone marrow transplantation is organized;
- tissue type patient and family (genotyping) for potential donors;
- bone marrow transplantation:
    - sibling (identical),
        - parent (haploidentical),
        - matched unrelated (MUD),
        - stem cell;
- cytoreductive conditioning of recipient (to prepare space for incoming stem cells);
- T-cell depletion of donor marrow (for mismatched grafts);
- gene therapy
    - experimental,
        - single-gene defects only (ADA).

Outcome

The outcome is dependent on the promptness of the diagnosis and what infections are present at the time of diagnosis. Poor prognostic indicators are late diagnosis and chronic viral infections (especially parainfluenza pneumonitis).

Meticulous care is required during the aplastic phase between conditioning and engraftment: this will require cell support (platelets, red cells), infection prophylaxis and treatment (fungi, viruses, and bacteria), management of the complications of conditioning (veno-occlusive disease of the liver; pneumonitis) and of graft-versus-host disease (mismatched donors).

Survival should be >80 per cent with early diagnosis, good matching of donors, and no pretransplant infections. This falls to <40 per cent with late diagnosis, chronic infections, and poorly matched donors.

Monitoring of post-BMT SCID

Regular monitoring post-BMT is required to follow engraftment and development of immune function. This should include:

- lymphocyte subpopulations: the return of T and B cells, expression of activation markers in association with GvHD, effectiveness of immunosuppression;
- T-cell proliferation: this is only valuable when T cells have returned to the circulation. The return of a PHA response defines probable safety for release from laminar flow confinement;
- NK-cell function and numbers may correlate with graft survival;
- immunoglobulins: adequacy of replacement IVIg therapy, return of IgA and IgM synthesis, IgG subclass development (off IVIg);
- specific antibodies: return of functional antibodies—isohaemagglutinins, immunization responses;
- genetic studies: chimerism of lymphocytes (DNA studies on separated T and B cells);
- biochemical reconstitution (ADA deficiency; enzyme deficiencies, e.g. ZAP-70 kinase).

COMBINED IMMUNODEFICIENCIES

This group of illnesses has features of both T- and B-cell defects, but the onset is much slower than in SCID. These diseases may not be benign, and management as for SCID may be required.

Combined immunodeficiencies: causes, presentation, and management

Purine nucleoside phosphorylase (PNP) deficiency

This is due to the rare genetic deficiency of another purine metabolic enzyme, PNP, leading to a build-up of the toxic metabolite dGTP, which preferentially damages T cells in the early stages, but later damages B cells also. The disease is an autosomal recessive; the gene is located at 14q13.1.

Neurological signs (spasticity, tremor, and mental retardation) occur early. Infections are common, especially disseminated varicella. Haemolytic anaemia and thyroiditis are also common.

Immunoglobulins are normal or low, B cells are normal in numbers until late disease, but there is a progressive decrease in T-cell numbers over years. A *low* serum urate is a useful marker. The diagnosis is made by enzymatic studies and by detection of elevated levels of the metabolite dGTP.

The disease is rare (about 50 cases worldwide), so the optimum treatment is unknown. BMT is probably best, although gene therapy is a future possibility.

MHC class II deficiency

This disease is found predominately in North Africa. It is an autosomal recessive; CIITA and RFX-5 transcription factors are abnormal.

Presentation is with diarrhoea, hypogammaglobulinaemia, and malabsorption; other infections may occur. Rarely it is asymptomatic.

Immunoglobulins are normal or low. B-cell numbers are normal; T-cell numbers may be normal but there may be low CD4+ T cells. Class I expression is variable; class II expression will be absent but may be inducible with γ-IFN. The diagnosis is made by the absence of expression of class II on lymphocytes.

BMT is the treatment of choice, but is surprisingly difficult to do successfully.

MHC class I deficiency

Deficiency of expression of MHC class I molecules has been reported in association with mutations in the TAP2 gene, which is essential for the correct assembly of MHC class I in the endoplasmic reticulum. The clinical picture may vary from asymptomatic to a severe combined immunodeficiency.

Reticular dysgenesis

This is a rare defect of the maturation of stem cells for both lymphoid and myeloid lineages. There is marked granulocytopenia, lymphopenia, and thrombocytopenia. It presents with early overwhelming infections and often death before the diagnosis is made. Materno-fetal engraftment is common. Bone marrow transplantation is required.

CD8 + T-cell deficiency

Defects due to lack of ZAP-70 kinase and the CD3 ζ-chain have only recently been described. They are autosomal recessive; mutations may occur in the ZAP-70 kinase (2q.12) gene which codes for an intracellular tyrosine kinase involved in signal transduction via the CD3–Tcr complex; ζ-chain deficiency has a similar effect. It presents with recurrent infections (as SCID), but survival for several years is possible. Normal immunoglobulins, normal B cells, very low CD8+ T cells, and normal/low CD4+ T cells are characteristic. Treatment is by bone marrow transplantation.

CD3 deficiency

Deficiencies of CD3 γ- and ε-chains have been described; there is variable expression of CD3. They present as mild combined immunodeficiency, with later onset than SCID, and accompanied by autoimmune phenomena. BMT is probably the treatment of choice.

Other rare defects

- CD7 T-cell deficiency
- Idiopathic CD4 lymphopenia occurs in adults (HIV-1 and HIV-2 negative); risk factor for opportunistic infections
- Multiple cytokine deficiency
- Lack of nuclear factor of activated T cells (NF-AT)
- IL-2 deficiency: presented as SCID, no transcription of IL-2
- Other signal-transduction defects, including T-cell calcium flux defects
- Fas-ligand deficiency: massive lymphadenopathy, autoimmunity and infections
- Undefined

T-CELL DEFECTS

Several disorders have traditionally been called T-cell defects; however it will be appreciated that these frequently also cause humoral immune defects.

Disorders with a predominant T-cell disorder

- DiGeorge syndrome
  - Including all the variants: CATCH-22 (see below)
  - Chronic mucocutaneous candidiasis
  - With and without family history
  - With and without endocrinopathy
- Wiskott–Aldrich syndrome
  - Also includes X-linked thrombocytopenia
- Ataxia telangiectasia
- Cartilage-hair hypoplasia
- Miscellaneous
  - Also consider some forms of CID (CD4+ T-cell lymphopenia)

DiGeorge syndrome (CATCH-22 syndromes)

DiGeorge originally described one phenotype of what is now realized to be a broad and complex array of developmental defects, probably due to more than one genetic lesion.

The range of defects is large and includes the CATCH-22 syndrome (cardiac abnormalities, abnormal facies, thymic hypoplasia, cleft palate, and hypocalcaemia, associated with 22q11 deletions), Shprintzen syndrome, velocardiofacial syndrome (VCF), conotruncal face anomaly syndrome, CHARGE associations, Kallman syndrome, and arrhinencephaly/holoporencephaly. Similar features may also arise in the fetal alcohol syndrome, maternal diabetes, and retinoid embryopathy.

Cause

Microdeletions at 22q11, possibly affecting a zinc-finger (DNA-binding) protein involved in early development have been associated with many of the phenotypic variants; other mutations, including 10p deletions, may give a similar phenotype.

There is abnormal development of branchial arch-derived structures, including heart, thymus, and parathyroid glands.

Presentation

Presentation may involve hypocalcaemic tetany, often occurring in first 48 hours after delivery, and due to parathyroid gland maldevelopment. The other major early presentation is with the cardiac abnormalities, typically those of a truncus arteriosus type, interrupted aortic arch or tetralogy of Fallot. The severity of the cardiac abnormalities often determines outcome. There is often a dysmorphic face with cleft palate, low-set ears, and fish-shaped mouth.

There is a highly variable immunodeficiency, associated with absence or reduction of thymic size; this often improves with age. Severe forms may present as SCID with absent T cells. Partial syndromes may occur without any immunological features (VCF and Shprintzen syndromes).

GvHD from blood transfusions may occur if the diagnosis is not thought of during surgery for cardiac abnormalities.

Diagnosis

The diagnosis is by clinical suspicion, based on the facial features, typical cardiac abnormalities and abnormally low calcium in full-blown cases. Partial variants may be more difficult to identify. All children with relevant cardiac abnormalities should be screened for 22q11 deletions and for other cytogenetic abnormalities.

Patients with an identified 22q11 deletion should be screened for immunological defects, both humoral and cellular (Igs, IgG subclasses, specific antibodies, lymphocyte surface markers, and proliferation assays).

Immunology

The immunology is highly variable and tends to improve with age. There may be a variable reduction in T cells, with normal or low T-cell proliferation. Immunoglobulins may be normal or reduced and specific antibody production may be poor, with low immunization responses.

Treatment

The optimum treatment is uncertain: the cardiac abnormalities define prognosis and repair of these takes priority. Irradiated blood should be used until it is known how severe the immunological abnormality is. Children with normal T-cell function are probably at very low risk of developing transfusion-related GvHD. As mild immune defects may improve, simple measures such as prophylactic antibiotics may be all that is required. If there is evidence for significant humoral deficiency, then IVIg may be required. Severe defects, with absent T cells, should be considered for BMT, although in the absence of a thymus it is interesting to speculate how it will work! Thymic transplants have been tried but are of uncertain value.

Wiskott–Aldrich syndrome

Cause

This is an X-linked disease; the gene is located at Xp11.22–11.3 and has been identified as WASP (Wiskott–Aldrich-associated protein). The function of the protein is currently unknown; it is a 501 amino acid protein with little homology to other known proteins. It interacts with certain cytoplasmic kinases. The gene for X-linked thrombocytopenia is identical with the WASP gene.

Abnormal O-glycosylation of surface proteins of both lymphocytes and platelets is well described. One such surface antigen is CD43 (sialoglycophorin). However, the gene for CD43 is normal in WAS. N-linked glycosylation is normal.

Presentation

The presentation is early in childhood with severe eczema, which has an atypical distribution compared to atopic eczema. Abnormal bleeding is due to the low platelet count. Infections develop more gradually, usually affecting the respiratory tract, and are bacterial. Autoimmunity (vasculitis and glomerulonephritis) is well described. There is often a family history.

A mild variant with thrombocytopenia alone (X-linked thrombocytopenia), but without eczema and immune deficiency is recognized. Two forms of WAS exist: a severe form culminating in early lymphoma, and a milder form compatible with survival to adult life. These probably represent different genetic abnormalities within the WASP gene (as for XLA).

Diagnosis

The clinical features and family history give the best clues. There is thrombocytopenia with abnormally small platelets. The immunological features on routine screening of humoral and cellular function are not diagnostic in their own right. However, the periodate proliferation test, which works through O-linked sugars is more useful, being absent in WAS.

Genetic and protein tests are likely to be available soon, now that the gene has been identified.

Immunology

There is a progressive reduction of T cells with poor proliferative responses to CD3, CD43 and periodate (specific for O-linked sugars). Proliferation to galactose oxidase and neuraminidase, which act via N-linked sugars, are normal.

There are reduced IgM and IgA with a normal or high IgG and elevated IgE. There is a progressive loss of antipolysaccharide responses (including isohaemagglutinins) with poor/absent responses to test immunization with polysaccharide antigens.

CD43 on lymphocytes and gpIb on platelets are unstable and tend to fall off cells when kept *in vitro*. Abnormalities of the cytoskeleton in T cells and platelets, with failure of actin bundling, have also been described.

Treatment

Splenectomy may be beneficial for thrombocytopenia, which is usually resistant to steroids. IVIg should be used for poor antipolysaccharide responses, if recurrent bacterial infections are a problem. Early BMT should be considered to prevent the development of lymphoma: it cures all the features of the disease, including eczema.

Outcome

Death may occur from infection or intracranial haemorrhage. Studies have shown that there is a very significant risk of death in late adolescence/early adulthood from high-grade lymphoreticular malignancy—this may be preventable by early BMT. Mild variants exist and may have fewer problems with bleeding or infection in adulthood.

Ataxia telangiectasia

Cause

Cells from AT patients have a disorder of the cell cycle checkpoint pathway, resulting in extreme sensitivity to ionizing radiation. Lymphocytes show frequent chromosomal breaks, inversions, and translocations; the major sites affected are the genes for the T-cell receptors and Ig heavy chains. The disease is an autosomal recessive; six genetic complementation groups (A, B, C, D, E, V1, V2) have been described and all but V2 map to 11q22–23. One of the genes has now been identified and appears to be a DNA-dependent kinase related to phosphatidylinositol kinase-3 (Ataxia telangiectasia mutated protein (ATM)).

Presentation

There is a progressive cerebellar ataxia, with typical telangiectasia, especially of the ear lobes and conjunctivae. This is accompanied by recurrent bacterial sinopulmonary infections.

Diagnosis

The clinical history is usually diagnostic, although the disease may be difficult to identify in the early stage when signs are minimal. The α-fetoprotein in serum is usually raised. Genetic tests will undoubtedly make life much easier.

Immunology

Immunoglobulins are variable: there is often a reduction of IgG2/IgG4, IgA, and IgE, with poor antipolysaccharide responses. There is an increased incidence of autoantibodies. T-cell numbers and function are usually reduced.

Treatment

No treatment is effective in what is a relentless disease with progressive neurological deterioration. IVIg reduces the incidence of infections and improves quality of life but does not affect the outcome.

Outcome

The ataxia is progressive and patients become wheelchair-bound early. There is a high incidence of malignancy, especially high-grade lymphoma, and the incidence of malignancy is raised in other family members (fivefold increase breast cancer). Death usually ensues in early adult life from infections or neoplasia. Heterozygotes for abnormal ATM genes may have an increased risk of chronic lymphocytic leukaemia.

Chronic mucocutaneous candidiasis (CMC)

Cause

The cause of CMC is unknown. Autosomal dominant and recessive forms as well as sporadic cases are all documented. A recently identified gene on chromosome 21 (21q22.3) is abnormal in auto-immune polyglandular syndrome type I (see Chapter 5), which is one of the forms of CMC.

Presentation

There is early onset of superficial candidiasis affecting nails and mouth and occasionally the oesophagus; persistent; invasive candidiasis is very rare and should raise questions of other diagnoses. There may be a family history.

Some patients also have an endocrinopathy causing hypo-calcaemia due to parathyroid insufficiency, hypothyroidism, and adrenal insufficiency.

There is an increased susceptibility to bacterial infections (particularly of the respiratory tract), tuberculosis, herpesviruses, and toxoplasmosis. Severe forms may progress to a more generalized combined immunodeficiency.

Diagnosis

There is no unequivocal diagnostic test. *In vivo* and *in vitro* T-cell responses to *Candida* antigens are poor or absent but anticandida IgG antibodies are high. The presence of superficial candidiasis with an endocrinopathy, either overt or cryptic (autoantibody positive without symptoms), is highly suspicious.

Immunology

Anticandida antibodies (IgG) are raised, often with multiple precipitin lines on double diffusion tests. IgG2/IgG4 are often reduced and there are poor antipolysaccharide responses with low immunization responses.

There is poor *in vitro* proliferation to *Candida* antigens, with abnormal cytokine production (high IL-6). T-cell responses to mitogens are usually normal. Cutaneous reactivity to *Candida* is absent, although other DTH responses are often normal. T-lymphocyte subsets are usually normal.

Autoantibodies may be detectable to endocrine organs (parathyroid, adrenal, ovary, thyroid).

Treatment

Treatment is difficult: *Candida* will respond well to antifungals (fluconazole or itraconazole) but inevitably relapses when the antifungal is withdrawn. Resistance to these antifungals may occur.

IVIg should be considered for patients with recurrent bacterial infections. Continuous antibiotics tend to exacerbate the candidiasis. γ-Interferon may have some beneficial effect. Bone marrow transplantation should be considered for severe forms but the procedure is difficult in heavily infected patients.

It is essential to maintain regular surveillance for significant endocrine disease, in particular adrenal insufficiency, which may be insidious in its onset.

Outcome

CMC is not as benign as the books would have you believe. Cases may die from overwhelming sepsis, in addition to deaths from unrecognized adrenal insufficiency.

Cartilage hair hypoplasia (CHH)

Cause

The inheritance is autosomal recessive and linked to chromosome 9, but the gene is unknown. It occurs particularly in Finland and old-order Amish in America.

Presentation

There is short-limbed skeletal dysplasia, with fine sparse hair and ligamentous laxity. Recurrent bacterial infections are a problem. Megacolon and macrocytic anaemia are reported.

Immunology

There is a neutropenia, together with a T- and B-cell lymphopenia.

Major defects of phagocytic cells

- Chronic granulomatous disease
  - X-linked
  - autosomal recessive
- Leucocyte adhesion defects (LAD)
  - LAD-1: defects of CD18, common β-chain for LFA-1, Mac-1, and CR4 (CD11a, CD11b, CD11c); defect in CD11c (?)
  - LAD-2: defects in synthesis of fucose from GDP-mannose; lack of expression of Lewis X ligand
- Glucose 6-phosphate dehydrogenase (G6PD) deficiency
- Myeloperoxidase deficiency
- Secondary granule deficiency
- Chediak–Higashi syndrome and Griscelli syndrome
- Schwachman syndrome
- Cyclic neutropenia

Chronic granulomatous disease (CGD)

This is the most significant neutrophil defect, although not the most common. It is also the easiest to diagnose.

Cause

There is a defect of intracellular bacterial killing in neutrophils and monocytes, due to a failure of superoxide, oxygen radical, and peroxide production. X-linked and autosomal recessive forms are described. There is a deficiency of components of cytochrome $b558$: 91 kDa protein (X-linked; Xp21.1), 22 kDa protein (16q24) or NADPH oxidase p47 (7q11.23) or p67 (1q25).

As phagocyte hydrogen peroxidase is normal, organisms that are catalase negative are killed normally, whereas catalase-positive organisms (*Staphylococcus aureus*, *Aspergillus*, *Nocardia*, and *Serratia*) cause major problems.

Presentation

Infections with catalase-positive organisms, especially deep-seated abscesses, osteomyelitis, and chronic granulomata (including oro-facial granuloma), are the hallmark of this disease. It may mimic inflammatory bowel disease and lead to malabsorption and obstruction of the bowel. Liver abscess is a common first presentation, and any child with a liver abscess has CGD until proven otherwise.

It usually presents initially in childhood but, rarely, first presentation may occur in adults.

Immunology and diagnosis

Neutrophil oxidative metabolism is abnormal (see Part 2). The easiest screening test is the nitroblue tetrazolium reduction (NBT test), but this may miss some cases. Bacterial killing will be absent.

Treatment

Long-term antibiotics (co-trimoxazole ± itraconazole) are the mainstay of treatment. In the USA low-dose prophylactic γ-interferon tends to be used instead. Acute infections should be treated promptly with intravenous antibiotics, supplemented with high-dose γ-interferon. Drainage of large abscesses may be required.

The inflammatory bowel disease may be significantly helped by high-dose steroids, particularly where there are obstructive lesions due to granulomata.

Bone marrow transplantation appears to be the treatment of choice and should be carried out early before infective complications become a threat to life.

Outcome

The outcome has been much improved by use of prophylactic antibiotics and γ-IFN, but it is still a life-shortening illness.

Leucocyte adhesion defects (LAD)

Cause

LAD-1 is due to a deficiency of the β-chain (CD18) for LFA-1 (CD11a), Mac-1 (CD11b) and CR4 (CD11c). The gene is located at 21q22.3. There may be variable expression: the severe phenotype has <1 per cent expression, while in the moderate (incomplete) phenotype there may be as much as 10 per cent of control expression.

Rare cases may be due to defects in other chains (CD11c?) and the Lewis X ligand (LAD-2), caused by an inability to synthesize fucose.

Presentation

The presentation is variable, depending on the phenotype. Delayed umbilical cord separation is a significant feature (>10 days). Skin infections, intestinal and perianal ulcers and fistulae are typical. Periodontitis occurs in older children and may lead to loss of teeth. Immunizations may leave scarred nodules. There is a lack of inflammatory change at the sites of infection and an absence of pus formation.

Diagnosis

Diagnosis is dependent on the demonstration of reduced/absent molecules on lymphocytes and granulocytes. PMA stimulation of granulocytes may be necessary to identify the moderate phenotype in which some up-regulation occurs.

There is usually a peripheral blood neutrophilia, which is often extreme.

Treatment

Prompt antibiotic therapy is required. BMT is necessary for the severe phenotype: graft rejection is not possible in the absence of LFA-1. This observation led to the use of anti-LFA-1 monoclonal antibodies as antirejection therapy. Moderate phenotypes may be more difficult to transplant.

Neutrophil G6PD deficiency

Cause

This is an X-linked (Xq28) condition; the gene is prone to frequent mutations (200 variants have been recorded). The absence of functional G6PD (1–5 per cent of normal activity) impairs the NADPH system of oxidative metabolism, with similar effects to CGD. However, most variants have enzyme activity of 20–50 per cent normal and have no phagocytic defect.

Presentation and diagnosis

The presentation is similar to that of CGD. Anaemia is often present. The NBT test is diagnostic.

Myeloperoxidase deficiency

This deficiency is not uncommon (the gene is located at 17q21.3-q23). The prevalence is between 1/2000–1/4000 in the USA. Cases are usually asymptomatic, although occasional defects in killing *Candida* have been reported.

Schwachman syndrome

This is an autosomal recessive syndrome of hereditary pancreatic insufficiency, accompanied by neutropenia, abnormal neutrophil chemotaxis, thrombocytopenia, and anaemia.

Hypogammaglobulinaemia with recurrent sinopulmonary infections may also occur. Responses to polysaccharide antigens may be absent. Treatment with IVIg may be helpful.

2 Primary immunodeficiency

Neutrophil G6PD deficiency
Myeloperoxide deficiency
Schwachman syndrome

Secondary (specific) granule deficiency

Neutrophil structure is abnormal with bilobed nuclei. Secondary (lactoferrin) granules are absent and there is a deficiency of other neutrophil enzymes (alkaline phosphatase). This leads to defective neutrophil oxidative metabolism and bacterial killing, resulting in skin and sinopulmonary infections.

The diagnosis can be made by careful examination of the blood film, supplemented by cytochemical studies for neutrophil enzymes (NAP score).

Cyclic neutropenia

This is a rare syndrome characterized by cyclic reductions in neutrophils, but it is perhaps more common than previously thought, with milder variants escaping notice. The cycle is usually 21 days ± 2–3 days. The defect is at the level of stem-cell regulation and a similar disease is found in collie dogs.

Mouth ulceration typically occurs at the neutrophil nadir; more significant invasive infection may occur. A mood change just before the nadir is often marked. Symptoms may improve with age.

The clue is usually a low neutrophil count during an infective episode. Diagnosis is confirmed by serial full blood counts with full differential, three times weekly over 4 weeks. Neutrophils may disappear completely. Symptoms usually occur if the count drops below 1×10^9/l. There is a compensatory monocytosis at the time of the neutrophil nadir.

G-CSF prevents a dramatic drop but does NOT abolish the cycle, which shortens to approximately 14 days. There is, however, a risk of myeloid leukaemia with chronic G-CSF therapy and this should be used with circumspection. Prophylactic co-trimoxazole either side of the predicted nadir may be valuable in preventing infection.

2 Primary immunodeficiency
Secondary (specific) granule deficiency
Cyclic neutropenia
Kostmann's syndrome

81

Kostmann's syndrome

This is a congenital severe neutropenia due to a neutrophil maturation defect with arrest at the pro-myelocyte stage. It presents with
recurrent severe infections. Immunoglobulins are raised; there is a
compensatory monocytosis, eosinophilia, and a thrombocytosis.
Bone marrow transplantation may be used as treatment. Co-
trimoxazole prophylaxis is necessary.

OTHER IMMUNODEFICIENCY SYNDROMES

Immunodeficiency has been described in a wide variety of other syndromes.

Chromosomal instability or defective repair

Bloom's syndrome

Gene located at 11q23; probably a DNA ligase deficiency. The immunodeficiency is characterized by low IgM, poor T-cell function, poor B-cell IgM production, and NK-cell defects. Malignancy is a complication.

Fanconi anaemia

This is an autosomal recessive disease with chromosomal breaks. There are multiple organ defects, bone marrow failure, radial hypoplasia, abnormal face, and leukaemic transformation. There are decreased T cells, NK cells, and low IgA.

ICF (immunodeficiency, centromeric instability, and abnormal facies)

This is due to abnormalities of chromosomes 1, 9, and 16, marked by a dysmorphic face, mental retardation, and malabsorption with failure to thrive. The immunodeficiency is mainly humoral but occasional patients have shown additional T-cell defects.

Nijmegen breakage and Seemanova syndromes

These are syndromes of microcephaly, mental retardation (not in the Seemanova syndrome), bird-like face, and recurrent infections. There is increased chromosomal sensitivity to ionizing radiation and immunoglobulins are reduced.

Seckel syndrome

An autosomal recessive syndrome characterized by 'bird-headed' dwarfism, mental retardation, hypoplastic anaemia, and hypo-gammaglobulinaemia.

Xeroderma pigmentosa

Extreme sun sensitivity leading to bullae, keratoses, and squamous cell carcinoma are the features of this syndrome, which is a DNA repair defect. There is an immunodeficiency with low CD4+ T cells in some patients; low IgG levels may also occur.

Chromosomal defects

Down's syndrome

This is due to trisomy 21. There is a progressive decrease IgM, dysplastic thymus, low NK activity, and an unusual sensitivity to γ-interferon, whose receptor is located on chromosome 21. There is an increase in Tcr $\gamma\delta$ cells at the expense of Tcr $\alpha\beta$ cells. T-cell proliferation to mitogens is reduced, with poor IL-2 production. There is an increase in infections and also in malignancy and autoimmune disease.

Turner's syndrome

The genetic abnormality is XO. Fifty per cent of patients have low IgG and IgM.

Chromosome 18 syndromes

Ring chromosome 18 and deletions of the long and short arms of chromosome 18 are associated with facial hypoplasia, mental retardation, and low/absent IgA.

Immunodeficiency with generalized growth retardation

Schimke immuno-osseus dysplasia

An autosomal recessive syndrome characterized by nephropathy, skeletal dysplasia, and lentigenes. There is a lymphopenia of CD4+ T cells with poor T-cell mitogen responses.

Immunodeficiency with absent thumbs (TAR syndrome)

There is radial dysplasia, ichthyosis and anosmia in this syndrome. Recurrent infections and chronic mucocutaneous candidiasis occur. There are poor T-cell mitogen responses and absent IgA, with low IgG and IgM.

Others

- Dubowitz syndrome (autosomal recessive; dwarfism, eczema, bone marrow failure)
- Growth retardation, facial anomalies, and immunodeficiency
- Progeria (Hutchison–Gilford syndrome): premature ageing

These syndromes have all been reported with variable immunodeficiencies.

Immunodeficiency with dermatological defects

Chediak-Higashi syndrome

This is an autosomal recessive disease: benign and aggressive presentations occur. Characteristic features are partial oculocutaneous albinism (due to abnormal melanocytes), leading to silver streaks in the hair (prematurely!). Recurrent infections, CNS abnormalities, and hepatosplenomegaly occur frequently.

There are giant cytoplasmic granules in leucocytes and platelets. Granulocyte and monocyte chemotaxis is abnormal with delayed intracellular killing (correctable by ascorbate *in vitro*). Defective NK-cell function is common.

The outcome is poor in the aggressive form with neurological deterioration and a lymphoproliferative syndrome like familial lymphohistiocytosis. This should be treated with BMT.

Partial albinism (Griscelli syndrome)

This is similar to Chediak–Higashi syndrome but is distinguished from it by the absence of giant granules. Poor T-cell and NK-cell function are typical.

Dyskeratosis congenita

Dyskeratosis congenita is characterized by cutaneous pigmentation, nail dystrophy, and oral leukoplakia, and is complicated by malignancy and bone marrow failure. Autosomal dominant or recessive and X-linked forms occur. Variable immune defects are found: hypogammaglobulinaemia and poor delayed-type hypersensitivity.

Netherton syndrome

There is trichorrhexis, ichthyosis, and atopy; some patients have low IgG.

Acrodermatitis enteropathica

This is caused by zinc deficiency, leading to eczema, diarrhoea, malabsorption, and sinopulmonary infections. T-cell numbers and function are reduced and immunoglobulins are low. All the defects are correctable with supplemental zinc.

Anhidrotic ectodermal dysplasia

Autosomal recessive or X-linked forms of this syndrome occur. Hypohydrosis and faulty dentition are the key features. Upper respiratory infections occur. There is variable T- and B-cell function; specific antibody responses may be poor.

Papillon–Lefèvre syndrome

Abnormal neutrophil chemotaxis has been reported in this syndrome of hyperkeratosis and pyoderma.

Metabolic disorders

Transcobalamin II deficiency

Autosomal recessive deficiency of TC II, a vitamin B12-binding protein essential for transport of B12, has been reported in association with diarrhoea, failure to thrive, megaloblastic anaemia, lymphopenia, neutropenia, and thrombocytopenia. Abnormal neutrophil function and hypogammaglobulinaemia are present. All the features are reversible with B12 therapy.

Methylmalonic acidaemia

The features are similar to TC II deficiency. It is treated with folic acid.

Type I hereditary orotic aciduria

This is an autosomal recessive disease of retarded growth, diarrhoea, and megaloblastic anaemia. Fatal meningitis and disseminated varicella may be complications. There is a T-cell lymphopenia and impaired T-cell function.

Biotin-dependent carboxylase deficiency

An autosomal recessive condition characterized by convulsions, ataxia, alopecia, candidiasis, and intermittent lactic acidosis. The severe neonatal form presents with severe acidosis and recurrent sepsis. There is increased urinary β-hydroxypropionic acid, methyl citrate, β-methylcrotonglycine, and 3-hydroxyisovalerate excretion. Decreased T and B cells with low IgA are noted. It is treated with biotin.

Mannosidosis

This is a lysosomal storage disease which is associated with abnormal neutrophil and lymphocyte function.

Glycogen storage disease Type Ib

Recurrent infections, including severe oral ulceration and abscesses, are associated with a neutropenia and neutrophil dysfunction in this syndrome.

Hypercatabolism of immunoglobulin

Familial hypercatabolism

Familial hypercatabolism of IgG has been associated with bone abnormalities, abnormal glucose metabolism, and recurrent infections. IgG is very low with a very short half-life; serum albumin may be normal or low.

Intestinal lymphangiectasia

This is due to a failure of normal lymphatic development in the bowel, with abnormally dilated lymphatics. Similar abnormalities may occur elsewhere, causing localized oedema, effusions, and ascites. There is enteric loss of lymphocytes and malabsorption, particularly of fats.

There is a profound lymphopenia, with hypoalbuminaemia and hypogammaglobulinaemia; IgM may be in the normal range and infections may be less severe than the IgG level might predict. Specific responses may be normal but very short-lived.

IVIg may be given but weekly therapy may be required to maintain adequate levels. Fat malabsorption may be severe and medium-chain triglyceride supplements may be required.

Splenic disorders

Congenital asplenia and Ivemark syndrome

Here asplenia is associated with partial situs inversus and cardiac defects. Early infections, especially with capsulated organisms, are a typical feature. Initial poor polysaccharide responses may improve after the first 3 years of life. However, there remains a risk of overwhelming sepsis and lifelong prophylactic antibiotics should be administered, together with regular immunizations against pneumococci, *Haemophilus influenzae* type b (Hib), and meningococci.

COMPLEMENT DISORDERS

Complement deficiency

Cause

Genetic deficiency of all complement components have been described, including the regulatory inhibitors, C1 inhibitor, Factor I, and Factor H. Properdin deficiency is X-linked, all the others are autosomal recessives, except C1-inhibitor deficiency which is autosomal dominant. Factors B, C2, and C4 form part of the extended MHC complex (short arm of chromosome 6, located between HLA-D and HLA-B loci).

Presentation

There is an increased susceptibility to pyogenic infections in C3, Factor I, and Factor H deficiency, while there is an increased susceptibility to neisserial infections in C5, C6, C7, C8α, C8β, C9, Factor D, and properdin deficiency. Recurrent neisserial infection, especially meningitis, should always prompt a screen for complement deficiency; the disease may be milder than in complement replete individuals. C9 deficiency is common in Japan and may be asymptomatic, as slow lysis through C5–C8 may take place without C9. There is an increased susceptibility to SLE-like syndrome in C1q, C1r/C1s, C4, C2, C5, C6, C7, C8α, and C8β. Complement deficiencies are common in South Africa and in the countries of the north African coast and eastern Mediterranean. C2 and C4 deficiencies are relatively common. An increasing number of C4 null alleles increase substantially the risk of developing lupus. C2-deficient lupus is often atypical with marked cutaneous features.

Diagnosis

The diagnosis is by the screening for classic, alternate, and terminal lytic sequence by functional complement assays (classic and alternate pathway CH50—see Part 2), followed by measurement of individual components, as indicated by the screening tests.

Treatment

No specific treatment is available. Recurrent neisserial infection may be prevented by prophylactic antibiotics and meningococcal vaccination may help, although there are concerns that disease may be more severe if it occurs in a complement-deficient person after vaccination. Autoimmune disease is treated in the normal way.

Hereditary angioedema (HAE, C1-inhibitor deficiency)

Cause

Two types of HAE are recognized: type I (85 per cent; gene deletion, no protein produced) and type II (15 per cent; point mutation in active site of enzyme). The gene is located on chromosome 11. The condition is an autosomal dominant as one normal gene is insufficient to protect against symptoms. There is failure of inactivation of the complement and kinin systems, but the angioedema is most likely to be due to the latter rather than the former.

Presentation

There is an angioedema (deep tissue swelling) of any part of the body, including airway and gut; the latter presents with recurrent abdominal pain and repeated laparotomies may be undertaken before the diagnosis is made. There is no urticaria or itch, although patients often describe an uncomfortable prodromal tingling.

Attacks begin in later childhood/teenage years and may be precipitated by trauma (beware dental work and operations) and infections. The frequency of attacks may be increased by oral contraceptives and by pregnancy There is an increased risk of immune complex disease.

Diagnosis

Typically C4 and C2 are undetectable during an acute attack and low/absent in between. In type I there will be a low C1-inhibitor level immunochemically and this will become undetectable in an acute attack. In type II there will be a normal or high level of inhibitor measured immunochemically, but function will be low or absent.

Angioedema may be acquired secondary to SLE or lymphoma and these may be distinguished from HAE by the reduction in C1q, although this is not always reliable (see Chapter 3).

Treatment

Treat major attacks with purified (steam-treated) inhibitor (1000–1500 IU, i.e. 2–3 ampoules). Fresh frozen plasma (FFP) may be an emergency alternative but there are the usual risks of transmitted infection and it is also possible for FFP to exacerbate attacks by providing more substrate. Tracheostomy may be required if there is significant laryngeal oedema.

Prophylaxis may be obtained with modified androgens (danazol, 200–600 mg/day; or stanozolol, 2.5–10 mg/day) or antifibrinolytics (tranexamic acid 2–4 g/day). Regular liver function tests are required for monitoring therapy with all these agents.

Prophylactic purified inhibitor should be used before high-risk surgical procedures, although tranexamic acid may be adequate for minor procedures. Dental work should always be carried out in hospital in view of the risk of developing oral oedema and airway obstruction.

Abdominal attacks respond poorly to purified inhibitor—treatment should be conservative: analgesia (NSAIDs), IV fluids, and avoidance of unnecessary laparotomies (unless there is good evidence for other pathology).

3 Secondary immunodeficiencies

Introduction

Many disease states have been associated with immune dysfunction of varying degrees of severity and significance: some rare secondary disorders have already been covered in Chapter 2. In this and subsequent chapters, the immunological abnormalities will be discussed, together with the value of immunological tests (if any): there will not, however, be a detailed discussion of the clinical and non-immunological features of the diseases and the reader is advised to consult other standard textbooks.

Classification of secondary immunodeficiency

- Viral infections
  - HIV, CMV, EBV, rubella, ? enteroviruses (echoviruses, coxsackieviruses), measles, influenza
- Acute bacterial infections
  - Septicaemia
- Chronic bacterial and parasitic infections
  - Tuberculosis, leishmaniasis
- Malignancy
- Plasma cell tumours and related problems
  - Myeloma, plasmacytoma, Waldenström's macroglobulinaemia
  - Amyloidosis (see Chapter 8)
- Lymphoma/leukaemia
  - Hodgkin's disease, non-Hodgkin's lymphoma, chronic lymphocytic leukaemia, other chronic and acute leukaemias
- Extremes of age
  - Prematurity, old age
- Transfusion therapy
  - Whole blood; clotting factors
- Drugs and biologicals
  - As an undesirable side-effect; immunosuppressive drugs (see Chapter 10)
- Physical therapies
  - Plasmapheresis and variants, radiation (see Chapter 10)
- Nutrition
  - Starvation, anorexia (see also Chapter 2 for immunological effects of certain inborn errors that affect nutritional status); iron deficiency
- Chronic renal disease
  - Uraemia, dialysis, nephrotic syndrome
- Gastrointestinal disease
  - Protein-losing enteropathies; secondary to cardiac disease
- Metabolic disease
  - Diabetes mellitus, glycogen storage disease, mannosidosis
- Toxins
  - Cigarettes, alcohol, other chemicals
- Splenectomy
  - In conjunction with other diseases (lymphoma; coeliac disease; sickle-cell disease); traumatic (see Chapter 2 for congenital asplenia)
- Burns
- Myotonic dystrophy

VIRAL INFECTIONS

Human immunodeficiency virus 1 and 2

Immunological features

The virus binds to CD4+ T cells via envelope glycoprotein gp120. It also infects other CD4+ cells (macrophages, dendritic cells) and other cells expressing CD4-like surface proteins (neuronal cells). Uptake of virus into phagocytic cells may be augmented by antibody and complement. High levels of viral replication may take place in lymph nodes.

Other surface molecules may be involved in binding (MHC class II) and formation of multinucleate giant cells (syncytium), e.g. LFA-1 (CD11a).

The initial viraemia after infection is controlled by CD8+ cytotoxic T cells (increased cell numbers). The asymptomatic phase is characterized by strong cytotoxic responses, but viral replication still detectable intermittently, i.e. HIV is not a true latent virus.

The antibody response to major viral proteins appears after a lag phase of up to 3 months and persists through the asymptomatic phase but declines in late-stage disease.

In the seroconversion illness there is a dramatic fall in CD4+ T cells and rise of CD8+ T cells. The levels of CD4+ T cells may drop to a level at which opportunist infections may occur at this early stage (poor prognostic indicator). Levels then usually recover to within the low normal range. There is then a slow decline of absolute CD4+ T-cell count over time (years) following infection.

The passage to the symptomatic phase is characterized by a rapid drop in CD4+ T cells, loss of cytotoxic activity, and switch of virus type from slow-growing, non-syncytial-forming strains to rapidly growing, syncytial-forming strains (quasi species evolving through lack of replicative fidelity and under immunological selection pressure). This is accompanied by the occurrence of opportunist infections.

Activation of T cells enhances viral replication and hence CD4+ T-cell destruction. Therefore opportunist infections enhance the self-destruction of the immune system. Cause and effect in determining the transition from asymptomatic to symptomatic is not known for certain yet.

Diagnosis and monitoring

Diagnosis depends on the detection of antiviral antibody ± viral antigen, NOT on immunological markers. The most accurate monitoring of disease is now available through measurements of viral load by quantitative PCR.

In the acute seroconversion illness, there is a sharp fall in absolute CD4+ T-cell numbers and increase in CD8+ T-cell numbers with T-cell activation markers increased (IL-2 receptor (CD25) and MHC class II (DR)); this normally returns rapidly to normal as evidence of viral replication disappears. Persistent CD4+

lymphopenia after seroconversion illness is a poor prognostic sign indicating rapid progression to terminal illness

The drop in CD4+ T cells and elevation of CD8+ T cells is NOT specific for HIV infection, and may be seen in most acute viral infections. Lymphocyte surface marker analysis is NOT a surrogate for proper viral testing (with informed consent).

Sequential monitoring of the CD4+ T-cell numbers provides guidance on the rate of progression of disease and identifies levels at which therapeutic interventions may be indicated (e.g. *Pneumocystis* prophylaxis at $0.2 \times 10^9/l$ CD4+ T cells).

Once the CD4+ T-cell count falls below $0.05 \times 10^9/l$, further monitoring is of little clinical value (except psychologically to patients, who view cessation of monitoring as doctors giving up).

Serum immunoglobulins are usually polyclonally elevated (IgG levels > 50 g/l may be recorded); serial measurements have no clinical utility. Most of the antibody is either 'junk' or relates to an anamnestic response. Autoantibodies may be detected (including anti-neutrophil cytoplasmic antibody (ANCA) and anti-cardiolipin).

Rare patients, usually children, may suffer from panhypo-gammaglobulinaemia or specific antibody deficiency, presenting with recurrent bacterial infections: these patients may derive significant benefit from IVIg. It has been more difficult to demonstrate specific antibody defects in adults, although a subpopulation of adult patients do have recurrent sinopulmonary infections with *Haemophilus* and *Pneumococcus*. IVIg seems to be less helpful.

Serum β2-microglobulin levels may be elevated, as a marker of increased lymphocyte turnover; however, the range of elevation in HIV+ patients is small compared to that seen in lymphoproliferative disease, and its value (except where CD4+ T-cell counts are unavailable) is small. Likewise, serum and urinary neopterin, a marker of macrophage activation, may also be elevated. There is little to choose between these two surrogate markers.

Immunotherapy

The mainstay of therapy at present is the use of antiretroviral agents. Single-agent chemotherapy has a limited role and combination chemotherapy is likely to offer the best way forward, although the optimum combinations are not yet known. However, significant improvements have been noted with current triple-therapy regimes, although the rise in CD4+ T-cell counts do not seem to indicate a restoration of cellular immune function.

As noted above, IVIg may be helpful in certain HIV+ infants, although not in adults.

Other immunotherapies (interferons, interleukin-2) have been uniformly disappointing and are not used routinely. α-Interferon enjoyed a vogue in the treatment of Kaposi's sarcoma, but the latter responds better to cytotoxic therapy and radiation.

Considerable hype has surrounded claims of benefit from passive serotherapy, using sera containing high levels of anti-HIV antibodies: until the findings have been widely replicated there is no justification for this approach.

No reliable vaccine is yet available, although trials are continuing on a number of candidate vaccines.

Epstein–Barr virus

Immunological features

EBV is a transforming B-lymphotropic virus of the herpes family binding to the cells via CD21 (C3d) receptor. This receptor is also expressed on follicular dendritic cells, pharyngeal, and cervical epithelium. All these tissues are targets. Pharyngeal epithelium is usually affected first, with infection spreading to B cells in the adjacent lymphoid tissue of Waldeyer's ring.

Following infection there is a B lymphoproliferation that is controlled rapidly by cytotoxic T cells, which form the 'atypical mononuclear cells' seen on smears. Both MHC-restricted and unrestricted cells are produced, with the latter directly recognizing a virally induced antigen on the cells (LYDMA, lymphocyte-determined membrane antigen).

Viral persistence occurs, with reactivation of infection in the immunocompromised (immunosuppressed patients, transplant recipients, HIV-infected patients), giving oral hairy leukoplakia, lymphocytic interstitial pneumonitis, and lymphoma. Nasopharyngeal carcinoma also occurs, although other co-factors are likely to be involved.

In some patients with a genetic predisposition (Duncan's syndrome, see Chapter 2) severe or fatal infection occurs on first exposure to EBV.

Although infectious mononucleosis (glandular fever) is usually a self-limiting illness, some patients fail to clear the virus and develop an appropriate sequence of IgG antibodies: such patients have persistently positive IgM antibodies to EBV and have chronic symptoms (fatigue, malaise, sore throats).

In the acute phase of EBV infection there is suppression of mitogen and allogeneic responses. NK function is also abnormal even though cell numbers are increased. It has been shown that EBV-transformed cells secrete a homologue of IL-10. Monocyte chemotaxis is also abnormal.

Immunological diagnosis

The usual screening test for acute EBV infection relies on the production of heterophile antibodies that agglutinate sheep cells. IgM antibodies are detected and are then succeeded rapidly by IgG antibodies to early antigen (EA) and viral capsid antigen (VCA); antibodies to EBV nuclear antigen (EBNA) appear weeks to months after infection

Initial lymphopenia is followed by lymphocytosis of CD8+ T cells, which give rise to the atypical lymphocytes seen on blood films. However, monitoring of lymphocyte subpopulations is of little value, except in unusual variants of EBV infection.

There is usually an acute polyclonal rise in immunoglobulins which may be associated with the production of autoantibodies.

Immunotherapy

None is required. However, in patients with a persistent EBV syndrome, high-dose acyclovir (800 mg 5 times daily for 14 days) may lead to remission of symptoms and disappearance of the IgM anti-EBV antibodies.

Cytomegalovirus

CMV behaves similarly to EBV, with an early CD8+ T-cell lymphocytosis giving atypical lymphocytes on a blood film. Proliferative responses are reduced during acute infections. CMV infection of monocytes with production of an IL-1 inhibitor may be important. However, congenital CMV infection leads to a prolonged suppression of T-cell function and may also suppress antibody production. In bone marrow transplant recipients, there may be prolonged suppression of myeloid differentiation. High-titre anti-CMV antibodies in the form of IVIg may help to prevent infection, although once infection is established treatment with antivirals is necessary.

Rubella

Congenital rubella, but not acute infection, causes poor lymphocyte responses (reduced PHA proliferation) and may lead to long-term depressed humoral immune function. Rubella appears to directly infect both T and B cells.

Measles

Measles virus is capable of infecting both lymphoid and myeloid cells. Acute measles depresses cutaneous type IV reactivity (tuberculin reactivity); this is transient. Similar effects occur with measles vaccines. There is also suppression of NK activity and immunoglobulin production. It is possible that acute measles may lead to reactivation of TB due to immunosuppression. Acute measles may cause a transient lymphopenia; PHA- and PPD-driven proliferation is reduced. Neutrophil chemotaxis may be impaired transiently (? significance). Early inactivated measles vaccines led to a response predominantly against viral haemagglutinin but not to the fusion protein, sometimes leading to an atypical wild-type infection as a result of the inappropriate immune response.

3 Secondary immunodeficiencies

Cytomegalovirus
Rubella
Measles

Influenza virus

Acute influenza may give a marked but transient lymphopenia accompanied by poor T-cell proliferative responses.

Post-viral fatigue syndromes

* Chronic fatigue syndromes, accompanied by muscle/joint pains and neuropsychiatric symptoms may occur after a range of viral infections, including enteroviruses
* Immunological abnormalities include: variable lymphopenia IgG subclass abnormalities
* May be transient or persistent
* See Chapter 8 for fuller discussion

3 Secondary immunodeficiencies

Influenza virus
Post-viral fatigue syndromes

Acute bacterial infections

Immunological features

Acute bacterial sepsis may lead to profound changes in immune function on a temporary basis. Neutrophil migration and chemotaxis are increased, while phagocytosis is normal or decreased Lymphopenia affecting CD4+ and CD8+ cells may be marked Significant and temporary hypogammaglobulinaemia may be present (?release of immunosuppressive components from bacteria).

There will invariably be a massive acute-phase response with elevation of C-reactive protein (CRP) and other acute-phase proteins (complement, fibrinogen, protease inhibitors, α2-macroglobulin (IL-6 carrier) and a reduction in albumin (a negative acute-phase protein).

Complement components will be consumed rapidly, but synthesis will be increased (all are acute-phase proteins), so measurements may be difficult to interpret. Functional assays of complement are usually highly abnormal.

Toxic shock may follow certain types of bacterial infections (staphylococci, streptococci), due to release of 'superantigenic' toxins, which activate many clones of T cells directly, bypassing the need for MHC on antigen-presenting cells by binding directly to the T-cell receptor. Effects are likely to be due to cytokine excess.

Immunological investigation

The most important investigations are microbiological. Monitoring of the acute-phase response (CRP) gives a good indication of response to therapy.

Acute measurement of immunoglobulins and complement is usually misleading and may lead to erroneous diagnoses of antibody or complement deficiency. It is best to leave these investigations until convalescence. Functional assays of complement may take 2–3 weeks to normalize after acute sepsis.

Acute measurement of cytokines in toxic shock is currently impractical and the diagnosis is a clinical one.

3 Secondary immunodeficiencies

Acute bacterial infections

Chronic bacterial sepsis

Immunological features

Hypergammaglobulinaemia is usual, often with small and some times multiple monoclonal bands developing, representing the immune response against the pathogen. Chronic antigenaemia will cause immune complex reactions and secondary hypocomple mentaemia (e.g. subacute bacterial endocarditis, SBE).

The acute phase becomes a chronic phase: anaemia of chronic disease, iron deficiency due to sequestration (defence against pathogen), see below. There is the risk of amyloid development (see Chapter 8).

T-cell function may be significantly impaired. The best example is mycobacterial infection, with anergy to PPD and third-party anti gens. Ten per cent of TB cases do not respond to tuberculin Mycobacterial products (arabino-D-galactan) interfere with *in vitro* proliferative responses to PHA, PWM, and PPD; the effect is poss ibly via macrophages and may involve prostaglandins (inhibitable by indomethacin). There is often a lymphopenia. Persistently raised CRP may also be suppressive. Miliary TB may cause neutropenia generalized bone marrow suppression, and leukaemoid reactions.

Untreated leprosy is a potent suppressor of cell-mediated immu nity: T-cell responses to mitogens and antigens are reduced. This defect disappears with appropriate antibiotic therapy and appears to be mediated by a glycolipid. The underlying bias of the immune system towards either Th1 (cellular) or Th2 (antibody) responses determines whether the response to leprosy is tuberculoid (Th1) or lepromatous (Th2). Other immunological features include the development of vasculitis (erythema nodosum) and glomerulonephritis (assumed to immune complex, with IgG and complement).

Immunological monitoring

Acute-phase markers provide the best guide to progress and response to therapy (but beware of elevations from drug reactions). The erythrocyte sedimentation rate (ESR) is less useful because of its long half-life.

Low complement (C3) and elevated C3d indicates immune-complex reaction (renal involvement likely); monitoring of func tional haemolytic complement is not valuable.

Immunoglobulins are usually high (polyclonal stimulation ± monoclonal bands). Electrophoresis also shows elevated $\alpha2$-macroglobulin, reduced albumin; beware apparent monoclonal 'bands' from very high CRP (use specific antisera on immuno-fixation to demonstrate this).

Hypogammaglobulinaemia is rare: consider underlying immuno-deficiency.

Measurement of *in vitro* T-cell function and lymphocyte markers is not valuable unless there is a suspicion that the infections are due to an underlying immunodeficiency.

Immunotherapy

γ-Interferon offers some possibilities for modifying the Th1:Th2 balance in chronic mycobacterial infections and in leishmaniasis.

Fungal infections

Except for cutaneous infections, invasive fungal infections are usually the markers of, rather than the cause of, immunodeficiency, indicating defective neutrophil/macrophage and T-cell immunity.

Parasitic infections

Immunological features

Malaria has no overt effect on cell-mediated immunity but reduces the humoral immune responses to bacterial antigens (tetanus toxoid, meningococcal polysaccharide, and *Salmonella* O antigen), presumably through effects on the spleen. There appears to be little interaction between HIV infection and malaria, where the two diseases overlap. Tropical splenomegaly due vivax malaria is associated with a CD8+ T-cell lymphopenia and raised IgM.

Trypanosomes suppress cellular responses, but there is often a polyclonal increase of non-specific immunoglobulin, especially IgM.

Visceral leishmaniasis is characterized by a polyclonal hypergammaglobulinaemia, often massive, but with absent cell-mediated immunity until after treatment. Splenomegaly may be massive and there is often lymphopenia. The cachexia and lymphopenia are mediated by release of tumour necrosis factor-α (TNF-α) by infected macrophages.

Immunological monitoring

There is little value in monitoring anything other than the acute-phase response.

3 Secondary immunodeficiencies

Fungal infections
Parasitic infections

MALIGNANCY

Immunological features

Malignancy, especially lymphoid, is very common in primary immunodeficiencies (Wiskott–Aldrich syndrome, CVID, DNA repair defects; see Chapter 2) and in secondary immunodeficiencies (HIV, EBV). Some viruses are directly oncogenic (hepatitis B, EBV). Malignancy is also increased in patients with autoimmune disease, possibly secondary to immunosuppressive drug therapy, and in transplant patients who are immunosuppressed (skin tumours, carcinoma of the anogenital tract).

Abnormalities of T-cell and NK-cell function have been described in patients with solid tumours, leading to the suggestion that impaired immune surveillance is related to the development of tumours, although they might equally be a consequence, not a cause. T-cell defects include reduction of IL-2 and TNF-α production, and activation markers such as CD71 (transferrin receptor). Cancer cells may alter immune function through the release of TGF-β, which reduces T-cell proliferative responses and macrophage metabolism, and through inhibitors of complement.

Some tumours have a propensity to generate autoimmune responses due to inappropriate expression of antigens; these may lead to paraneoplastic phenomena, such as the Lambert–Eaton myasthenic syndrome (small cell lung carcinoma) due to an auto-antibody against voltage-gated calcium channels, and neuronal and retinal autoantibodies in breast, ovarian, and colonic tumours.

Major immunosuppression may result from radio- and chemo-therapy. This may be prolonged and lead to secondary infective complications.

Immunological monitoring

There is little value in immunological monitoring of aspects such as NK-cell numbers or function. However, patients with significant and persistent infective problems post-treatment may warrant investigation of cellular and humoral immune function, depending on the type of infections. Lymphocyte surface markers, immunoglobulins, IgG subclasses, and specific antibodies to bacteria and viruses may be appropriate.

Paraneoplastic phenomena may suggest a search for unusual autoantibodies (voltage-gated calcium channels, cerebellar Purkinje cells, retinal antigens).

Immunotherapy

Immunotherapy of solid tumours has a chequered career. IL-2 therapy has been proposed for certain tumours (renal and melanoma) but there are no good controlled trial data to support this and it is very toxic. *In vitro* stimulation of non-specific killers (LAK cell therapy) by IL-2, using either peripheral blood cells or tumour-infiltrating cells, has also been claimed in small open trials to be beneficial but is even more toxic.

Other immunotherapies tried have included the use of non-specific immunostimulants such as BCG, *Corynebacterium parvum*, and *Bordetella pertussis*, often given intralesionally. Occasionally spectacular results have been achieved. α-Interferon has been used with success in certain lymphoid disorders (hairy-cell leukaemia, plateau-phase myeloma).

A major benefit of immunotherapy has been in the use of colony-stimulating factors to protect the bone marrow, allowing higher doses of conventional cytotoxic agents to be used. However, there are concerns that this approach may increase the risk of secondary myeloid leukaemias.

Plasma cell tumours and related conditions

Immunological features

Myeloma is tumour of plasma cells, leading to clonal proliferation. A single isolated lesion in bone is referred to as a plasmacytoma.

Waldenström's macroglobulinaemia is a clonal proliferation of IgM-producing lymphocytes. Staging of disease depends on bone marrow features, paraprotein level, calcium, and haemoglobin.

There may be a genetic background (HLA-Cw2, -Cw5) and IgA paraproteins may be associated with a translocation t(8;14). Ig gene rearrangements are detectable. Myeloma cells often express both lymphocyte and plasma cell antigens simultaneously. Abnormal B cells may be detectable in the peripheral blood, expressing high levels of CD44 and CD54. Cells also express CD56 (NCAM), an adhesion molecule, and soluble levels of NCAM are elevated in myeloma.

IL-6 plays a key role as either autocrine or paracrine factor stimulating proliferation. CRP may be raised in consequence. Osteoclast activating factors are also produced, leading to bone destruction (IL-1, IL-6, TNF-β).

Monoclonal immunoglobulin production parallels the frequency of B cells: 52 per cent IgG, 22 per cent IgA, 25 per cent free light chain only, and 1 per cent IgD. IgE myeloma is exceptionally rare and is found with plasma cell leukaemia. Biclonal myeloma and non-secreting tumours may be found. The synthesis of heavy and light chains is often discordant and whole paraprotein may be accompanied by excess free light chains. Free light chains are readily filtered but nephrotoxic. IgD myeloma often presents in renal failure.

Hyperviscosity is common with high levels of IgM and IgA paraproteins but is rare with IgG and free light-chain paraproteins. IgA frequently polymerizes *in vivo* (dimers and tetramers). Paraproteins may have autoantibody activity and may be cryoglobulins (types I and II). Complexes of paraproteins (especially IgM) with coagulation factors may cause bleeding.

Although myelomatous change probably arises in spleen or lymph node, these are unusual sites for disease, which is usually found in bone and bone marrow. Excess clonal plasma cells will be found in the bone marrow. Normal humoral immune function is impaired and there is suppression of non-paraprotein immunoglobulin (arrest of B lymphocyte maturation). Specific antibody responses are poor. T-cell function is also impaired, leading to viral infections.

Low levels of monoclonal paraproteins are found in other lymphoproliferative conditions, chronic infections, connective tissue diseases, and old age. Where a paraprotein is present without other features of myeloma (no increase plasma cells in bone marrow), the term 'monoclonal gammopathy of uncertain significance' is applied. A proportion of these patients develop myeloma with time and all should be monitored at intervals.

Heavy-chain disease is rare (μ, γ, and α). α-Heavy-chain disease is the most common. All are associated with lymphoma-like disease.

POEMS syndrome (polyneuropathy, organomegaly, endocrine abnormalities, monoclonal gammopathy, and skin rashes) appears to be a plasma-cell variant of Castleman's disease, a hyperplasia of lymph nodes, which may occur with autoimmune diseases (see also Chapter 5).

Immunological diagnosis and monitoring

The diagnosis of a paraproteinaemia depends on accurate electrophoresis of serum AND urine, followed by immunofixation. Immunochemical measurements of immunoglobulin levels (by radial immunodiffusion (RID) or nephelometry) may be misleading due to polymerization or, in the case of IgM, monomeric paraprotein. Paraprotein levels are best determined by scanning densitometry, provided that the total protein in serum can be measured accurately. There are difficulties if the M-band overlaps the β-region.

Urinary light-chain excretion may be helpful as a prognostic monitor of tumour cell burden, but there are difficulties in the calculation of this (see Part 2) and renal function affects the output.

Serum β2-microglobulin is a valuable marker of tumour-cell activity. CRP may be a surrogate for IL-6 production and soluble NCAM may be of prognostic value.

The degree of humoral immunodeficiency should be assessed by measurement of exposure and immunization antibodies, followed by test immunization with protein and polysaccharide antigens.

Immunotherapy

The disease is probably not curable at present. Standard chemotherapy includes melphalan and prednisolone; other agents used include vincristine, doxorubicin (or related drugs), and carmustine (BiCNU®). α-Interferon has a major effect in prolonging the plateau phase. Bone marrow transplantation (allogeneic and autologous purged marrow) may also prolong remission but it is doubtful if it is curative. Colony-stimulating factors should be used with caution as they may enhance tumour cell growth.

IVIg may be beneficial in dealing with secondary infective problems but should be used with great caution in patients with renal impairment and those with rheumatoid activity of their paraproteins (both may lead to renal failure). Prophylactic antibiotics may be an alternative.

Plasmapheresis may be required to deal with hyperviscosity and/or cryoglobulinaemia.

Lymphoma—Hodgkin's disease

Immunological features

Hodgkin's disease (HD) is a lymphoma seen predominantly in the young. It is characterized by the presence of typical Reed–Sternberg cells (CD15, CD30 positive).

Three major types (nodular sclerosing, mixed cellularity, and lymphocyte depleted) are recognized. Lymphocyte predominant may well be a separate disease, as it occurs later and often relapse to non-Hodgkin's lymphoma. Staging depends on the number of sites affected and by the presence or absence of constitutional symptoms

EBV genome is often found in HD, and Reed–Sternberg (RS) cells are usually positive. RS cells are thought to be the true neoplastic cell, possibly derived from interdigitating reticulum cells.

T- and B-cell numbers are reduced. Immunoglobulins are often raised, especially IgE. Ten per cent of patients will have hypogammaglobulinaemia (severe disease). There may be poor specific responses, with reduced T-cell proliferation (reversible by indomethacin, suggesting a possible macrophage defect) and poor primary antibacterial responses. Secondary antibody responses may be normal. Cutaneous anergy is common. Responses to Pneumovax® may be present even if there is a lack of DTH responses. In some cases the defects have been shown to precede the development of the disease and also to persist long-term after successful treatment (although the role of the cytotoxic regimes in this is poorly understood). It is difficult then to distinguish from a primary immunodeficiency complicated by lymphoma.

Bacterial infections are common (*Pneumococcus* and *Haemophilus influenzae*), related to poor humoral function and possibly also to poor neutrophil function.

Before CT scanning became widespread, splenectomy for staging was common. This is now only undertaken for symptomatic hypersplenism. Splenectomy has a very significant effect on immune function in lymphoma, and patients may become unresponsive to bacterial vaccines.

Immunological diagnosis and monitoring

The diagnosis is made on histological examination of excised lymph node, supplemented by the use of immunocytochemistry to identify populations of cells. This may be useful in the identification of scanty RS cells. However, RS cells may also be found in association with glandular fever, reactive hyperplasia, and some non-Hodgkin's lymphomas. There is usually a reactive expansion of CD4+ T-cells. Molecular techniques should be used to look for evidence of EBV genome.

HD is associated with an acute-phase response, with elevated ESR, CRP, and caeruloplasmin. This may be a poor prognostic indicator

All patients with lymphoma should be monitored for evidence of humoral immune deficiency: serum immunoglobulins, IgG subclasses, and specific antibodies. Test immunization is appropriate. Particular attention should be paid to apparently cured patients, who may still have a persisting immunodeficiency.

Immunotherapy

Treatment is with radiotherapy and/or chemotherapy. The latter is used for patients with constitutional ('B') symptoms. There are many regimes for combination chemotherapy. Most regimes are myelosuppressive and impose a temporary secondary defect through neutropenia. Relapse may be treated with autologous bone marrow transplant (harvested in remission) or with a stem-cell transplant. Secondary neoplasms may occur (myelodysplasia, acute myeloid leukaemia) and the risk is related to the intensity of treatment.

IVIg may be required for those with a persisting symptomatic humoral defect after treatment.

Non-Hodgkin's lymphoma

Immunological features

This category includes all those lymphoid and histiocytic lymphoid malignancies that are not Hodgkin's disease. There are many classifications, but the two used most often in the UK are Kiel and the Working Formulation. Morphology and cellular origin play a major role in classification. Tumours are also divided on the basis of their clinical grade (= aggressivity). Low-grade B-cell tumours overlap with chronic lymphocytic leukaemia. Waldenström's macroglobulinaemia is often referred to as an immunocytic lymphoma. Both T- and B-cell lymphomas are recognized, as well as tumours derived from histiocytic elements.

The retrovirus, HTLV-1 has been associated with T-cell lymphomas in areas where it is endemic (Japan and the Caribbean). EBV has been associated with certain B-cell lymphomas, particularly associated with immunosuppression and endemic Burkitt's lymphoma, which is found in malarial areas. This tumour, but also others, is associated with chromosomal abnormalities, normally translocations t(14;8). Many other translocations have been identified. It is thought that these translocations allow dysregulated activity of cellular oncogenes by placing them in proximity to active promoters. In Burkitt's lymphoma it is the oncogene c-*myc*. Often sites of translocations involve the heavy- and light-chain genes for immunoglobulin and the genes for T-cell receptors.

Secondary lymphomas are usually non-Hodgkin's lymphoma (NHL). These are found with primary immunodeficiencies (WAS, CVID, AT, Chediak–Higashi, DNA repair defects), connective tissue diseases (rheumatoid arthritis, Sjögren's syndrome, SLE), phenytoin therapy, post-transplant (cyclosporin therapy). In the case of primary immunodeficiency, it is likely that the chronic infections lead to an abortive immune response which predisposes to lymphoma. Perhaps earlier diagnosis and better treatment will prevent this.

Studies of humoral and cellular function have shown abnormalities that have not always correlated with the type of lymphoma. Abnormalities are more likely in high-grade tumours. Both hypo- and hypergammaglobulinaemia may occur and may persist after treatment. Monoclonal bands, often IgMκ may be found in association with B-cell tumours. Autoantibody activity may be noted. Acquired angioedema is often associated with an underlying B-cell lymphoma with a paraprotein. The paraprotein binds to and inhibits C1-esterase inhibitor.

As in Hodgkin's disease, splenectomy may have been undertaken in the past, imposing an additional immunological defect. These patients require careful supervision.

Immunological diagnosis and monitoring

The diagnosis requires histological examination of lymphoid tissue, accompanied by immunohistochemistry, using panels of monoclonal antibodies to identify the predominant cell type. Clonality will be established by molecular techniques looking at Ig and Tcr gene rearrangements.

Humoral immune function should be monitored, as for Hodgkin's disease. Serial β2-microglobulin measurements may be helpful as a marker of lymphocyte turnover. Electrophoresis will demonstrate the presence of paraproteins. If autoimmune phenomena are present, then association with the paraprotein can be shown by light-chain restriction on immunofluorescence.

Sometimes abnormalities of immunoglobulins precede overt disease. In contrast to primary immunodeficiency, IgM disappears first, followed by IgG and IgA. Finding an isolated but marked reduction of IgM in an older person should lead to a review for evidence of lymphoma (selective IgM deficiency is vanishingly rare!).

Immunotherapy

Treatment depends on the type of treatment and its grade. Localized disease may be amenable to radiotherapy, while disseminated disease will require chemotherapy. Aggressive chemotherapy of high-grade tumours may result in some cures. Autologous bone marrow transplantation may be helpful in relapse. IVIg may be required if there are infective problems.

Chronic lymphocytic leukaemia (CLL)

Immunological features

CLL is a clonal proliferation of small lymphocytes. It is the most common form of lymphoid leukaemia. Ninety-five per cent are B cell in origin; 5 per cent are T cell in origin. Other variants include prolymphocytic leukaemia (B-PLL), hairy cell leukaemia (HCL), and splenic lymphoma with circulating villous lymphocytes (SLVL). Cell counts may become very high (>100×10^9/l). It is predominantly a disease of the elderly (95 per cent of patients are over 50).

The different variants may be distinguished by flow cytometry. B-CLL is usually CD5+, CD23+, FMC7-, CD22±, with weak surface Ig. Clonal restriction can usually be demonstrated with anti-light-chain antisera. B-PLL has the phenotype CD5±, CD23-, FMC7+, CD22+, sIg+. HCL is CD5-, CD23-, FMC7+, CD22+, sIg+. SLVL is CD5±, CD23±, FMC7+, CD22+, sIg+. Circulating lymphoma cells may be distinguished because they often express CD10 (CALLA). T-PLL is rare: cells are usually CD4+, CD8-, but dual positive or CD4-, CD8+ variants may occur. Large granular lymphocytic leukaemia has cells of the phenotype CD4-, CD8+, CD11b+, CD16/56+, CD57+. The cells may be highly active in an NK assay. Bone marrow examination shows an excess of lymphocytes.

Chromosomal abnormalities are common: trisomy 12 and deletions of the long arm of chromosome 13 in B-cell disease, and chromosome 14 abnormalities (inversion or tandem translocation) or trisomy 8q in T-cell disease. Recent studies have demonstrated that some CLL patients have an abnormal ATM gene (ataxia telangiectasia mutated).

Recurrent bacterial infections are a major problem. Humoral function is impaired and response to Pneumovax® is a better predictor of infection than total IgG. Studies of normal B-cell function is difficult *in vitro* due to the predominance of the aberrant clone. Electrophoresis may show small bands (usually IgM). T-cell numbers may be increased (CD4+ T cells), but function may be poor with low/absent PHA responses. Viral infections may be a problem (shingles with dissemination, HSV).

Autoimmune phenomena are common: ITP and haemolytic anaemia. Splenectomy may be required and this exacerbates the immune deficit. Vaccine responses are frequently entirely absent in this situation and patients must have prophylactic antibiotics. HCL may be associated with vasculitis.

Immunological diagnosis and monitoring

Diagnosis of straightforward CLL is usually possible from the white count and examination of the film. Confirmation requires flow cytometry and examination of the bone marrow.

Studies of humoral immune function are necessary and should include test immunization with Pneumovax®. As these diseases are chronic, monitoring should be carried out at regular intervals, to identify deterioration.

Immunotherapy

127

Treatment is with cytotoxic agents. Chlorambucil is the usual agent but, fludarabine, deoxycorfomycin, and 2-chlorodeoxyadenosine are highly effective. The last named produces a state similar to ADA deficiency. This leads to a profound immunosuppression, with T-cell lymphopenia and a significant risk of opportunist infections. Patients treated with these agents should have regular T-cell counts by flow cytometry and receive prophylactic co-trimoxazole and irradiated blood products (risk of engraftment). α-Interferon is very effective in HCL. The humanized monoclonal antibody Campath-1H® has been used in resistant cases with success. Younger patients may be candidates for bone marrow transplantation

Recurrent infections may require prophylactic antibiotics or IVIg. Monthly treatment is usually adequate (dose 200–400 mg/kg).

Chronic myeloid leukaemia (CML) and myelodysplastic syndromes

Immunological features

Chromosomal abnormalities occur in almost cases of CML and myelodysplastic syndromes. The Philadelphia chromosome (t(9;22)) is the most common, but others have been described, including the 5q- syndrome, monosomy 7, trisomy 8, 19, or 20, and deletions on other chromosomes (12 and 20). The deletions of chromosome 5 are of interest because they map to the region containing the genes for IL-3, -4, -5, G-CSF, and GM-CSF. There is a high incidence of progression to acute myeloid leukaemia.

Abnormal neutrophil function is well described: neutropenia is common in myelodysplasia. Even if the neutrophil count is normal, function is often not, with abnormalities of adhesion, chemotaxis, phagocytosis, and bacterial killing being well documented. This occurs particularly with monosomy 7 in childhood. Infections are common.

Acute leukaemias

Acute leukaemia is a common malignancy of childhood, and accounts for about 30–40 per cent of paediatric malignancy. Eighty per cent of cases are due to acute lymphoblastic leukaemia (ALL). Certain primary immunodeficiencies are risk factors for ALL (Bloom's syndrome, ataxia telangiectasia, Schwachmann's syndrome, xeroderma pigmentosa). Most ALLs are B cell in origin. T-ALL is associated strongly with HTLV-1 infection in areas where this virus is endemic. A number of chromosomal translocations have been described, including the Philadelphia translocation (t(9;22)), which is common in adult ALL. T-ALL is often associated with translocations involving the T-cell receptor genes.

ALL is classified according to the FAB classification, on the basis of cytological appearance, into L1, L2, and L3 types. Immunophenotyping allows the distinction of B, T, and null (rare) ALLs.

Immunological features

In acute lymphocytic leukaemia, the immune system is usually normal, although primary IgM responses to some antigens (viruses), may be poor. Secondary' responses are usually normal. Non-neoplastic cells are normally present in normal numbers. The leukaemic clones rarely have functional activity, although there have been reports of cytokine production. Rare cases may be hypogammaglobulinaemic at presentation.

Acute myeloid leukaemia has also been classified by the FAB group into M0–M7, depending on the predominant cell type identified by morphology and cytochemistry. Cases of AML may be secondary to Wiskott–Aldrich syndrome, Chediak–Higashi syndrome, and Fanconi anaemia, as well as to the use of cytotoxic drugs such as cyclophosphamide.

Occasionally biphenotypic leukaemias may be detected, defined as the presence of at least two markers from each lineage (e.g. lymphoid and myeloid). They account for 5–10 per cent of acute leukaemia and tend to have a poor prognosis. Often they present as AML, but have evidence of clonal rearrangements of immunoglobulin and Tcr genes.

The chemotherapy is profoundly immunosuppressive, affecting both T- and B-cell function and rendering patients neutropenic. Careful attention to prevention of infection (isolation, irradiation of food, gut decontamination) is essential.

Immunological diagnosis

The diagnosis of leukaemia is usually made on the basis of suspicious blood films, supplemented by immunphenotyping of both peripheral blood and bone marrow, to identify the characteristics of the leukaemic clone. This is supplemented by genetic analysis to identify any translocations: probes to the sites of recombination for these translocations give a very sensitive tool for detecting minimal residual disease in bone marrow after treatment.

Leukaemia phenotyping is best undertaken by haematologists who will have access to supportive evidence from blood films, bone marrow smears and trephines, as well as cytochemical enzymatic studies. They will also undertake the therapy.

Monitoring of humoral and cellular function post-treatment, and especially after bone marrow transplantation, is essential.

Immunotherapy

The management of ALL involves intensive chemotherapy and radiotherapy to sanctuary sites such as the nervous system (often with intrathecal methotrexate). For relapse or high-risk patients bone marrow transplantation is used, either matched unrelated donors or purged autologous if an HLA-identical donor is not available. There is a high risk of long-term development of non-Hodgkin's lymphoma and acute myeloid leukaemia.

AML is treated similarly with intensive chemotherapy, with the option for bone marrow transplantation when remission is obtained. Acute promyelocytic leukaemia associated with the t(15;17) translocation may be treated with all-*trans* retinoic acid, which allows differentiation of the blocked cells to mature neutrophils, although bone marrow transplantation is still required.

Certain cytokines may have a role as adjunctive agents, allowing intensification of chemotherapy.

Bone marrow transplantation

Bone marrow transplantation (BMT) is part of the treatment for a variety of inherited diseases (SCID and SCID variants, Wiskott–Aldrich syndrome, osteopetrosis, Gaucher's disease) in addition to its role in the acute leukaemias and CML with blast transformation. The process is discussed in more detail in Chapter 9.

BMT leads to an immediate severe immunodeficiency, due to the conditioning required to allow 'take'. All blood products must be irradiated to prevent viable lymphocytes engrafting and must be CMV-. There follows a period of gradually improving immune function while the immune system reconstitutes. This recapitulates immunological ontogeny. T-cell function reconstitutes early but full B-cell function may take up to 2 years. IgG2 levels may remain depressed and there are frequently poor responses to polysaccharide antigens. The degree of reconstitution is affected by the degree of mismatch and by graft-versus-host disease.

Return of T-cell function *in vitro* (positive PHA) is usually taken to define the time when release from isolation is safe.

While B-cell function is poor, during the acute phase and for the first year thereafter, IVIg prophylaxis is desirable. Return of B-cell function can be monitored by IgA and IgM levels and the development of isohaemagglutinins. Once off IVIg, a full programme of immunizations should be undertaken, starting with killed vaccines (killed polio, DPT, Hib, and Pneumovax®). The response to these can be assessed (pre and post levels are required, and remember that antibody from IVIg may persist for up to 6 months or longer). Once there is a good response to killed/subunit vaccines, then live vaccines can be administered (MMR).

Immunological function in chronic GvHD is markedly abnormal, with a persisting risk of invasive infections of all types. The gastrointestinal involvement superimposes a severe nutritional defect, which further reduces immune function.

Extremes of age: prematurity

At birth, infants are dependent for the first 6 months of life on maternally transferred immunoglobulin (IgG only). During this time the baby's immune function gradually develops, although there is usually a physiological trough in IgG levels around 6 months: if this is prolonged, then transient hypogammaglobulinaemia of infancy results (Chapter 2). Additional protection to the neonatal gut is provided by breast feeding, particularly in the first few days when the IgA-rich colostrum is produced.

Maternal antibody transfer is an active process in the placenta that begins around 14 weeks' gestation and accelerates markedly after 22 weeks. The process can take place against a concentration gradient and is selective for some IgG subclasses: IgG2 is transferred relatively less well. Antibody-deficient mothers will also be at risk of producing hypogammaglobulinaemic infants, who will require IVIg for the first 6 months of life. Good replacement therapy during pregnancy will obviate the need for this.

Premature delivery interrupts the placental transfer and leaves the infant deficient in immunoglobulins and with a relatively less mature humoral and cellular immune system. Breast feeding is rarely possible, but oral administration of colostrum is desirable to prevent necrotizing enterocolitis. Infections are often problematic, although other factors, such as ITU nursing, venous and arterial lines, and lung immaturity, all contribute. Group B streptococcal infections are particularly troublesome.

Immunological features and diagnosis

All immunoglobulins will be low, as will be IgG subclasses. However, the 'normal' ranges are calculated from full-term delivery. Provided that there are no major complications, the immune system rapidly catches up after delivery and there are rarely long-term sequelae.

Immunotherapy

The role of IVIg replacement as routine for premature infants has been investigated extensively, with conflicting results, and a consensus as to the value is difficult to obtain. Differences in products and batches may relate to highly variable levels of anti-group B streptococcal antibodies. Better products, enriched for specific antibodies to the problem pathogens, may be required. Oral, IgA-rich products have also been used to reduce the risk of enterocolitis.

Immunization of the premature causes problems in timing, as there may be very poor responses if routine immunizations are given at intervals calculated from date of delivery uncorrected for gestational age.

Extremes of age: elderly

Immunological changes in the elderly are multifactorial, relating to the decline in normal immunoregulatory processes, the increased incidence of disease, and the increased use of drugs. There is no relationship to chronological age.

Immunological features

There is no significant change in lymphocyte numbers or subsets in the healthy elderly, although lymphoid organs show a reduction of germinal centres. Mucosal immunity seems to be reasonably intact, although the non-specific inflammatory response is reduced. Aged lymphocytes have metabolic abnormalities such reduced 5'-nucleotidase activity (also associated with CVID), and there are changes in the expression of surface antigens.

Immunoglobulin levels change with age: IgG and IgA tend to rise while IgM and IgE fall. Primary humoral responses are reduced and secondary responses give lower peak titres and a more rapid fall with time. Antibody affinity may also be poorer. However, some studies have shown that vaccine responses in the elderly may be as good as in younger people.

CVID may present for the first time post-retirement, but this diagnosis should only be entertained when other secondary causes have been eliminated.

With increasing age there is an increasing incidence of small monoclonal bands on electrophoresis, such that 20 per cent of 95-year-olds will have bands. These are present at low levels and are rarely of great significance. There is a parallel increase in autoantibodies of all types. These are usually present at low titres and are not associated with disease. Normal ranges for antibody titres should be adjusted to take account of these changes.

Cell-mediated immunity, as tested by mitogen responses and by DTH testing, are also reduced in the elderly.

Biologically, the healthy very elderly (>85 years old) represent a special group. There may be combinations of MHC genes that can be associated with survival (in Japan, a high frequency of DR1 and low frequency of DR9), but this might be due to selection out of those individuals with less favourable MHC types associated with autoimmune disease.

Co-existing disease imposes additional strains on the immune system; for example, chronic lung disease from smoking, cardiac failure with pulmonary oedema and malnutrition. These often tip the balance away from the immune system in favour of invading pathogens.

Diseases such as influenzae have a disproportionate effect on the elderly through the risks of secondary bacterial infection and exacerbating pre-existing underlying diseases. Infections common in early childhood, such as meningitis, are also more common in the elderly

Immunological diagnosis

The investigation of the elderly for immunodeficiency should be symptom-driven.

Immunotherapy

Preventative vaccination of at-risk groups is thought to be helpful, for instance with influenza vaccine and Pneumovax®. Risk groups are those with underlying significant disease, particularly chronic lung disease. However, protection may be poor because of the underlying decay of immune function. Consideration should also be given to ensuring that other vaccines such as tetanus are kept up to date (this tends to be forgotten in the elderly) as tetanus antibodies may fall below protective levels. Keen gardeners are at most risk.

Immunoglobulin therapy may be required for those with significant symptomatic hypogammaglobulinaemia. Occasional elderly patients may prefer the simplicity of weekly IMIg at their GP's surgery rather than regular hospital trips.

Transfusion therapy

In addition to immediate reactions to blood products due to transfused white cells, preformed antibodies (to HLA or IgA), etc., there is evidence for an immunosuppressive effect. This is most noticeable in the effect on renal allograft survival (Chapter 9). Intravenous immunoglobulin has complex immunoregulatory properties when used in high doses (Chapter 10). Crude Factor VIII concentrates were immunosuppressive, although this may relate as much to chronic hepatitis due to hepatitis C. High-purity FVIII is much less immunosuppressive. Other infections may be transmissible by blood, such as HIV and CMV, which can have major immunosuppressive effects. The use of unirradiated blood in the immunocompromised (with poor/absent cell-mediated immunity; CMI) may lead to engraftment of viable lymphocytes and the development of graft-versus-host disease. Lymphocytes may be viable for up to 2 weeks in bank blood.

The transfusion effect in solid organ transplantation is discussed in Chapter 9. Effects of high dose IVIg are discussed in Chapter 10.

Chronic renal disease

Renal protein loss should always be considered when investigating hypogammaglobulinaemia. In the nephrotic syndrome there is an increased susceptibility to *Pneumococcus* and other streptococci. The typical pattern is loss of immunoglobulins in order of ascending molecular weight, depending on the selectivity of the proteinuria, with preferential loss of IgG, then IgA, and preservation of IgM until gross nephrosis ensues. The IgG synthetic rate is normal or increased and the IgM catabolic rate is normal. There are poor responses to Pneumovax® but normal responses to influenza. Poor neutrophil chemotaxis and opsonization are also described. Investigation of humoral function is important if there is significant proteinuria. Loss of complement proteins such as C3 and Factor B may also contribute to poor bacterial handling through decreased opsonization.

Chronic uraemia is immunosuppressive with poor humoral and cellular immune responses. The molecules responsible for this are uncertain. Lymphopenia is common, affecting CD4+ and CD8+ T cells, and DTH and mitogen responses are reduced. Immunoglobulins and specific antibody responses to pneumococcal and hepatitis B vaccines may be low. Lymph nodes show a loss of secondary follicles. Neutrophil function shows defective chemotaxis and phagocytosis, with impaired oxidative metabolism, leading to poor bacterial killing.

Certain types of dialysis membrane (cellophane, now no longer used) activated the alternate pathway of complement, with release of anaphylotoxins and neutrophil activation leading to severe circulatory and respiratory problems. Dialysis patients often have a CD4+ T-cell lymphopenia.

The immunosuppression required in renal transplantation significantly affects cellular immune function, leading to opportunist infections and malignancy. Monitoring of lymphocyte subpopulations will identify at-risk individuals.

Protein-losing enteropathy

Causes

Secondary hypogammaglobulinaemia may be due to protein-losing enteropathy, for which there are many causes:

- Ménétrier's disease (giant rugal hypertrophy);
- coeliac disease and other types of sprue;
- inflammatory bowel disease (Crohn's disease);
- infections—hookworm, TB;
- fistulae; post-gastrectomy syndrome;
- neoplasms;
- allergic gut disease (eosinophilic gastropathy);
- secondary to constrictive pericarditis and gross right heart failure;
- Whipple's disease;
- chylous effusions;
- intestinal lymphangiectasia (dilated lymphatics).

Immunological features

Immunoglobulins are low, with a short half-life, but the synthetic rate may be increased. Specific antibody responses may be normal, although they may decline rapidly. Lymphopenia is associated with dilated or blocked lymphatics (intestinal lymphangiectasia, constrictive pericarditis, right heart failure). This may lead to poor mitogen responses and DTH reactions.

Diagnosis

Proof that the bowel is the source of immunoglobulin and cellular loss is difficult as most laboratories are singularly unkeen on trying to measure faecal immunoglobulin excretion! Whole bowel perfusion studies may make this more tolerable.

Full studies of humoral and cellular function are required, together with investigation for the underlying cause (radiology, endoscopy, and biopsy).

Metabolic diseases

A number of metabolic diseases are associated with concomitant immunological impairment:

- Glycogenosis type Ib: neutropenia and neutrophil migration defect. Recurrent infections a problem: septicaemia, wound infections, osteomyelitis, and sinusitis.
- Mannosidosis: recurrent severe infections; impaired neutrophil chemotaxis. Poor T-cell responses to PHA and concanavalin A (ConA).
- Galactosaemia: increased risk of Gram-negative septicaemia due to abnormalities of neutrophil motility and phagocytosis.
- Myotonic dystrophy: hypercatabolism of IgG but not albumin, IgA, or IgM may occur, although infections are not usually a major problem..
- Sickle-cell disease: increased susceptibility to meningitis and septicaemia. There is an acquired splenic dysfunction, due to infarction. Tissue hypoxia also contributes to bacterial infection. Serum immunoglobulins and vaccine responses are usually normal, even to polysaccharide antigens. It is recommended that all patients should be treated as other asplenic or hyposplenic patients and should receive Pneumovax® and Hib vaccines, and be considered for prophylactic antibiotics.
- Coeliac disease: this may be accompanied by splenic atrophy and these patients should be investigated and treated as other asplenic patients.

Diabetes mellitus

Diabetes interferes with immune function through two mechanisms. First, there is the underlying genetic susceptibility to type I diabetes (the MHC type is shared with CVID) and consequent immune dys-regulation. As a result of the association with the A1, B8, DR3, C4Q0 haplotype, there is an increased incidence of C4 deficiency in diabetes. Secondly, in established disease, the raised glucose itself interferes with both innate and specific immune functions. Most of the research has been done on chemically induced or genetic diabetes in mice, much less work has been done on human diabetes.

Immunological mechanisms

Humoral function is impaired: IgG levels may be reduced, while IgA may be increased. Specific antibody responses may show poor primary immune responses and the non-enzymatic glycation of immunoglobulin may interfere with function. Both T-dependent and T-independent antigens are affected.

Lymphoid organs are essentially normal but peripheral blood lymphocytes may show variable abnormalities. CMI may be depressed with poor DTH responses and abnormal mitogen responses and poor cytokine production (IL-2). Macrophage and neutrophil function is also reduced.

Infections with *Candida* and other fungi, TB, and pneumococci are more common in diabetes. Staphylococcal colonization of the skin is higher in diabetics than in normal individuals.

Abnormalities of immune function are more marked in type I diabetes but correlate poorly with blood glucose levels. It is possible that immune dysfunction relates to glycation of surface antigens on immunologically important cells.

Diagnosis and treatment

Recurrent infections in diabetics should be investigated in the normal way and not merely accepted, particularly if diabetic control is not bad. This should include humoral and neutrophil function.

In the USA, regular pneumococcal vaccination is recommended, but this policy has not been adopted in the UK.

Iron deficiency

An induced sideropenia due to sequestration is part of the body's response to chronic infection, as iron is essential to bacteria. However, it is also essential to host defences. Iron deficiency due to loss or inadequate intake impairs neutrophil bactericidal activity, as it is essential for the activity of myeloperoxidase. There is often a T lymphopenia. Immunoglobulins are usually normal but specific antibody production is reduced. All the changes are reversible with iron.

Nutritional status

The immunodeficiency of malnutrition is difficult to disentangle because it is usually accompanied by multiple other health problems, which make identification of cause and effect impossible. Marasmus is total nutritional deficiency while kwashiorkor is protein deficiency in a high-calorie diet. Both are usually accompanied by vitamin deficiency. Increased susceptibility to infection seems to be the rule. Non-specific barriers are impaired (especially in vitamin A deficiency). There may be variable abnormalities of neutrophil bactericidal activity, but these may well be secondary to infection. Immunoglobulins are often normal or high, even if the albumin is low. IgE levels may be elevated, even in the absence of significant parasitic infections, suggesting dysregulation of the Th1:Th2 axis. Mitogen responsiveness is reduced in kwashiorkor. Lymph nodes show germinal centre depletion and there is thymic atrophy, although the latter is also a feature of infection.

Asplenia

Acquired asplenia (surgery, trauma) or hyposplenia (sickle-cell disease, coeliac disease) is associated with an increased susceptibility to overwhelming infection with capsulated organisms and problems in handling malaria and babesiosis. This risk appears to be lifelong, and is not limited to the first 2–3 years after splenectomy, as was previously thought. The degree of compromise also depends on the reason for splenectomy. For example, individuals splenectomized for lymphomas often have a more severe defect than those splenectomized for trauma. Ideally all patients undergoing elective splenectomy should be immunized with Pneumovax® and Hib vaccine and probably with the meningococcal A&C vaccine preoperatively. If this is not possible, then immunization prior to discharge may be adequate, although responses immediately post-surgery will be reduced. All asplenic patients should be on prophylactic antibiotics (penicillin V, 500 mg twice a day, for choice) and should have their antibodies to Pneumovax® and Hib measured. Those with suboptimal levels should be (re)-immunized. Asplenic patients may also not maintain adequate levels following vaccination for more than 3–5 years and regular checks should be carried out to ensure that protection is adequate. Note that the licence for Pneumorax® does not indicate that it can be given this frequently. However, provided steps are taken to avoid immunizing patients with high antibody levels, the risk of adverse events appears to be low.

Drugs

In addition to the drugs discussed in Chapter 10, the major therapeutic action of which is immunosuppression, other drugs have also been reported to cause immunodeficiency. In many cases the evidence is poor, because pre-existent immunodeficiency has not been excluded. However, anticonvulsants, especially phenytoin and carbamazepine, both have strong associations with humoral immune deficiency, which may or may not resolve on withdrawal of the drugs.

Smoking suppresses mucosal immune responses, improving some allergic diseases such allergic alveolitis. Illegal drugs have considerable immunosuppressive potential, in part due to contaminants. Cannabis is particularly dangerous to severely immuno-compromised patients as it may contain fungal spores.

Alcohol in excess suppresses macrophage function, and as result increases the risk of tuberculosis.

Burns

Burns cause a highly significant acquired T- and B-cell immunodeficiency. A major factor is the disruption of the integrity of the normal cutaneous barriers and associated non-specific defences. However, in severe burns neutrophil function is impaired and there is a lymphopenia, with depletion of lymphoid organs. DTH, mitogen and allogeneic responses are reduced. These changes may be stress related, due to excessive endogenous steroid production (Curling's ulcer is also associated) or to the release at the burned site of bacterial products. Immunoglobulin levels fall, often dramatically, due to reduced synthesis and increased loss through exudation. However, there is no benefit from IVIg replacement therapy. The best treatment is good intensive care and rapid grafting to re-establish normal barrier function.

Myotonic dystrophy

Hypogammaglobulinaemia due to hypercatabolism of IgG has been recorded in this syndrome. This is rarely of clinical significance as specific immune responses are normal.

4 Allergic disease

Introduction

Allergic diseases are common: it has been estimated that 15 per cent
of the population will suffer from some sort of allergic reaction during their lifetime. It is clear that there has been an increase in atopic
diseases since the Second World War. The precise cause of this
change is unknown but undoubtedly reflects changes in life style,
in particular 'improvements' in housing, rendering houses more
heavily colonized with dust mites. A reduction in breast feeding
may also have contributed, particularly to atopic eczema. The evidence for air pollution, particularly car exhaust fumes, contributing
to the increase is conflicting. It is also likely that the improvements
in public health, leading to elimination in the Western world of
parasitic infections, may contribute through a lack of physiological
function for the IgE-mast cell axis. In the mind of the public,
allergy is responsible for all ills but in many cases the blame is
wrongly apportioned. This perception has led to a proliferation of
alternative practices pandering to these beliefs and using diagnostic
techniques and treatments that have little to do with allergy
as understood by immunologists and have more to do with the
gullibility of members of the public. That these practitioners can
flourish indicates that we are failing our patients in being unable to
cure their perceived illnesses, either through lack of knowledge or
through lack of appropriate allergy facilities.

Anaphylaxis

Anaphylaxis represents the most severe type of allergic reaction and a medical emergency. The usual features are:
- generalized giant urticaria;
- angioedema, often involving face, lips, tongue, and larynx, causing stridor;
- bronchospasm;
- hypotension with loss of consciousness;
- gastrointestinal symptoms (nausea, vomiting, abdominal cramps, diarrhoea).

Not all symptoms will be present during an attack and only 50 per cent of patients will have a rash.

The onset is rapid after exposure, usually within minutes, although some agents (foods and latex) may lead to a slower onset. Agents that are injected (drugs, venoms) give the fastest responses. The reaction is a type 1 reaction, dependent on the presence of specific IgE. Other reactions may mimic the clinical symptoms but without the involvement of IgE (anaphylactoid reactions—see below).

Repeated challenge at short intervals may lead to progressively more severe reactions, but otherwise the severity of a reaction does NOT predict the severity of subsequent reactions.

Causes

Any substance may cause anaphylaxis, but the most common causes are biological proteins: bee and wasp venoms, peanuts (and related legumes, soya, etc.), true nuts (walnut, almond, cashew, hazelnut, etc.), shellfish (crustacea, prawns, shrimps, crab, lobster), fish, latex (and related foods, banana, avocado, kiwi, chestnut, potato, tomato), egg, milk, penicillin and other drugs (anaesthetic agents), peptide hormones (ACTH, insulin), heterologous antisera (antivenins, antilymphocyte globulins, monoclonal antibodies).

In some cases a co-factor is required for the reaction, such as concomitant aspirin ingestion with the food, or exercise. It is probable that these co-factors alter the amount of allergen entering the circulation.

Immunological features

The involvement of IgE requires prior exposure to sensitize the patient. In childhood sensitization to peanut may occur via formula milk, which may contain peanut oil. Following sensitization, only tiny amounts may be required to trigger subsequent reactions.

The reaction is triggered by cross-linking of mast-cell cytophilic IgE by the allergen, leading to degranulation and activation of the mast cell. The symptoms occur as a result of mast-cell release of histamine, which is responsible for bronchoconstriction, increased airway mucus secretion, stimulation of gut smooth muscle, hypotension due to increased vascular permeability, and vasodilatation and urticaria/angioedema.

Other mediators include mast-cell tryptase and chemotactic factors for eosinophils. Activated mast cells also synthesize prostaglandins and leukotrienes, which reinforce the effects on smooth muscle. Tosyl-L-arginine methyl ester (TAME) has a similar effect. Platelet activating factor causes the activation of platelets, leading to the release of histamine and serotonin and augmenting the effects on vascular tone and permeability.

Mast-cell numbers at sites of allergen exposure are critical. It is speculative that there are variations in the output of mast cells from bone marrow which influence the possibility of developing reactions.

The complement and kinin systems are activated (basophils release kallikrein when activated). Bradykinin, C3a, and C5a all act as smooth muscle constrictors and increase vascular permeability.

Reactions may recur after 2–4 hours, despite successful initial treatment, due to the continuing synthetic activity of mast cells and the release of leukotrienes.

Those with underlying atopic disease are said to be more at risk of developing serious allergic responses.

Immunological diagnosis

The history is all important, particularly the timing of reaction in relation to the suspected trigger. If the trigger is not clear, a detailed review of all exposures over the preceding 24 hours is required. The reaction should be graded:

- mild, a feeling of generalized warmth, with sensation of fullness in throat, some localized angioedema and urticaria but no significant impairment of breathing or features of hypotension;
- moderate, as for mild, but with more widespread angioedema and urticaria, some bronchospasm and mild gastrointestinal symptoms;
- severe, intense bronchospasm, laryngeal oedema, with severe shortness of breath, cyanosis, respiratory arrest, hypotension, cardiac arrhythmias, shock, and gross gastrointestinal symptoms.

Attention must be paid to other conditions that may appear similar clinically: pulmonary embolus, myocardial infarction (but this may follow anaphylaxis in those with pre-existing ischaemic heart disease), hyperventilation, hypoglycaemia, vasovagal reactions, phaeochromocytoma, carcinoid, and systemic mastocytosis. Rarely the symptoms may be factitious.

Confirmation of the nature of the reaction may be obtained by taking blood for mast-cell tryptase (levels will be elevated for up to 12 hours and it is stable); urinary methyl histamine is an alternative, but is less readily available. Evidence should also be sought for activation of the complement system (measurement of C3, C4, and C3 breakdown products). Measurement of C3a and C5a is possible but requires a special tube, which is unlikely to be available in time.

Total IgE measurements are of little value. Tests for specific IgE (RAST, etc.) may give negative results in the immediate phase, even

151

when it is quite clear what has caused the reaction. Repeating tests 3–4 weeks later may be helpful.

Skin-prick testing may be sufficient to trigger a further systemic reaction and should be undertaken with great caution and only in a situation in which full facilities for cardiopulmonary resuscitation are immediately available.

Management

Immediate management comprises adrenaline given intramuscularly in a dose of 0.5–1 mg for an adult. The dose can be repeated if required. If there is intravenous access, the adrenaline may be given in small aliquots of 0.1 mg every 2–3 minutes rather than as a bolus (arrhythmias and hypertension may result from a large bolus). Great care should be observed during IV administration to conscious patients: the rate of administration must not be exceeded.

An antihistamine should be given intravenously (chlorpheniramine 10 mg) and a bolus of hydrocortisone (200 mg) should be given. The latter has no effect on the immediate reaction but reduces the possibility of a late reaction.

Oxygen should be administered and the blood pressure supported with intravenous fluids (colloid). Persisting hypotension may require further vasopressor agents. Tracheotomy may be required if there is major laryngeal oedema. Admission for observation is required (risk of late reactions).

Great care must be taken with latex allergic patients, as hospital staff with latex gloves and resuscitation with latex-containing equipment (masks, catheters, etc.) may make the reaction paradoxically worse during resuscitation.

Patients who have had severe reactions should be trained to self-administer adrenaline using a self-injection aid and should carry a Medic-Alert bracelet or equivalent. Regular annual follow-up should be undertaken to ensure that patients remain competent in using the adrenaline injector. Carrying a supply of antihistamines may also be helpful (used prophylactically if entering a situation of unknown risk, e.g. eating out). Patients deemed to be at risk of further anaphylaxis should not receive treatment with β-blockers, as these agents will interfere with the action of adrenaline if required.

Patients should receive detailed counselling on how to avoid the triggering allergen; if a food is involved this should be undertaken by a dietician experienced in dealing with food allergy. Many foods may be 'hidden', so that the consumer is unaware of the contents. This applies particularly to pre-prepared foods and restaurant meals.

For bee/wasp anaphylaxis, patients should be warned to avoid wearing brightly coloured clothes and perfumes as these attract the insects. They should also stay away from fallen fruit and dustbins. Desensitization is possible (see Chapter 10). This is a process that requires considerable dedication on the part of the patient (and the hospital staff!). It should be reserved for those who have had a

systemic reaction and where the risk of further stings is considered
to be high.

Latex-allergic patients need to be warned about possible reactions to foods (banana, avocado, kiwi fruit, chestnut, potato, and tomato) and be given advice on avoidance. It is important that they tell doctors as reactions may be triggered during operations by surgeons' gloves or anaesthetic equipment and by investigations such as barium enema (rubber cuff on tubing)

Tests immediately	Tests later
Mast cell tryptase (up to 24 hours)	Specific IgE (may be undetectable at time
(Urinary methyl histamine is an alternative)	of acute reaction)
C3, C4, C3d	
(C1-inhibitor if angioedema with no urticaria)	

Anaphylactoid responses

These may be every bit as severe as IgE-mediated reactions. In most cases they are due to activation of mast cells directly or via other mechanisms that will indirectly activate mast cells.

Causes

The most common causes are:
- Direct mast-cell stimulation: drugs (opiates, thiamine, vancomycin, radiocontrast media, some anaesthetic agents, especially those dissolved in cremophor, tubocurarine), foods (strawberries), physical stimuli (exercise, cold, trauma), venoms.
- Immune complex reactions (types II and III), with release of anaphylotoxins C3a, C5a: reactions to IVIg, other blood products, heterologous antisera.
- Cyclo-oxygenase inhibitors: non-steroidal anti-inflammatory drugs (may also stimulate mast cells directly).
- Massive histamine ingestion: eating mackerel and other related fish that are 'off' (scombrotoxin due to breakdown of muscle histidine to histamine).

Immunological diagnosis

The history usually gives the clue. No tests are entirely specific. Challenge is very risky.

Management

The acute management is the same as for anaphylaxis.

For patients who require intravenous radiocontrast media and are known or suspected to react, then pretreatment with oral corticosteroids (40 mg prednisolone, 13, 7, and 1 hour prior to examination), together with an antihistamine (cetirizine or loratidine 10–20 mg orally 1 hour before) and an H2-blocker (cimetidine, 400 mg orally 1 hour before) should be used. Low-osmolality dyes should be used as these have a lower incidence of reactions.

Angioedema

Angioedema is a deep-tissue swelling that must be distinguished from urticaria. It is rarely itchy, and tends to give discomfort from pressure. In hereditary angioedema there is often a premonitory tingling before the swelling occurs. Any part of the body (including gut) may be involved.

Causes

- Allergic (accompanied by other features such as urticaria, anaphylaxis, etc.)
- C1-esterase inhibitor deficiency (Chapter 2)
- Acquired C1-esterase inhibitor deficiency (autoantibody-mediated, SLE, lymphoma)
- Physical (pressure, vibration, water—often with urticaria)
- Drugs (angiotensin converting enzyme (ACE) inhibitors)
- Idiopathic (rarely involves larynx)

Immunological features

The mechanism is thought to involve activation of the kinin system, leading to tissue oedema. Histamine is not involved (unless there is accompanying urticaria). C1-esterase inhibitor is known to be a control protein for the kinin cascade in addition to its role in the complement and clotting systems.

The inhibition of ACE also interferes with the metabolism of kinins and explains the well-reported association of this class of drug with angioedema. There are polymorphisms of this enzyme but it is not known whether they correlate with the tendency to develop angioedema. Congenital ACE deficiency has also been associated with angioedema.

Diagnosis

The history will give useful clues: family history, connective tissue disease, lymphoma (may be occult), drug exposure, association with physical stimuli.

Angioedema with urticaria will not be due to hereditary angioedema. However, in angioedema without urticaria, C1-esterase inhibitor deficiency should be excluded. C4 will be low, even between attacks, C1-inhibitor will be low in type I but high in type II (Chapter 2). Levels of C2 are said to distinguish acquired from inherited C1-esterase inhibitor deficiency (low in inherited deficiency) but this test is not reliable.

The association with lymphoma requires a screen of immunoglobulins (there is often a paraprotein, usually IgM) and β2-microglobulin, followed by a search for clinical evidence (CT scan for lymphadenopathy). Connective tissue disease will usually be obvious, but detection of autoantibodies (antinuclear antibody (ANA), ds DNA and extractable nuclear antigen (ENA) antibodies) may be necessary.

Therapy

Treatment is dependent on the cause.

The management of C1-esterase inhibitor deficiency is discussed in Chapter 2. Acquired C1-esterase inhibitor deficiency due to lymphoma will be improved by effective treatment of the underlying disease, as will the autoimmune-associated angioedema. Control may be helped with antifibrinolytics (tranexamic acid, 2–4 g/day), or modified androgens (stanozolol, 2.5–10 mg/day; danazol, 200–800 mg/day).

The idiopathic form (other causes excluded) responds best to tranexamic acid and less well to modified androgens.

In acute attacks, adrenaline, anti-histamines, and steroids are less effective than in anaphylaxis. Laryngeal involvement is less common in the non-hereditary forms. FFP may be helpful but may also make symptoms worse. There is no role for purified C1-inhibitor in the absence of evidence of deficiency.

Patients with a history of angioedema should never be given ACE inhibitors, as these drugs may precipitate life-threatening events.

Urticaria ± angioedema

Urticaria is common, affecting 10–20 per cent of individuals at some time. Urticaria is dependent on mast cells and histamine is the principal mediator. The reaction may be due to IgE on mast cells or stimuli that directly activate mast cells (see above under Anaphylactoid reactions). Urticaria may occur alone or be accompanied by more systemic symptoms, including angioedema, although (as noted above) histamine is not involved in the latter. Patients with urticaria do not scratch (unlike atopic dermatitis).

Causes

Urticaria may be acute or chronic (more than 1 month's duration). Chronic urticaria is often idiopathic (75 per cent of cases) and rarely associated with allergy. Five per cent of the population may develop a physical urticaria. Idiopathic urticaria may disappear spontaneously after 1–2 years.

- Allergic: (ingested allergens, injected allergens, e.g. cat scratch; also contact).
- Autoimmune: autoantibodies to IgE and to FcεRI (probably rare); also in association with connective-tissue diseases (antibodies to C1q) SLE.
- Physical: sunlight (also think of porphyria), vibration, pressure (immediate and delayed, dermographism), aquagenic, heat.
- Cold: familial (autosomal dominant), acquired (cryoglobulins, cryofibrinogen).
- Cholinergic (much smaller wheals, often triggered by heat and sweating).
- Adrenergic: provoked by stress.
- Contact: (e.g. urticaria from lying on grass, wearing latex gloves, occasionally from aeroallergens).
- Urticaria pigmentosa: rare disease with reddish-brown macules in skin (accumulations of mast cells).
- Vasculitis: usually a leukocytoclastic vasculitis, painful not itchy; also serum sickness (immune complex).
- Hormonal: autoimmune progesterone-induced urticaria, related to menstrual cycle; occasionally other steroids may cause the same reaction; hypothyroidism.
- Infections: prodrome of hepatitis B, Lyme disease, cat-scratch disease; rarely acute or chronic bacterial infections; parasitic infections.
- Papular urticaria: related to insect bites (may last several days).
- Rare syndromes: Muckle–Wells (urticaria with fever, deafness, and amyloidosis); mastocytosis; PUPP (pruritic urticaria and plaques of pregnancy).

Immunological features

Mast-cell activation is the cause, with local release of mediators and activation of other pathways, complement, and kinin.

Autoantibodies against IgE and the IgE receptor (FcεRI) have been proposed as a mechanism in some patients with chronic urticaria. These lead to activation of mast cells by cross-linking surface IgE or receptors. How generally applicable this mechanism is, remains to be determined.

Mast cells can be stimulated through other pathways, either directly by drugs, etc. (see above) or by the anaphylotoxins C3a, C5a (type II) and by immune complexes (type III). In cholinergic urticaria mast cells are unusually sensitive to stimulation by acetylcholine released by local cholinergic nerves.

Diagnosis

The history is everything! The appearances of the lesions may give clues (distinctive lesions in cholinergic urticaria). Dermographism should be sought. Physical causes can usually be replicated in the clinic to confirm the diagnosis.

Other diagnostic tests should depend on likely cause. Allergy testing is rarely justified in chronic urticaria as the yield is low. Check thyroid function, acute-phase response, full blood count, and think of infective causes. For acute urticarias, foods may play a role, exclusion diets may help but only if there is a strong suspicion on clinical grounds. The role of natural dietary salicylates and/or preservatives in chronic urticaria is controversial.

In cold urticaria, seek family history and check for cryoglobulins and causes thereof (electrophoresis of serum, search for underlying diseases, infections, connective tissue disease, lymphoproliferation).

Autoantibodies (ANA, RhF) and complement studies may be relevant in some instances. In SLE with urticaria, think of autoantibodies to C1q.

Skin biopsy should be considered if there are atypical features.

Therapy

Urticaria may be difficult to manage, especially cold urticaria. Acute urticaria should be treated with potent antihistamines. Short-acting ones such as acrivastine may be appropriate for intermittent attacks. Long-acting non-sedating ones, such as loratadine, fexofenadine, and cetirizine (also said to have mast-cell stabilizing activity, of uncertain clinical significance), are useful for prophylaxis against frequent attacks. A few patients may still be sedated by these drugs.

If these are unsuccessful alone, then the addition of an H2-blocker may be helpful, although the evidence is weak. There is no evidence to suggest whether ranitidine or cimetidine is preferable.

Other therapeutic options include doxepin, an antidepressant with potent H1- and H2-blocking activity, and ketotifen and oxatomide, which have mast-cell stabilizing activity in addition to anti-H1 activity (both increase appetite and are sedating). Calcium-channel blockers may have some beneficial effect (nimodipine is said to be better than nifedipine). β2-Agonists (terbutaline) and phosphodiesterase inhibitors (theophylline) may help in rare cases. Oxypentifylline has been reported to reduce cytokine synthesis by macrophages and may be helpful. Colchicine is helpful in delayed pressure urticaria but is poorly tolerated. Leukotriene antagonists may also be helpful in some patients.

Cold urticaria may respond to cyproheptadine, calcium-channel blockers, β2-agonists, and phosphodiesterase inhibitors, although responses tend to be poor.

Urticarial vasculitis may respond to NSAIDs, antimalarials (hydroxychloroquine), dapsone, and sulphasalazine.

Steroids may be effective but should be used as a last resort as chronic therapy is not justified by the side-effects; danazol and stanozolol may be used as alternatives (with varying benefit). Short courses may be helpful for acute disease. Cyclosporin A may also be helpful, but the disease relapses once the drug is withdrawn. The side-effects (hypertension, nephrotoxicity) make it an undesirable drug for urticaria.

Whenever chronic therapy is started, it is important to withdraw it at intervals to see whether it is still required in the light of possible spontaneous remission.

Asthma

Asthma is one of the atopic diseases and is characterized by bronchospasm. It is also a chronic inflammatory disease. However, the cause is multifactorial, with a complex interaction of genetic background with environmental factors. There is also a complex interaction at the local level between changes in the airway (reactive airways disease), neurogenic components (particularly involving vasoactive intestinal polypeptide (VIP) and substance P), and the innate and specific immune system.

Causes

Many factors, including occupational exposures, combine to give the clinical pattern of asthma.

- Genetic background: there is no doubt that there is a familial tendency, with inheritance more obvious through the maternal line. The loci involved are controversial, with loci on chromosome 5 (mapping to the region containing the genes for IL-4, IL-5, and the β-adrenoreceptor) and on chromosome 11 being proposed.
- Allergy: inhaled allergens (aeroallergens) such as pollens, danders, dust mites, etc. are potent triggers: IgE will be involved. Allergy is less commonly demonstrated in late-onset asthma. Occupational allergens may cause symptoms, with small, reactive molecules such as platinum salts acting by reaction with self-proteins to produce neo-antigens: IgE may be difficult to demonstrate.
- Th1 : Th2 balance: an intrinsic bias towards Th2-mediated reactions will lead to higher IgE production and levels of Th2 cytokines (IL-4, IL-5) which, in turn, down-regulate potentially balancing Th1 responses.
- Irritants: some agents cause asthma without the involvement of IgE, e.g. sulphites (see below); in part the effects here may be due to non-specific inflammation with recruitment of eosinophils and an IgE-independent cycle of cytokine and mediator release. Smoking and viral infections may contribute through this mechanism and through direct epithelial damage. Cold air and exercise may also be non-specific triggers to the hyperreactive airway.
- Smooth muscle abnormalities: abnormally low numbers of β-adrenoreceptors have been documented in asthma. This may contribute to the reactivity of airways.
- Neurogenic: local axon loops involving C-type fibres releasing substance P and neurokinin A contribute to smooth muscle constriction. VIPergic neurones antagonize this response, and these neurones may be reduced in asthma.
- Chronic inflammatory response: unchecked acute inflammation in the lung proceeds via cytokine release to chronic inflammation, with damage to bronchial epithelium and increased collagen deposition, leading to end-stage irreversible airways disease.

Immunological features

Activation of mast cells leads not only to immediate and delayed mediator release but also to synthesis of cytokines (IL-3, IL-4, IL-5, which are chemotactic for and stimulatory to eosinophils). Lung eosinophilia may be marked. These, in turn, continue the inflammatory process through the release of cytokines. Lymphocytes are recruited and activated, releasing Th2 cytokines and stimulating further IgE production. The chronic phase may be considered to include a type IV reaction.

Diagnosis

The diagnosis is dependent on history and examination. There is frequently an atopic background and a family history of atopic diseases. Wheeze is less common in children who tend to cough instead. Serial peak flow measurements may show the typical asthmatic pattern. Chronic disease may show loss of reversibility and be difficult to distinguish from chronic obstructive pulmonary disease (COPD). Reactive airways may be demonstrated with challenge tests (methacholine—see Part 2).

A high total IgE makes asthma more likely but does not correlate well with symptoms. A low IgE only excludes IgE-mediated bronchospasm. Skin-prick tests to common aeroallergens may pick up positives, but the history will indicate whether these are relevant clinically. There may be an eosinophilia on full blood count, although this is rarely marked and is only present in about 50 per cent of asthmatics; sputum eosinophilia is much more common.

Other serum markers have been proposed for assessing the severity of disease and adequacy of therapy. These include soluble CD23 (a cytokine involved in IgE production) and eosinophil cationic protein (ECP), which is said to correlate well with the underlying chronic eosinophilic inflammation. These tests are expensive and their role in monitoring remains to be determined.

Therapy

The mainstay of treatment remains inhaled bronchodilators (β2-agonists, anticholinergics) together with inhaled corticosteroids. Our current view of the inflammatory nature of asthma makes the use of inhaled steroids more important in preventing long-term lung damage. β2-agonists relieve symptoms but have little/no effect on the underlying inflammation; long-acting drugs, such as salmeterol, may lead to a false sense of security as symptoms are suppressed, and should be used with care. Courses of oral steroids may be required. Research is focusing on inhibitors of other mediators, but inhibitors of PAF, which was thought to have a major role, have been disappointing. Leukotriene antagonists have now been introduced and may benefit some patients.

Disodium cromoglycate inhibits degranulation of connective tissue mast cells only and inhibits the activation of neutrophils, eosinophils, and monocytes. It is most effective in children and in exercise-induced asthma. Nedocromil sodium is similar but inhibits both mucosal and connective-tissue mast cells and is a more potent inhibitor of neutrophils and eosinophils.

Phosphodiesterase inhibitors (theophyllines) have a valuable adjunctive therapy, particularly in acute asthma. Care must be taken if administered intravenously to patients taking oral preparations.

Experimental immunosuppressive therapy with low-dose methotrexate or cyclosporin A has been used with success in severe disease.

Antihistamines have little effect in acute asthma.

Immunotherapy has been used where there is allergy to a single agent. This can be extremely dangerous, and current guidelines exclude asthmatics from consideration of desensitization. Other forms of immunotherapy, aimed at switching immune responses from Th2 to Th1 using peptides or genetically engineered BCG have shown considerable promise.

Environmental control is important both in the home and in the context of occupational asthma. Attempts should be made to reduce house dust-mite exposure by reducing ambient temperature and avoiding high humidity (fewer house plants). Avoid thick-pile carpets, heavy curtains, and other dust traps. Regular vacuuming with a high-efficiency vacuum cleaner is necessary (ones that do not spray dust back into the room may be better, although much more expensive). Mattress covers are desirable and all bedclothes should be washable (at high temperatures). De-miting mattresses is difficult: liquid nitrogen is effective but needs specialist services. Acaricides such as benzylbenzoate may also be effective but may be irritant. If animal danders are a problem, the animal should go, although this news is rarely popular with patients!

4 Allergic disease
Asthma

Sulphite sensitivity

Some individuals are unusually sensitive to sulphites. These agents include sulphur dioxide, sodium and potassium metabisulphite and sulphite. These agents are used widely in foods and drinks as antioxidants and preservatives. Reactions include severe wheeze accompanied by flushing, tachycardia, and, if severe, may mimic anaphylaxis.

The history is usually diagnostic, with reactions typically to white wine or beer, soft drinks, pickles, salami and preserved meats, dried fruits, shrimps/prawns, and prepared salads. Certain drugs for injection contain sulphites, particularly adrenaline-containing local anaesthetics used by dentists.

The mechanism is unclear but probably involves direct mast-cell stimulation and cholinergic stimulation. IgE antibodies have occasionally been detected. There does not appear to be any cross reactivity with other agents.

No tests are of particular value except for exclusion followed by re-challenge under controlled conditions (with facilities for resuscitation).

Management is by avoidance and proper dietary advice is required. Care must be taken with the prescription of drugs. Severe reactors may need to carry adrenaline (without sulphites).

Aspirin sensitivity

In addition to its propensity to cause angioedema, aspirin is also associated with a triad of asthma, nasal polyposis, and hyperplastic sinusitis. Each feature can occur without the others. The effect is due to a sensitivity to cyclo-oxygenase inhibition, and therefore occurs with other NSAIDs but not usually with choline or sodium salicylate or paracetamol. There is a loss of bronchodilating prostaglandins and a shunting of substrate to the lipo-oxygenase pathway with the production of bronchoconstrictor leukotrienes. Some patients with aspirin intolerance also react to tartrazine and related azo-dyes. There are no specific tests and aspirin challenge is not recommend unless there is doubt about the diagnosis as re-actions may be severe. Exclusion of natural salicylate from the diet may be helpful if asthmatic symptoms persist. Significance of avail-able specific IgE tests against acetylalicylic acid is uncertain. Leukotriene antagonists may be of benefit (unlicenced indication).

4 Allergic disease

Sulphite sensitivity
Aspirin sensitivity

Allergic rhinitis

Allergic rhinitis needs to be distinguished from non-allergic causes such as vasomotor rhinitis, rhinitis medicamentosa, and infectious cause. This is not always easy. Timing of symptoms (seasonal versus perennial) will give useful clues. Perennial rhinitis is often due to dust mite allergy: symptoms often worsen in October when windows are shut and the central heating switched on as mite numbers increase with rising humidity and temperature.

168

Causes of rhinitis

- Allergic
- Vasomotor
- Non-allergic rhinitis with eosinophilia (NARES)
- Drug-induced: α-agonist nasal sprays, cocaine abuse (direct), antihypertensives, chlormethiazole (indirect)
- Irritant: fumes, solvents
- Infectious: viral, bacterial, leprosy, cilial dyskinesia
- Vasculitis: Wegener's granulomatosis
- Mechanical: nasal polyps, septal deviation, foreign bodies, tumours, sarcoidosis
- Pregnancy: last trimester (related to oestrogen levels)
- CSF leak

Immunological mechanisms

The mechanisms in allergic rhinitis are very similar to those described above for asthma, although histamine release plays a more significant role and the role of neurogenic mechanisms is less well established. Histamines and leukotrienes are though to be responsible for the itch, sneezing, rhinorrhoea, and nasal obstruction, through swelling and hyperaemia. There is a predominant eosinophilia. Perennial rhinitis may be a manifestation of chronic antigen exposure and, like chronic asthma, may lead via type IV mechanisms to chronic tissue damage with connective tissue proliferation.

The allergens involved are similar to those involved in asthma, i.e. aeroallergens, although larger allergens will tend to be trapped preferentially in the nose.

Diagnosis

The diagnosis relies heavily on the history and on examination of the nose. Rhinoscopy may be necessary to obtain a good view. The eosinophil count is rarely elevated. Total IgE may hint at an allergic basis if elevated, but a normal IgE does not exclude allergy. Skin-prick tests (SPTs) demonstrate sensitization to aeroallergens, but the clinical relevance can be determined only from the history. RASTs should be limited only to confirming equivocal skin-prick tests, or when drugs such as antihistamines cannot be discontinued.

Both RASTs and SPTs may be negative even in the presence of significant local allergy if no specific IgE is free to spill over into the bloodstream.

Examination of nasal secretions for excess eosinophils may be helpful, although there is a condition of non-allergic rhinitis with eosinophilia (NARES). This is often associated with aspirin sensitivity and asthma; sinusitis is also common. Peripheral blood eosinophilia is variable and is a poor diagnostic marker.

If the suspect allergen is available, then nasal provocation tests may be possible (see Part 2).

Management

Topical or systemic antihistamines provide relief in mild cases. More severe cases may require topical steroids or mast-cell blocking agents such as disodium cromoglycate or nedocromil sodium. Ipratropium bromide is particularly helpful in vasomotor rhinitis. Decongestants should be used with caution because of a rebound increase in symptoms. Very severe cases may require courses of corticosteroids and long-acting steroid injections have been used in seasonal rhinitis.

If drug therapy fails at maximal levels, then immunotherapy may be appropriate if a single allergen is responsible and there are no contraindications such as severe asthma, pregnancy, β-blockers, or ischaemic heart disease. This should only be undertaken in hospital. It is most effective for seasonal rather than perennial rhinitis, and then only if commenced prior to the season of symptoms.

Surgery may be required for sinus involvement and for polyps, if topical steroid therapy fails to reduce them.

Environmental control may be important as adjunctive measures. Avoidance of allergens where possible should be tried. In the grass-pollen season avoid opening windows more than necessary during the day. Air filtration systems able to trap pollens are available for cars and for houses, although the latter are expensive to install. Masks are likely to be of little value. Cold air and spicy foods may exacerbate symptoms.

Allergic conjunctivitis

Allergic conjunctivitis often accompanies rhinitis (the two areas are connected by the lacrimal ducts). The mechanisms are identical. Typical features include itching and watering of the eye, with redness and swelling. More extreme forms include vernal conjunctivitis, in which giant papillae are seen on the tarsal surface of the eyelid. In this condition the allergic component is a trigger. This disease is difficult to treat but may burn out after 5–10 years.

The diagnosis follows similar principles to those of rhinitis. Specific IgE may be detected in tears but it is rarely of value as a diagnostic test. Challenge tests may be helpful in very rare circumstances.

Topical antihistamines and mast-cell stabilizing agents (disodium cromoglycate and nedocromil) may help to relieve symptoms. Lodoxamide is another mast-cell stabilizer specifically available for allergic eye problems. Topical steroids may be very valuable but should only be prescribed under ophthalmological supervision, as long-term use may lead to glaucoma and cataracts. Topical cyclosporin A and NSAIDs (flurbiprofen and diclofenac) have also been used successfully in vernal conjunctivitis.

Sinusitis

Sinusitis may be a consequence of allergy, with secondary infection due to allergic swelling closing off the drainage ostia. It is common in the aspirin intolerance syndrome (with asthma and nasal polyposis). Ethmoiditis may mimic acute conjunctivitis in children. Chronic sinusitis is also a feature of antibody deficiency, and has been associated specifically with IgG3 subclass deficiency. Inflammatory disease such as Wegener's granulomatosis and midline granuloma may also present in this way.

Radiology of the area will demonstrate opacification: CT scanning is most sensitive. Nasal smears will demonstrate eosinophilia if there is an allergic cause, but neutrophilia will be present in infective cases. Measurement of humoral immune function (immunoglobulins, IgG subclasses, and specific antibodies) and antineutrophil cytoplasmic antibodies should be considered in chronic sinusitis.

Obstructed sinuses can be washed out. This can be done by an endoscopic procedure, which allows the sinuses to be inspected. Nasal decongestants and topical steroids assist in reducing oedema and promoting free drainage. Antibiotics are required for infective problems. *Haemophilus influenzae* and pneumococcus are the most common organisms. Ciprofloxacin is appropriate as it penetrates well into sinus fluids.

4 Allergic disease

Allergic conjunctivitis
Sinusitis

Secretory otitis media (glue ear)

This has been suggested to be related to underlying allergy but there is little evidence for this in children, unless there is allergic disease elsewhere in the respiratory tract. Rarely, it may be related to specific antibody deficiency or a more widespread antibody deficiency. The history will reveal if there are other infective problems that would suggest such a diagnosis.

Secretory otitis media (glue ear)

Atopic eczema

Atopic eczema is the most common manifestation of atopic disease. It is usually worst in childhood, improving with age in 80 per cent and affects particularly the cheeks and flexures. It is a risk factor for the development of contact dermatitis in later life. Asthma or rhinitis will develop in 50–75 per cent of patients. It is on the increase. Eye involvement may occur, with an atopic keratoconjunctivitis and in severe cases subcapsular cataract may form.

Causes

There is a genetic basis, as demonstrated by twin studies, although whether the background is the same as for asthma (chromosome 1 or 5) has not yet been demonstrated.

In addition to the immunological factors, there are abnormalities of the lipids of the skin and evidence for autonomic nervous abnormalities (white dermographism). There is a reduce threshold for itch, which leads to a vicious cycle of itch and scratch, leading to the lichenification of chronic eczema.

Non-specific irritants make the disease worse, such as wool, heat and stress. Staphylococcal infection is common, and may play a role in exacerbating the disease: IgE against the bacterium may be detected, although the role is unclear. Staphylococcal superantigens have also been suggested to play a role. Cutaneous fungi may also exacerbate the disease.

The role of diet is controversial. It has been suggested that maternal diet during pregnancy may contribute, as may a lack of breast feeding. The contribution of diet to established symptoms is even more controversial, although some children are helped by exclusion diets.

Immunological features

The precise role of type I responses is unclear. IgE levels are often very high, and specific IgE may be detected against a variety of aero- and food allergens, although most of the IgE is 'junk', with no recognizable specificity. Langerhan's cells in the skin do have IgE receptors, although their role in atopic eczema is speculative. Keratinocytes release cytokines when damaged, which will excite the immune response (TNF-α, IL-1, IL-6, IL-8).

There is more evidence for a type IV reaction with an infiltrate of CD4+ T cells into the epidermis and dermis; most of these cells are of the Th2 phenotype which will support IgE production. As part of the inflammatory response, eosinophils, mast cells, and basophils are all increased in the affected skin, and mechanisms similar to those found in the chronic phase of asthma probably predominate.

Diagnosis

Blood eosinophilia is common. Eighty per cent of cases will have a high IgE, often >1000 kU/l. Specific IgE may be detected by SPT or RAST, but this rarely helps in management.

Atypical patterns of eczema with other infections should raise the possibility of the hyper-IgE syndrome. Here the IgE is even higher, usually >50 000 kU/l, and there may be evidence of other humoral abnormalities such as low IgG2, so a full investigation of humoral immunity is warranted.

Viral infections such as eczema herpeticum, molluscum contagiosum, and warts are common in atopic eczema and do not indicate a significant generalized immunodeficiency but are a manifestation of disturbed local immunity.

Management

Management is usually designed to reduce itch by the use of emollients, inflammation by the use of topical steroids, and staphylococcal superinfection by the use of appropriate oral antibiotics.

Cyclosporin A is helpful in severe disease as a temporary measure but the disease relapses as soon as the drug is withdrawn. Theoretically, γ-interferon should be helpful, by reducing the Th2 predominance, and this has been borne out in several small trials.

Where babies, by virtue of a strong family history, are at risk of developing atopic eczema, avoidance of cows' milk for the first 6 months of life and late weaning may be helpful. The addition of γ-linoleic acid and fish oil have been suggested to be helpful, the evidence from controlled trials is less supportive. In older children, the avoidance of foods as a control measure is controversial.

175

Contact hypersensitivity

Contact hypersensitivity is a localized type IV reaction due to contact with a triggering allergen. The pattern of rash together with a careful exposure history usually identifies possible allergens. For example, nickel allergy often leads to dermatitis affecting the ear lobes, under the back of watches, and where jean studs press on the skin. Aniline dyes in leather cause dermatitis affecting the feet and where leather belts come in contact with skin. It needs to be distinguished from straightforward irritant dermatitis due to a localized toxic effect that does not involve the immune system. Typical irritants are solvents, acids, alkalis, and other chemicals. However, the skin has a limited number of ways in which it can respond, and the appearance of irritant and allergic dermatitis can look clinically similar. Typical allergens eliciting an allergic reaction include certain plants, metals (nickel, chromium), rubber compounds (latex, hardening agents), resins, dyes, preservatives, fragrances, topical antibiotics, and colophony. Nickel is top of the list, especially in women (jewellery). Some allergens require concomitant exposure to sunlight for the effect to develop (plants; drugs, including sulphonamides and phenothiazines; and sunscreens). Here the rash only occurs on sun-exposed surfaces.

Immunology

Type I and type IV hypersensitivity may co-exist. In most cases the allergens are low molecular weight substances that penetrate the skin readily and lead to neoantigen formation. As with all T-lymphocyte-mediated responses, sensitization precedes reactivity. Active lesions show a sparse CD4+ T-lymphocytic infiltrate but few eosinophils.

Diagnosis

The history and examination give the most important information. This should be supplemented by patch testing (see Part 2). SPT and measurement of total IgE are of little value.

Management

This should be undertaken by a dermatologist. Antihistamines may be needed to control itch. Wet compresses may be required for weeping eczema, but potent topical steroids accompanied by avoidance of the offending agents usually leads to resolution.

Food allergy

Food allergy causes more trouble than any other aspect of immuno logy. Foods are blamed by the general population for a multitude of sins. However, the public perception of food allergy is not reflected by its true incidence when large-scale population studies are under taken. True food additive intolerance is very rare (<0.23 per cent of the population) when those claiming to be intolerant are formally tested. Food allergy (in which IgE is involved) must be distin guished from food intolerance, which may have a variety of causes, and from psychogenic causes.

Symptoms of true food allergy are invariably limited to the gut, the skin, and the respiratory tract. Symptoms outside these systems are much less likely to be due to true allergy. There is no convinc ing association with arthritis. There is no evidence that food allergy is a cause of chronic fatigue syndromes (Chapter 8), and thus 'desensitization' therapies have nothing to offer; equally there is no evidence to support *Candida* overgrowth as a cause of CFS.

Causes

True food allergy is very real and may be severe (see Anaphylaxis above). It is most common in children (up to 0.5 per cent may be allergic to cows' milk). Almost any food can cause true allergy mediated via IgE. Most allergens involved in food allergy are heat stable (resisting cooking) and acid stable (resisting stomach acid). There are exceptions to this, so that a food will be allergic cooked but not raw, or vice versa: these foods are typically fruit and vegetables.

Cows' milk is one of the most common foods causing allergy. The proteins responsible for the allergic response include β-lactoglobulin, α-lactalbumin, casein, bovine serum albumin, and bovine immunoglobulins. Often the response is against more than one antigen. This allergy usually disappears by the age of 5 years. Rarely, gastrointestinal haemorrhage may result (Heiner's syn drome is this complex accompanied by iron-deficiency anaemia and pulmonary haemosiderosis).

Egg allergy is also common in the under-fives, and often dis appears with age, although anaphylactic responses may occur. The major antigens are ovomucoid and ovalbumin. Cross-reaction with chicken meat is unusual.

Fish allergy may be severe, such that inhalation of allergens in the vapour from cooking fish or second-hand contact (e.g. kissing someone who has eaten fish) may be enough to trigger reactions. The allergens are species specific in 50 per cent and cross-reactive with all fish in the remainder. Fish allergy is usually permanent. Similar constraints apply to shellfish, both crustacea (prawns, crabs and lobster) and molluscs (mussels, scallops, and oysters).

The legumes, peanuts and soya, are major causes of severe aller gic reactions. These agents cause major problems because they are widely used as food 'fillers' and may not be declared on labels. ˙voidance may be difficult. Sensitization is often extreme, such that ˙ amounts of residual protein in peanut (groundnut) oil may be enough to trigger reactions. Sensitization may occur through the use of groundnut oil in formula milks. Arachis oil (groundnut oil) is used as a carrier in certain intramuscular injections. True nuts may be equally troublesome. These reactions are usually lifelong.

Cereals may cause direct allergic responses if ingested or cause symptoms via gluten intolerance (coeliac disease). Flour also causes baker's asthma as an occupational disease. Wheat, barley, and rye are all closely related. Symptoms are less extreme and this is hypothesized to be due to proteolysis reducing the allergenicity, although why this does not apply to other foods is unclear. Rice and maize allergy are rare.

There are links between some inhalant allergies and specific food allergies. The best described is the birch-pollen syndrome, where there is often food allergy to hazelnut, apple, pear, and carrot. Other described associations include latex with banana, avocado, and kiwi; ragweed with banana and melons; and mugwort with celery, parsley, and vermouth.

Occasionally trace contaminants may be responsible for allergy, as in the case of antibiotics in meat (used by farmers to improve the animals' weight gain), which may lead to reactions to meat and to therapeutic drugs.

True food allergy must be distinguished from food intolerance, which takes many forms:
- Pharmacological: caffeine and theobromine (tachycardias in heavy tea/coffee drinkers), tyramine (headaches, hypertension in patients on monoamine-oxidase inhibitors (MAOIs)), alcohol (obvious symptoms, plus beer drinkers' diarrhoea), NSAIDs (may include natural salicylates), figs (laxatives).
- Toxic: scombrotoxin (histamine from spoiled mackerel), green potatoes, aflatoxins (peanuts), lectins (PHA in undercooked kidney beans), food poisoning (*Bacillus cereus* (fried rice), staphylococcal toxins), monosodium glutamate (headaches, nausea, and sweating—Chinese restaurant syndrome).
- Enzyme deficiencies: lactase deficiency (common in Asians; diarrhoea due to laxative effect of lactose), also sucrase and maltase deficiency (excess undigested fructose causes diarrhoea, abdominal cramp, and bloating; high levels in onions, peppers, and fruit juices).
- Other bowel disease: Crohn's disease, coeliac disease, infections (*Giardia*, *Yersinia*), bacterial overgrowth (in association with reduced motility, e.g. systemic sclerosis), 'irritable bowel syndrome' (other causes must be excluded).
- Pancreatic insufficiency: cystic fibrosis, Schwachman's syndrome.
- Psychogenic: 'smells', somatization disorder.

Immunological mechanisms

For true allergic reactions pre-sensitization is required. The bowel contains a specific subset of mast cells (MC$_T$), which are capable of being armed by IgE. Activated T cells are also present. The pattern of reactions is probably very similar to mechanisms involving mast cells in other sites, although less well studied because of inaccessibility.

Abnormalities of mucosal immunity may contribute to the generation of IgE antibodies to foods. IgA deficiency may be a predisposing factor for allergic disease in general and also to coeliac disease, although cause-and-effect has not been proven beyond reasonable doubt. Exposure of an immature mucosal immune system may also be a factor, hence the lower rates of food allergy in babies breast fed and weaned late.

It has been suggested that some of the slower-onset food reactions may involve type III (immune complex reactions): this is difficult to prove as IgG anti-food antibodies are not uncommon in healthy individuals.

Diagnosis

The history may give good clues about particular foods that cause problems. Skin-prick tests tend to be helpful mainly for foods causing severe reactions (milk, egg, fish, peanuts, true nuts) while being less useful for other food groups. If commercial reagents do not work, then the fresh food should be tried (stab lancet into food then into patient). However, SPT may be dangerous in those who have had severe anaphylactic reactions. RAST tests are less sensitive. Total IgE is not especially helpful.

The allergy practitioner will need to have a good understanding of the biological families in which plants are grouped, as this often helps explain patterns of reactivity: members of the same biological family often share common antigens.

Dietary manipulation plays an important role in diagnosis, but is time consuming and should be undertaken only in collaboration with a dietician. Elimination diets (oligoallergenic diets), with gradual reintroduction of foods in an open but controlled manner, may be helpful in identifying troublesome foods. Formal confirmation requires a double-blind placebo-controlled food challenge, in which the suspect food is disguised in opaque gelatine capsules.

The differentiation of food intolerance requires careful history taking. Patients should be investigated for evidence of malabsorption (iron, B12, folate, clotting, calcium, and alkaline phosphatase), and for coeliac disease (endomysial antibodies); if there is diarrhoea, do stool microscopy and culture. Acute-phase proteins will indicate likely inflammatory bowel disease. Bacterial overgrowth, lactose intolerance, and pancreatic insufficiency can be diagnosed on appropriate radioisotopic tests or by measuring breath hydrogen production. Radiology of the bowel may be revealing and biopsy should always be considered: enzyme levels can be measured and coeliac disease confirmed rapidly. In early coeliac disease, histology may show only a lymphocytic infiltrate without complete villous atrophy.

Management

The most important facet of the management of food allergy is the identification of true food allergy and its distinction from other causes of food intolerance. It is also important to educate the patient about their symptoms and the cause. This may be hard if the patient already has a well-established preconception that they have 'food allergy'.

Management of food allergy is mainly avoidance, while maintaining a nutritious diet: specialist dietetic support is required. Antihistamines (H1 and H2) are of little benefit (except possibly as prophylaxis against severe reactions). There is little positive evidence to support the use of oral disodium cromoglycate. A short course of steroids may be necessary for severe disease (eosinophilic gastropathy). At present there is no value in attempting desensitization for food allergy, and enzyme-potentiated desensitization (EPD) is also not of proven value despite claims by some practitioners to the contrary. The management of food intolerance depends on the underlying cause.

Drug allergy

Drugs may cause allergic reactions due to all four mechanisms of hypersensitivity, or combinations thereof. For example, penicillin may cause anaphylaxis (type I), a haemolytic anaemia (type II), serum sickness (type III), and interstitial nephritis (type IV). As noted above, drugs may also cause reactions through other mechanisms, such as direct histamine release (opiates, radiocontrast media), undue sensitivity to the pharmacological effect (NSAIDs), and direct complement activation. Drug fever may be the primary manifestation of an adverse reaction to antibiotics. This may be difficult to detect when the drug is an antibiotic being used to treat an infective condition, where the reappearance of fever may lead to further investigation for an infective focus. The CRP will also be elevated during a drug fever.

Penicillin allergy

Penicillin allergy is very common, perhaps occurring in up to 8 per cent of treatment courses. However, most of the reactions are trivial. Severe reactions are rare and occur mainly after parenteral administration. Occasional patients react on apparent first exposure and it has been suggested that sensitization may occur through antibiotics occurring in food. As noted above, all four types of Gell and Coombs' hypersensitivity reactions may occur with penicillin, together with reactions of uncertain significance such as Stevens–Johnson syndrome. There are major antigenic determinants (benzylpenicilloyl nucleus) and minor determinants (benzylpenicillin, benzylpenicilloate, and others), although both are capable of causing severe immediate reactions. Unfortunately the currently available tests (RAST and SPT) detect only major determinants, although benzylpenicillin may detect some minor-determinant-only reactions if suitably diluted and used for SPT. Tests for IgE (i.e. RAST and SPT) have no predictive value for other types of reactions, and indeed up to 3 per cent of SPT-negative patients may subsequently have reactions, although the reaction rate falls if both major and all minor antigens are used for testing. Some recent studies have claimed very few false negative results with SPT. Conversely, not all SPT-positive patients will react when subsequently challenged. Unfortunately, comprehensive testing kits with all major and minor determinants are not readily available commercially, which limits the utility of testing. Up to 75 per cent of patients who have had a reaction to penicillin will tolerate the drug subsequently. This probably applies to patients with non-specific reactions of dubious allergic aetiology (nausea, vomiting, diarrhoea) but more care should be taken in patients with a history of angioedema, Stevens–Johnson syndrome, etc.

There is a high level of cross-reactivity with other semisynthetic penicillins with a β-lactam ring, such as the carbapenems and the monobactams (up to 50 per cent in the case of imipenem), for IgE-mediated reactions. The related cephalosporins and cephacarbams also cross-react, but at a lower level: up to 20 per cent of penicillin-allergic patients may also react to cephalosporins.

However, anaphylaxis to cephalosporins is said to be very unlikely if there are no responses to major or minor determinants of penicillin. In some cases the IgE is directed not at the nucleus but at the side-chain, which may be shared between a penicillin and a cephalosporin (e.g. aztreonam and ceftazidime). One should remember the specific rash associated with the administration of amoxycillin to patients with acute EBV infection. This does not indicate a likelihood of subsequent true penicillin allergy.

The management of the penicillin-allergic patient depends on obtaining a clear history from the patient. For patients with severe reactions, avoidance is the best course, including other semi-synthetic β-lactam antibiotics. SPT and RAST testing is of limited use because of its suspect predictive value for further reactions. If penicillin or equivalent is essential, rush desensitization schedules may be used, although there is a high risk of reactions, for which supportive therapy will be required. The desensitization must be followed by the treatment course and there is no lasting tolerance. Desensitization should NOT be attempted in those who have had a Stevens–Johnson reaction.

Other antibiotics

Little is written about true allergy to other antibiotics. Patients with AIDS have a very high reaction rate to trimethoprim-sulphamethoxazole. This has been associated with IgE to a derivative of the sulphamethoxazole, while abnormal metabolism with generation of toxic intermediates has been proposed as a mechanism for the generation of erythema multiforme and Stevens–Johnson syndrome. Cross-reactivity to sulphonamides may also affect other drugs that are closely related such as frusemide, hydrochlorothiazide, and captopril.

Insulin

Insulin allergy may occur due to changes in the tertiary structure of insulin engendered in the manufacturing process for human insulin, or previously due to the sequence differences in bovine and porcine insulin, with the production of IgE antibodies. These do not recognize natural human insulin. Other components such as protamine and zinc may also contribute. There is urticaria at the site of injections and frequently induration. Rarely, systemic reactions occur. Treatment is difficult: local reaction may be amenable to the prophylactic use of antihistamines or the inclusion of a tiny dose of hydrocortisone (1–5 mg) with the insulin. 'Desensitization' regimes have been used where there are major problems and diabetic control has failed.

Anaesthetics

The major difficulty of the investigation of anaesthetic reactions is that multiple drugs are administered nearly simultaneously. Some of the drugs used (opiate derivatives) are capable of inducing mast-cell degranulation, while solvents such as cremophor, used to dissolve lipophilic drugs, may activate the complement system. Problems of severe reactions peroperatively may also arise from synthetic plasma expanders and blood products and in patients with unrecognized (or ignored) sensitivity to latex. RAST tests for specific IgE are currently limited commercially to suxamethonium and thiopentone, although research centres may have tests for IgE to other agents. Opinion is divided as to the value of SPT or intradermal testing and whether it should be used to positively identify the offending agent or to screen potential alternative agents for non-reactivity. Either way, challenge testing should only be carried out with full resuscitation facilities to hand. However, patients should be referred to a specialist interested in drug reactions for formal evaluation and challenge testing as felt appropriate.

Complex protocols for the investigation of anaesthetic reactions have been suggested by some authorities. These involve repetitive blood sampling through the 24 hours following, with samples taken immediately and at short intervals in the first 4 hours. Unfortunately, it rarely proves possible to collect all the necessary samples, in particular the early ones, when most attention is being spent on dealing with the consequences of the reaction. In practice, one sample as soon as possible after the reaction and one at 24 hours (both clotted and EDTA) give almost as much information. Important measurements are C3d for evidence of complement breakdown and mast-cell tryptase, a stable marker of mast-cell degranulation. If either suxamethonium or thiopentone have been used, then measurement of specific IgE is helpful; total IgE measurements are not useful. It may be necessary to repeat the tests for specific IgE at 3–4 weeks after the reaction, as testing immediately after the reaction may give a false negative result.

Local anaesthetics

Local anaesthetics may cause both type I and type IV reactions, so a careful history is required to identify the nature of the reaction and guide subsequent testing. As overdose of local anaesthetic may cause significant adverse reactions, it is essential to exclude this possibility. Local anaesthetics divide into two groups: group I are the benzoic acid esters, including benzocaine and procaine; group II are the amides, including lignocaine, bupivacaine, and prilocaine. There is little cross-reactivity between the two groups, but there is often cross-reactivity within the groups. SPT is of uncertain value, but incremental challenge is valuable.

Local anaesthetics may contain sulphites (particularly if adrenaline is present) and other preservatives such as parabens, which may causes adverse reactions in their own right.

Diagnosis

In general, the diagnosis of drug reactions requires a good history. Specific *in vitro* tests are available to only a few drugs and in some cases are of little help in the management of the patient. Challenge tests are of more value but are time consuming and potentially dangerous. During the investigation of an acute reaction, measurement of complement breakdown products, mast-cell tryptase or urinary methyl histamine assist in identifying some of the mechanisms involved. Complement breakdown products are moderately labile and require EDTA samples. Measurement of C3a and C5a is of even more help, but measurement requires samples taken in Futhan-EDTA, which is unlikely to be available at the right time and right place. Measurement of other components is complicated by changes in plasma volume, either through leakage of plasma into the extravascular space or by infusion of colloid or crystalloid.

Therapy

The therapy of all drug reactions involves removal of the drug and, if the reaction is severe, resuscitation as for anaphylaxis (see above). It is important that the patient is informed of the cause of their reaction and if it is thought likely to recur, then they should be advised to wear a Medic-Alert bracelet or equivalent.

Extrinsic allergic alveolitis (EAA)

The typical features of EAA are fever, shortness of breath, and cough within 4–6 hours of allergen exposure, i.e. much slower than for type I reactions. Rhonchi are present and there is acute hypoxaemia. About 10 per cent of patients are also asthmatic and then show both an immediate (type I) and a later (type III) reaction. For occupational allergens, features are often most marked on Monday morning (after a weekend free of exposure) and improve somewhat later in the week: this is 'Monday morning fever'. Chronic allergen exposure leads to a more insidious deterioration in lung function, often without much in the way of fever, but a steadily progressive shortness of breath.

Cause

EAA is a hypersensitivity reaction mediated by IgG, mainly through a type III reaction, although there may well be a type IV reaction in addition. The antigens are inhaled and must be of such a size ($<5 \mu m$) to enable them to penetrate to the alveolus. Many different antigens have been associated with this type of disease, including animal, fungal, bacterial, plant, and chemical allergens. Many are associated with occupational exposure. In the UK, the most widely recognised diseases are bird-fancier's lung (pigeons, caged birds) and farmer's lung (thermophilic fungi).

Curiously, smoking appears to have a protective effect against the development of EAA. This may be due to the inhibition of macrophage function.

Immunology

Total IgG is often raised and precipitating IgG antibodies to the offending allergen may be detected. However, these specific antibodies are a marker of exposure and do not correlate with the presence of disease. Precipitins may also decline with time, so that a negative test does not exclude the diagnosis. IgE levels are not usually elevated, and specific IgE is not detected; SPT has no role in the diagnosis of type III reactions. In the acute stage, there is a peripheral blood neutrophilia, rather than the eosinophilia seen in type I reactions. Bronchoalveolar lavage (BAL) studies typically show a lymphocytosis with a reversal of the normal CD4:CD8 ratio, due to an expansion of the CD8+ T-cell population. The CD8+ T cells show evidence of activation, expressing CD25 and VLA antigens. However, as with precipitins, BAL also shows changes in exposed but asymptomatic individuals, although the most extreme elevations of CD8+ T cells are seen in those with active disease.

Diagnosis

The diagnosis is based on typical symptoms together with evidence of allergen exposure. Precipitin tests provide supportive evidence only. The chronic disease, with interstitial changes, may be difficult to diagnose, but BAL may help differentiate EAA from sarcoidosis.

and idiopathic pulmonary fibrosis. In the occupational setting, challenge tests within an environmental chamber may be required as proof positive of the causal link. Pure allergens are required and the process may make the patient seriously unwell.

Treatment

Avoidance is the mainstay. This may require difficult decisions if the patient's livelihood is affected, hence the need for positive evidence of causation through a challenge. If the disease is identified early and the allergen exposure terminated, no permanent harm will be done. However, in chronic cases, if fibrotic lung damage has occurred, then this will be irreversible. Oral corticosteroids may help to deal with acute symptoms.

Allergic bronchopulmonary aspergillosis (ABPA)

ABPA is a specific entity in which there are both type I and type III reactions to *Aspergillus*. The presentation is with bouts of wheeze, fever, cough, and haemoptysis. Bronchiectasis may develop. Chest radiographs show transient infiltrates. Symptoms are often most marked in the winter.

Similar features of a mixed type I and type III response to *Aspergillus* may occur in some patients with cystic fibrosis. This appears to be a poor prognostic sign.

Cause

The causative fungus, *Aspergillus*, is usually present in the sputum of patient with ABPA, and can be seen on microscopy and often cultured from serial specimens.

Immunology

Both IgE and IgG precipitins to the relevant strain of *Aspergillus* can be detected. SPTs against *Aspergillus* are also strongly positive and give both an immediate and a late response. Total IgE is usually very high and there is a marked peripheral blood eosinophilia during acute episodes. Both fall during remission.

Treatment

Acute flares are treated with high-dose corticosteroids; some patients require continuous low-dose steroids to maintain remission. Bronchodilators are also required. Immunotherapy with extracts of *Aspergillus* is unhelpful!

4 Allergic disease
Allergic bronchopulmonary aspergillosis (ABPA)
Other pulmonary eosinophilic syndromes

Other pulmonary eosinophilic syndromes

Pulmonary eosinophilia may also be caused by drug reactions, parasitic infestations (*Ascaris*, *Strongyloides*, filariasis), vasculitis (Churg–Strauss vasculitis, see Chapter 7), and idiopathic eosinophilic pneumonias, including Löffler's syndrome and hypereosinophilic syndromes.

189

Allergy and renal disease

A seasonal nephrotic syndrome has been described in atopic patients, corresponding to the pollen season. IgE has been documented in the glomeruli. This appears to be rare.

ENDOCRINE SYSTEM

Thyroid disease

Graves disease

Graves disease usually presents with thyrotoxicosis and a diffusely enlarged thyroid gland. It is often accompanied by exophthalmos and occasionally by thyroid acropathy. There is a strong female predominance, $M:F = 1:7$ and the disease runs in families. It is associated with HLA-A1 B8 DR3, although less strongly than some other autoimmune diseases, although some studies have suggested that possession of this haplotype increases the risk of relapse. In Asians the disease has been associated with HLA-Bw35 and Bw46; linkage to IgG Gm allotypes has also been reported.

The disease has been associated with aberrant MHC class II expression on thyrocytes, which is thought may play a role in the induction of the autoimmune response. One study has suggested that a viral infection with a human spumaretrovirus may be the initial trigger.

Patients with Graves disease have elevated levels of antibodies to thyroid peroxidase (present in 50–80 per cent) and antibodies to thyroglobulin (20–40 per cent). These autoantibodies are not specific for Graves disease but also occur in other thyroid diseases (see below). Other anti-thyroid antibodies are also present: these include thyroid stimulating antibodies, both growth promoting (TGSI, 20–50 per cent) and stimulating (TSI, 50–90 per cent), and antibodies that compete with the binding of thyroid stimulating hormone (TSH) (TBII, 50–80 per cent). These autoantibodies are directly involved in the pathogenic process. The Graves goitre has been associated with stimulating autoantibodies to both the TSH receptor (TSH-R) and to the insulin-like growth factor receptor (IGF1-R), which both promote growth of the gland. Studies with recombinant TSH receptor have shown multiple binding sites for these autoantibodies, which may lead to the different functional activities. The human TSH-R has some homology to HIV-1 Nef protein, and retroviral sequences have been reported in thyroid tissue from patients with Graves disease. The presence of TSI and TBII correlate with risk of relapse and of neonatal hyperthyroidism if present in pregnancy. The exophthalmos may be due to a separate autoantibody directed against unknown antigens expressed on retro-orbital connective tissue, probably fibroblasts or fat cells, leading to a localized inflammatory response, with plasma-cell infiltrate, and consequent hypertrophy and hyperplasia. There is a strong association of exophthalmos with HLA-DR3. The diagnosis is a clinical one, supported by tests of thyroid function, thyroid isotope scans, and autoantibody detection.

Control of the thyrotoxicosis is undertaken with drugs, surgery, or radioiodine or an appropriate combination. Long-term use of suppressive doses of thyroxine with antithyroid drugs has led to prolonged remissions, with a putative mechanism of decreased thyrocyte autoantigen expression. Treatment of the thyrotoxicosis does not usually involve immunotherapy, but the eye disease may require treatment with steroids, cyclosporin A, or irradiation to control the inflammatory process. Surgical intervention may be required. I^{125} ablation of the thyroid to control the thyrotoxicosis may be associated with a flare of the eye disease, and pretreatment with steroids may be helpful. The eye disease and the thyroid disease proceed independently.

Hashimoto's thyroiditis

This is an acute inflammatory thyroiditis, accompanied by a lymphocytic infiltrate of the gland, of unknown aetiology. The lymphocytic infiltrate comprises all types of cells and may result in germinal centre formation within the gland. Patients are usually hyperthyroid initially and then progress to hypothyroidism as fibrosis of the gland occurs. There is usually a goitre. It also tends to occur in families with other thyroid disease and has a predilection for older females. It is strongly associated with other autoimmune diseases, including SLE, chronic active (lupoid) hepatitis, primary biliary cirrhosis, vitiligo, Addison's disease, diabetes mellitus type I, myasthenia gravis, dermatitis herpetiformis, and scleroderma. There is an association of DR5 with goitrous Hashimoto's disease. DR3 and DR4 are also associated.

Anti-thyroid peroxidase antibodies will be present in 80–95 per cent of patients, usually at extremely high titres (higher than in Graves disease). Autoantibodies to multiple other thyroid antigens, including thyroglobulin, can be detected. Up to 20 per cent of patients may have antibodies directed at the TSH receptor, both stimulatory and blocking antibodies.

No immunotherapeutic manoeuvres are used.

Subacute thyroiditis syndromes

These include transient thyroiditis syndromes such as granulomatous thyroiditis (de Quervain's syndrome) and postpartum thyroiditis. De Quervain's thyroiditis may be caused by viral infections (mumps, measles, adenovirus, Epstein–Barr virus, coxsackievirus, and echovirus), which leads to an acute, painful thyroiditis; no single agent has been unequivocally linked to the disease. Patients are initially hyperthyroid but may become transiently hypothyroid in recovery before the euthyroid state is restored. Antithyroid antibodies, against thyroglobulin and thyroid peroxidase, are present, usually in lower titres in 10–50 per cent of patients.

Postpartum thyroiditis usually occurs within 3 months of delivery and is usually painless. There is usually a hyperthyroid phase followed by hypothyroidism then a return to the euthyroid state. Although only recently described, it appears to be common (1–11 per cent of pregnant women) and is associated with HLA-DR5. It is associated with high titres of antibodies against thyroid peroxidase, and the presence of such antibodies during or after pregnancy in otherwise well women has a predictive value of sub-sequent thyroid dysfunction.

Primary hypothyroidism

This may well be due to occult thyroiditis, leading eventually to pre-sentation with overt hypothyroidism years later. There may be a lymphocytic infiltrate of the gland, with marked fibrosis. Eighty per cent of patients will have antibodies to thyroid peroxidase, and a lower proportion will have antibodies to thyroglobulin. Some specific cases may have antibodies that block the TSH-R, prevent-ing normal function.

Thyroid disease and other symptoms

It is worth remembering that thyroid disease, both hypo- and hyper-thyroidism, can be a cause of significant arthropathy. The detection of thyroid antibodies in a patient with joint pain may therefore be significant and should not be ignored.

Occult hypothyroidism has also been associated with the development of urticaria, although the reasons are unclear. Unfortunately the urticaria does not always settle when the hypothyroidism is treated.

The wider use of autoantibody testing has led to the detection of anti-thyroid antibodies in fit euthyroid patients. The Wickham com-munity survey has demonstrated that a significant number of these patients go on to develop overt thyroid disease subsequently. The detection of such antibodies in asymptomatic patients should there-fore lead to a high index of suspicion for thyroid disease and a low threshold for requesting thyroid function tests when the patient re-presents with symptoms. It may be worth screening the thyroid function annually.

Autoimmune thyroid disease is strongly associated with perni-cious anaemia and vice versa. Gastric parietal cell antibodies may therefore be detected in patients with thyroid disease. Such patients should be monitored for the subsequent development of B_{12} defi-ciency. More rarely, thyroid disease may be accompanied by Addison's disease, in addition to pernicious anaemia (Schmidt's syndrome).

Sporadic goitre

This has been associated with stimulating autoantibodies to the IGF1-R, in the absence of other antibodies, leading to glandular growth.

Tests for diagnosis	Tests for monitoring
Thyroid function (TSH, FT4, FT3)	Thyroid function
Free thyroglobulin (carcinoma)	Immunological tests not helpful
Antibodies to thyroid microsomes (thyroid peroxidase)	Watch for signs of pernicious anaemia and other endocrinopathies
Thyroid-binding, thyroid-stimulating antibodies	
Consider gastric parietal cell antibodies (and B$_{12}$)	

Diabetes mellitus

There are two types of diabetes, type I or insulin-dependent diabetes mellitus (IDDM) and type II or non-insulin-dependent diabetes mellitus (NIDDM). The latter may be a misnomer, as NIDDM may require insulin therapy. Type II is mainly a disease of older people, although there is considerable overlap with type I. Type II does not have an immunological basis.

Type I diabetes (insulin-dependent)

This is a disease characterized by immunological destruction of the islets of Langerhans in the pancreas, with subsequent insulino-paenia. It has been postulated that, as for autoimmune thyroid disease, there is an initial viral infection, leading to subsequent autoimmune damage in a genetically susceptible host. Twin concordance for IDDM is only 30–40 per cent, confirming the role of environmental agents, and there is a seasonal fluctuation in the presentation. Viruses that have been proposed include coxsackievirus, reovirus, mumps, influenza, rubella, and cytomegalovirus. There is a clinical association of type I diabetes with coeliac disease.

Males and females are almost equally affected, unlike other autoimmune diseases. Much work has been done on the genetics of diabetes. Early studies of the genetic background showed an association with HLA-B8, DR3 and B15, and DR4, while DR2 seemed to protect. More recently the susceptibility gene has been identified as mapping to DQ8. DQ7, which shares the same α-chain, but has a β-chain with very small amino acid differences, is not associated with diabetes. The key change appears to be polymorphisms at residue 57, substituting an uncharged amino acid for aspartate, in the β-chain, at least in Caucasians, although in other racial backgrounds, such as Japanese, this does not apply. Polymorphisms in the DQ α-chain have also been associated with an increased risk. The protection conferred by DR2 also appears to be linked to DQ β-chain polymorphisms (DQ6): this protection is dominant over risk DQ8 polymorphisms. Conversely, possession of DQ2 with DQ8 appears to synergistically increase the risk, hypothesized to be due to the formation of unique heterodimers of α- and β-chains. No polymorphisms in the Ig or Tcr V-region genes have been identified, although a Tcr β-chain constant region polymorphism has been identified in diabetes: this is of uncertain significance.

In the early stages of the disease there is a lymphocytic infiltrate, predominantly of CD8+ T cells, but with small numbers of other types too. Autoantibodies are detectable, which are directed against the islet cells. These include antibodies recognizing cell types in the islets other than the insulin-producing β-cells. These antibodies are not involved in the autoimmune destruction, but are merely a marker of the disease process (secondary autoantibodies). These antibodies are present in 65–85 per cent of newly presenting IDDM, but disappear within 1–2 years. They also occur in the first-degree relatives of patients with IDDM, who have a high risk of developing the disease. β-cell-specific antibodies have been detected that recognize glutamic acid decarboxylase (GAD). This antigen occurs in both nerve and pancreas in two isoforms (65 kDa and 67 kDa), encoded by separate genes. Autoantibodies against this antigen have also been described in the stiff-man syndrome (see below). The primary target appears to be the 65 kDa protein, and antibodies to this are found in up to 80 per cent of newly presenting IDDM, although antibodies to GAD-67 are also found. There is sequence homology between GAD and a coxsackievirus antigen. A range of other putative target antigens have been described:

- insulin autoantibodies (30–50 per cent IDDM positive by radio-immunoassay, RIA), which seem more common in children developing IDDM;
- gangliosides, GT3, GM2 and others, antigens that are again shared between β-cells and neuronal tissue;
- an autoantigen that cross-reacts with a rubella capsid antigen (? peripherin);
- a glucose transporter (GLUT-2, not β-cell specific);
- ICA p69, which has sequence homology with bovine serum albumin;
- ICA-512, a protein whose intracellular sequence has some homology to other protein tyrosine phosphatases; the complete molecule is known as insulinoma antigen-2 (IA-2); another closely related antigen is known as IA-2β;
- heat-shock protein 65 (Hsp65);
- insulin receptor;
- carboxypeptidase H.

The relevance of these other autoantibodies, if any, remains to be determined.

The diagnosis is a clinical one, based on evidence of elevated blood sugar. The presence of anti-islet cell antibodies is helpful in distinguishing type I and type II diabetes in the older patient, but does not have any predictive value in the patient. Screening of first-degree relatives for ICA may be more valuable in identifying those at risk of developing diabetes. Identification of patients in the pre-diabetic phase may well become more important, as trials of immunoregulatory therapies become more widespread. Here the aim is to prevent damage to the islets, as the presentation with overt diabetes clearly represents the end stage of the disease when insufficient islet tissue remains.

Other than the obvious replacement of insulin, interest is focused on immunosuppressive therapy. Aggressive therapy with corticosteroids, azathioprine, cyclosporin A, tacrolimus (FK506), and anti-thymocyte globulin (ATG) has been tried with some success in newly presenting patients and has staved off the requirement for insulin for some time. Monoclonal antibody therapy (anti-CD3, -CD5, and -CD25) has also been tried. Novel therapies include MHC class II blockade with peptides, and tolerance induction. Early insulin treatment may also assist by β-cell rest, and perhaps by decreasing MHC class II expression, although the role of this in diabetes is controversial. Studies of immunotherapy are aided by the existence of a mouse model (NOD mouse). Clearly, these

Diabetes mellitus *(cont.)*

therapies need to be commenced early before too much immune-mediated damage to the islets has occurred.

Immunological complications of insulin therapy

As noted in Chapter 3, reactions may occur to administered insulin. While these are less common now that diabetics are treated with human insulin, rather than that from pigs or cattle, they still occur, and it appears that the manufacturing process for the human insulin is capable of altering the tertiary structure of the molecule in a way that can render it immunogenic. Other agents such as zinc and protamine, used to alter the pharmacokinetics of the drug, may also contribute. Reactions may include local or generalized urticaria and, very rarely, severe systemic reactions. Both immediate and late reactions may occur. Oral antihistamines and the inclusion of 1–5 mg of hydrocortisone in the syringe with the insulin may be helpful. Desensitization may be possible, but should only be attempted where severe reactions are occurring that compromise diabetic control. Development of antibodies to protamine in diabetics may lead to major systemic reactions if intravenous protamine is used to reverse anticoagulation with heparin (e.g. after cardiac bypass surgery). IgE antibodies have been documented.

Insulin resistance may occur due to IgG anti-insulin antibodies. These may arise spontaneously or as a result of attempted desensitization where reactions have occurred. Resistance to insulin action may occur as a result of abnormalities of the peripheral insulin receptor (type A, severe insulin resistance, hirsutism, and acanthosis nigricans) or due to IgG insulin-receptor-blocking antibodies (type B, often associated with other autoimmune diseases).

Tests for diagnosis	Tests for monitoring
Blood sugar and HbA1c	Blood sugar and HbA1c
Urinalysis	Urinalysis
Islet-cell antibodies (anti-GAD)	Immunological tests unhelpful but consider regular
IgA endomysial antibodies	IgA EMA

Autoimmune polyglandular syndromes (APGS)

Type I (autoimmune polyendocrinopathy candidiasis ectodermal dysplasia; APCED)

The diagnosis requires at least two from: Addison's disease, hypoparathyroidism, alopecia, chronic active hepatitis, hypogonadism, pernicious anaemia, and candidiasis. Onset is early, usually in childhood; slight male predominance. It is thought possible that it is a Th2-type disease. It forms part of the spectrum of chronic mucocutaneous candidiasis (see Chapter 2). There is no strong HLA linkage, although several reports have suggested a link to HLA-A28. There is an autosomal recessive inheritance and the gene has been identified on the long arm of chromosome 21 (21q22.3), coding for a protein known as AIRE (autoimmune regulator), thought to be a transcriptional regulator with homology to the Mi-2 autoantigen.

Type II (Schmidt's syndrome)

This comprises Addison's disease plus autoimmune thyroid disease (Graves disease), and/or IDDM. Pernicious anaemia, chronic active hepatitis, vitiligo, and hypogonadism may also occur. Onset can be at any age (peak 20–30 years of age) and it affects females more than males (2:1). It may be a Th1-type disease. There is an association with HLA-B8, DR3, and with certain subtypes including DQA1*0501, DRb1*0301, and DQB1*0201. Both autosomal dominant and recessive patterns of inheritance have been identified. Abnormal cellular immune function may occur.

Type III

This comprises autoimmune thyroid disease with IDDM and/or pernicious anaemia. Non-endocrine autoimmune disease may also occur, for example myasthenia gravis. Vitiligo and alopecia may also be present. There is a very strong female predominance and an association with HLA-DR3.

Anti-GAD antibodies are found in up to 4 per cent of patients with APGS, but most of these patients do not develop diabetes.

Autoimmune polyglandular syndromes (APGS)

Tests for diagnosis	Tests for monitoring
Endocrine function tests	Endocrine function tests
Autoantibodies (parathyroid, thyroid, adrenal, islet cell, gonads, gastric parietal cells)	Watch for development of cellular or humoral immune deficiency
Humoral immune function	
Cellular immune function	
Lymphocyte surface markers	
Anti-candida antibodies	

Addison's disease

The major worldwide cause of adrenal insufficiency is tuberculous adrenal destruction (prevalence 100/million). Other causes include malignancy, sarcoidosis, haemochromatosis, haemorrhage (pregnancy), and infections (fungi, viruses). However, in the UK, autoimmune disease is more common.

The adrenal target antigens include multiple adrenal proteins, identified by immunoblotting: the major antigen is 55 kDa 17α-hydroxylase in type I autoimmune polyglandular syndrome; in idiopathic Addison's the target is 55 kDa 21-hydroxylase (localized to the endoplasmic reticulum of zona glomerulosa cells), but antibodies are also found in types I and II APGS. There are conserved epitopes at the site of hormone binding and antibodies interfere with enzyme function. Antibodies to adrenal cell membranes are also found and cross-reactive antibodies that react with steroid-producing cells of other organs, e.g. ovary, may be detected.

Lymphocytic infiltrate in the adrenal gland is confined to the cortex and comprises mainly activated CD4+ T cells, with some B cells and CD8+ T cells. It has been suggested that Addison's disease is a Th2 disease in APGS I and a Th1 disease in APGS II.

The diagnosis depends on the demonstration of adrenal-cell antibodies; because of the strong association with autoimmune ovarian disease, females with Addison's should also be checked for the presence of ovarian antibodies. Checks should also be made for other features of the APGS syndromes.

Tests for diagnosis	*Tests for monitoring*
Endocrine function tests Antibodies to adrenal, steroid-producing cells, thyroid microsomes, gastric parietal cells	Endocrine function tests Watch for development of other endocrinopathies and screen as appropriate

Cushing's syndrome

In Cushing's syndrome due to pigmented nodular dysplasia, stimulating IgG antibodies have been described, which are thought possibly to bind to the ACTH receptor, analogous to thyroid-stimulating antibodies.

Pernicious anaemia

Pernicious anaemia causes deficiency of B12 and hence a megaloblastic anaemia and, in severe cases, subacute combined degeneration of the cord. It occurs in older patients with a slight female predominance and there is also an excess of blood group A. In the UK it is more common in Scotland. It is associated with HLA-B8, B12, and B15. Patients often have prematurely grey hair and blue eyes. It is strongly associated with thyroid autoimmune disease and may be associated with the APGS. There is an increased risk of both gastric carcinoma and carcinoids. Treatment is with intramuscular B_{12} (given initially in high doses with supplemental potassium, having checked that other haematinics, especially iron, are adequate, and then 3-monthly).

Histology demonstrates the loss of parietal and chief cells in the stomach; in the early stage there is an infiltrate of CD8+ T cells and IgA- and IgG-secreting B cells. There is interest in the triggering role of *Helicobacter pylori*. The target antigens for the autoimmune process are the α- and β-subunits of H^+,K^+-ATPase (the β-subunit is the major T-cell target in an experimental mouse system). These give rise to the typical gastric parietal cell (GPC) antibodies found in 90 per cent of patients. Other antibodies detected include blocking antibodies to the gastrin receptor and antibodies to intrinsic factor (IF). Two types of intrinsic-factor antibodies are recognized: type I, which binds to IF and prevents binding of B_{12} (50 per cent of patients); and type II, which blocks the uptake of the B_{12}–IF complex by the terminal ileum (35 per cent of patients). IF antibodies are only found in pernicious anaemia, although GPC antibodies may be found in asymptomatic patients with gastric atrophy. Antibodies may appear long before B_{12} levels fall: if antibodies are detected then monitoring of Fbc and B_{12} should take place so that treatment is not delayed.

Tests for diagnosis	Tests for monitoring
Fbc and MCV	Fbc and MCV (when on B_{12})
Thyroid function	Thyroid function
B_{12} level	
Schilling test	
Gastric parietal cell antibodies	
Intrinsic factor antibodies	

Gonadal autoimmunity and infertility

Gonadal autoantibodies are found in patients with Addison's and hypogonadism. They react with steroid-producing cells of the adrenal cortex, syncytiotrophoblast, Leydig cells of the testis, and the theca interna/granulosa cell layer of the ovary. They are associated with type I APGS. The target antigens are 17α-hydroxylase and P450 side-chain-cleavage enzyme. Steroid-cell antibodies are found in 15 per cent of Addison's without hypogonadism, but in >80 per cent with hypogonadism. They rarely disappear and infertility is usually lifelong. Another target enzyme appears to be 3β-hydroxysteroid dehydrogenase, which may be a more sensitive and specific marker of premature ovarian failure than standard immunofluorescence techniques.

Premature ovarian failure affects 1 per cent of women (defined as a menopause <40 years of age). Twenty per cent of these are associated with Addison's and anti-steroid-cell antibodies, but the remainder are not associated with APGS. Antibodies have been described against the follicle-stimulating hormone (FSH) receptor and other unidentified surface receptors in premature ovarian failure, although this appears still to be controversial. The significance of these antibodies, if any, remains to be determined. Screening of patients with premature ovarian failure should include a search for ovarian-, adrenal-, and steroid-cell antibodies by immunofluorescence.

Infertile women may have anti-oocyte antibodies (approximately 9 per cent of patients) which inhibit adherence and penetration of spermatozoa through the zona pellucida. ZP3, the primary sperm receptor, has been identified as a target antigen in an experimental mouse system. Antibodies have also been described against spermatozoa, causing agglutination or immobilization. However, it is not now thought that these antibodies play a major role in the genesis of the infertility, as they may also be detected in 12 per cent of fertile women. There is little to be gained by measuring them.

5 Organ-specific autoimmunity

Gonadal autoimmunity and infertility

Pituitary

Anterior hypophysitis may be associated with type I APGS; target antigens are unknown at present but a possible target is the prolactin-secreting cell. Also, antibodies may be detected against vasopressin-producing cells, associated with autoimmune diabetes insipidus. A lymphocytic hypophysitis associated with pituitary failure has been found in young women during or after pregnancy; this may be associated with pituitary-reactive autoantibodies. Care needs to be taken to exclude a rare presentation of Wegener's granulomatosis. Pituitary antibodies may also be found in some patients with Sheehan's syndrome (pituitary infarction).

Parathyroid

Antibodies may be detected that recognize parathyroid gland surface membrane antigens and which may inhibit parathyroid hormone (PTH) secretion *in vitro*. They recognize the external domain of the calcium-sensing receptor and are associated with CMC and APGS. Other antibodies to mitochondria of parathyroid chief cells have been described. Blocking antibodies to the parathyroid hormone receptor have been described in secondary hyperparathyroidism of renal failure. Detection is by immunofluorescence on parathyroid sections, but normal mitochondrial and antinuclear antibodies must be excluded first, using a standard multiblock slide, as these will interfere with the detection of parathyroid antibodies.

Vitiligo and alopecia

Vitiligo is due to melanocyte loss and occurs in isolation or in association with other autoimmune diseases, typically thyrogastric autoimmunity and type II APGS. The target antigen of the immune response is tyrosinase and antibodies are present in most patients; this enzyme is an important target antigen in melanoma and patients with vitiligo and melanoma who have detectable antibodies do better than those without. Anti-tyrosinase antibodies are only found in patients with type II but not type I autoimmune polyglandular syndromes or sporadic vitiligo.

Although alopecia frequently accompanies autoimmune diseases, especially thyroid, vitiligo and, SLE, there is no conclusive evidence for autoantibodies to the hair follicles, although this would not preclude a T-cell-mediated disease process.

NERVOUS SYSTEM

Myasthenia gravis (MG)

MG is a syndrome characterized by undue fatiguability of the muscles, leading to severe weakness. The cause is unknown but the disease is strongly associated with thymomas (benign and malignant), thymic hyperplasia, and other autoimmune diseases such as SLE, polymyositis, haemolytic anaemia, and thyroid disease (especially in those less than 40 years old). Prevalence is 2–10/100 000. Patients with thymoma are usually older and both sexes are affected equally; about 10 per cent have thymomas, but removal of the tumour does not always affect the course of the disease. In younger patients there is an association with HLA-A1, B8, and DR3, and with a strong female predominance. The disease may also be induced by penicillamine, and is mostly found in those who are HLA-Bw35/DR1 positive. The muscle weakness is due to impaired action of acetylcholine (ACh) at the muscle endplate. IgG anti-ACh-receptor (AChRAb) are detected in 90 per cent of patients, but 10 per cent are seronegative (the figure is 50 per cent for pure ocular myasthenia). Evidence that the seronegative patients are clinically different is scant, and this is likely to be a failure of the assay to identify the antibodies (? IgM antibodies).

Disease is caused by direct receptor blockade, complement-mediated endplate damage, and enhanced recycling of the receptor off of the endplate surface membrane. AChRAb levels are variable, but high titres are found in those less than 40 years old with thymic hyperplasia. As the antibodies are IgG isotype, they can be transmitted across the placenta, causing neonatal myasthenia. The presence of striated muscle antibodies is a marker for the presence of a thymoma. Cardiac arrythmias may occur in the presence of anti-cardiac muscle antibodies.

Treatment

Treatment is with oral anticholinesterases. Immunosuppressive therapy may be required: prednisolone (1–1.5 mg/kg), azathioprine, cyclophosphamide, methotrexate, or cyclosporin A. Thymectomy may be required to prevent local extension and to exclude malignancy. Plasma exchange may be helpful in myasthenic crisis, but must be coupled with other immunosuppressive therapy. High-dose IVIg (hdIVIg) has also been demonstrated to be helpful in acute crises.

Tests for diagnosis	Tests for monitoring
Tensilon (edrophonium) test	AChRAb
AChRAb	
Striated muscle antibodies	
Cardiac muscle antibodies	
Immunoglobulins	

Lambert–Eaton myasthenic syndrome (LEMS)

LEMS is associated with small cell lung cancer as a paraneoplastic phenomenon; some cases occur without cancer (especially children and some adults) and are associated with HLA-B8. Proximal muscle weakness is marked but bulbar and ocular muscles are spared with autonomic signs. It is associated with other auto-immune diseases, especially thyroid and vitiligo.

There is a decrease of voltage-gated calcium channels on presy-naptic nerve terminals due to an autoantibody reactive with the channels. The tumour cells have been shown to express this antigen on their cell surface.

Treatment of the tumour with chemotherapy may give temporary benefit but 3,4-diaminopyridine (blocks potassium channels) or guanidine may be needed to control the weakness. Plasma exchange or hdIVIg may be of significant (but temporary) benefit. Immunosuppressive therapy is required for non-cancer LEMS.

Acquired neuromyotonia

This syndrome is marked by acquired spontaneous and continuous muscle contraction, stiffness, twitching, cramp, and sweating. Some cases are due to autoantibodies against voltage-gated potassium channels at presynaptic nerve terminals. It is treated with phenytoin, carbamazepine, or immunosuppression.

5 Organ-specific autoimmunity
Lambert–Eaton myasthenic syndrome (LEMS)
Acquired neuromyotonia
Stiff-man syndrome

Stiff-man syndrome

This rare neurological syndrome is also associated with anti-GAD antibodies. It causes a fluctuating and progressive muscular rigidity, which is painful. The finding of the autoantibody ties in with the neurological conclusion that GABAergic neurones which regulate muscle tone should be involved. It is much more common in men, although anti-GAD antibodies are said to be more common in affected women; up to a third will develop diabetes and there may be features of other autoimmune glandular disease. Treatment is with muscle relaxants such as diazepam, baclofen, and valproate, although the autoimmune nature has led to interest in the use of immunosuppressive agents in severe disease.

217

Rasmussen's encephalitis

This rare syndrome usually presents in children with hemiparesis and fits; based on an animal model, it may have an autoimmune basis related to the presence of antibodies to glutamate receptors.

Paraneoplastic syndromes

A paraneoplastic cerebellar degeneration has been associated with carcinoma of the breast and carcinoma of the ovary. These are associated with anti-Yo antibodies directed against the cytoplasm of cerebellar Purkinje cells, and recognizing two antigens, of molecular weight 34 kDa and 62 kDa. Patients with a paraneoplastic neurological syndrome in association with carcinoma of the breast may have anti-Yo or an anti-neuronal nuclear antibody, anti-Ri. The latter antibody is associated with a syndrome of ataxia and myoclonus. Anti-Hu is found in patients with small cell carcinoma who also have a paraneoplastic ataxic sensory neuropathy or paraneoplastic encephalomyelitis. Anti-Hu is an anti-neuronal nuclear antibody (ANNA), recognizing a group of proteins of molecular weight 35–40 kDa. Anti-Hu is one of the autoantibodies now known to penetrate intact cells containing the Hu antigen in their nucleus, indicating that it may have a primary pathogenic role. All these antibodies are usually detectable in both serum and CSF, but it is easier to test serum.

5 Organic-specific autoimmunity

Rasmussen's encephalitis
Paraneoplastic syndromes

Demyelinating disease

Multiple sclerosis

The cause of multiple sclerosis (MS) is unknown, although there are strong indications that it is triggered by infection. It affects any age, but predominantly the young and with a 2:1 female predominance. The pattern of illness is difficult to predict and may be chronic and progressive, relapsing and remitting, or episodic. MHC susceptibility loci have been identified, although these differ in different racial groups; DR2, DQ1 and DQ6 seem to be particularly important. The disease seems to involve abnormal T cells reactive to myelin basic protein. Animal studies suggest that the disease can be transferred with CD4+ T cells. Macrophages and microglia are involved, with local release of inflammatory cytokines and upregulation of MHC class II antigens. Plasma cells also localize to lesions, increasing local synthesis of IgG. Clinical presentations are highly variable and include visual disturbance (optic neuritis), ataxia, weakness, and sensory signs, which usually, at least in initial attacks, resolve completely over a few days. There are no specific diagnostic immunological tests. Examination of serum and CSF demonstrates increased intrathecal immunoglobulin synthesis, with a CSF IgG/albumin ratio of >22 per cent. Isoelectric focusing and immunoblotting demonstrate the presence of oligoclonal IgG bands, but these are not specific for MS, being also found in neurosarcoid, neurosyphilis, acute viral infections of the CNS, SLE, and Sjögren's syndrome. Other helpful tests include evoked potentials (visual, auditory, peripheral) and MRI scanning to show typically placed demyelinating lesions. The differential diagnosis is wide and the immunological studies form only a small part. Rarely, patients with MS develop a uveitis as well as an optic neuritis: this may be associated with autoantibodies to the retinal S-antigen.

Acute attacks may respond to high-dose steroids, but chronic steroid therapy does not prevent relapses. The cytotoxic agents azathioprine and cyclophosphamide have also shown some benefit. β-Interferon (8 mU/alternate days subcutaneously) has shown considerable promise in decreasing the relapse rate in the relapsing–remitting form. This drug has significant immunomodulatory effects, including reducing T-cell proliferation, decreasing induced MHC class II antigen expression, and reducing the production of inflammatory cytokines (TNF-α and γ-IFN). Another drug undergoing trials is copolymer-1, which may have immunomodulatory action in MS. Both plasmapheresis and hdIVIg are beneficial, although the role of these agents has yet to be fully determined; how the effectiveness of these agents fits into a T-cell-mediated central disease remains speculative.

Guillain–Barré syndrome (GBS) and Miller Fisher variant

GBS is an inflammatory demyelinating peripheral neuropathy that frequently follows 1–3 weeks after infection, particularly with *Campylobacter jejuni*. It is known that the enterotoxin of the latter organism binds the ganglioside GM1. In full-blown GBS, the disease begins with ascending weakness, which may progress with alarming rapidity and involve bulbar and respiratory muscles, including the diaphragm, leading to respiratory failure. Sensory symptoms are mild. There may be marked autonomic instability. Demyelination may progress for up to 4 weeks before remyelination begins. Recovery may be very prolonged. There are a number of recognized limited variants, including the Miller Fisher variant, with ophthalmoplegia, ataxia, and areflexia. Although there is some evidence for a cellular immune response, most evidence points to an autoantibody-mediated disease process. GBS is characterized by the presence of antibodies to membrane gangliosides (glycolipids including GM1, LM1, and GD1b); antibodies to GQ1b are present in 90–100 per cent of cases of the Miller Fisher variant and seem to be specific for this condition, related possibly to the very high expression of this antigen in the third cranial nerve. Anti-GM1 antibodies are known to cross-react with lipopolysaccharides from *C. jejuni*.

221

Treatment is best undertaken with plasmapheresis or hdIVIg, which appear to be equally effective if begun early. There is a suggestion that the relapse rate may be higher with hdIVIg. Steroids are of no benefit, and may make symptoms worse.

Chronic inflammatory demyelinating polyneuropathy (CIDP)

CIDP is a chronic form of GBS and is characterized by mainly distal weakness and areflexia as well as marked sensory signs. There is usually no history of antecedent infection. The diagnosis is confirmed by the course, exclusion of other diseases, and by typical electrophysiological studies, compatible with demyelination. Complement-fixing IgG and IgM antibodies may be demonstrated in affected nerves, and autoantibodies to the gangliosides GM1, LM1, and GD1b can be found in some patients. Treatment is with steroids, cytotoxic agents, plasmapheresis, and with hdIVIg; it is said that response to hdIVIg is most likely in ganglioside-antibody-positive patients, although personal experience suggest that this is a poor marker. Current practice is to give three courses of hdIVIg at monthly intervals and a further three courses if there is benefit. Treatment is then discontinued, to see whether patients maintain a remission. Some patients require long-term hdIVIg therapy.

Other related conditions which may have an autoimmune basis include amyotrophic lateral sclerosis and multifocal motor neuropathy with conduction block; treatment is the same as for CIDP.

Paraproteinaemic neuropathy

Demyelinating polyneuropathies may be associated with para-proteins of all classes, which may be due to amyloid or to an autoimmune mechanism. The latter is particularly associated with IgM paraproteins directed against myelin-associated glycoprotein (MAG), a 100 kDa glycoprotein of central and peripheral nerves. Paraproteinaemic neuropathy is also associated with the POEMS syndrome (polyneuropathy, organomegaly, endocrinopathy, mono-clonal gammopathy, and skin changes). The skin changes tend to be a sclerodermatous thickening, and the endocrine diseases include diabetes, thyroid disease, gonadal failure, and hyperprolactinaemia. Lymph nodes may show the changes of Castleman's syndrome, or angiofollicular lymph node hyperplasia (with 'onion-skin' lesions), which is of itself also associated with a polyneuropathy; the lesion is not thought to be malignant. IL-6 levels are said to be raised, explaining the plasma-cell abnormalities. Treatment of para-proteinaemic neuropathies should include treatment of the under-lying plasma-cell clone with steroids, melphalan, or chlorambucil; plasmapheresis and hdIVIg are useful as for CIDP

CARDIAC

Myocarditis and cardiomyopathy

Myocarditis is associated with connective tissue diseases, especially SLE. It may present with congestive heart failure, arrhythmias, and chest pain. There appears to be an association with anti-ribonucleoprotein (RNP) antibodies. There is a good response to steroids.

Anti-cardiac antibodies are associated with dilated cardiomyopathy, which may also have features of myocarditis on biopsy. Anti-cardiac antibodies are also found in 20 per cent of cases of type II autoimmune polyglandular syndrome, but in this case are not associated with cardiomyopathy, but with an increase in blood pressure. The antibodies here are directed against cardiac atrial cells producing atrial natriuretic peptide.

Rare eosinophilic syndromes may affect the myocardium, leading eventually to endomyocardial fibrosis.

Recurrent pericarditis and Dressler's syndrome

Recurrent pericarditis may occur as a disease in its own right, although it is a common feature of connective tissue diseases including SLE and rheumatoid arthritis (RhA). The pericardium is thickened, with an infiltrate of inflammatory cells. NSAIDs are the first line of treatment; steroids may be required, and colchicine has been suggested as a useful agent. Pericardectomy may be required. There are no specific immunological tests.

Dressler's syndrome is (myo-)pericarditis following 2–3 weeks after a myocardial infarction and presenting with typical pericarditic pain. Antibodies to cardiac muscle are often present. It is very rare since thrombolytic therapy has been introduced. Post-pericardotomy syndrome is similar but follows cardiac surgery. NSAIDs and steroids may be required but the syndromes settle spontaneously

5 Organic-specific autoimmunity

Myocarditis and cardiomyopathy
Recurrent pericarditis and Dressler's syndrome

Rheumatic fever

Rheumatic fever is now on the increase again, after a period of retreat. It can affect any age but is mainly a disease of children. Clinical features include carditis, polyarthritis, chorea, cutaneous nodules, erythema marginatum, prolonged PR interval on ECG, raised CRP/ESR, together with evidence of previous streptococcal infection with group A streptococci.

The immunopathology of the process appears to be due to an aberrant immunological response to the streptococcal M-proteins (M-proteins 5, 14, 24), some of which generate antibodies that are cross-reactive with human sarcolemmal proteins and with myosin. Other streptococcal M-proteins cause cross-reactive antibodies reacting with the vimentin of glomerular mesangial cells, and are therefore associated with glomerulonephritis, and M-protein types 1, 5, and 18 cross-react with cartilage epitopes, thus potentially leading to arthritis. In addition, the M-proteins may act as bacterial superantigens, enhancing the autodestructive immune response.

Diagnosis is clinical, supported by elevated acute-phase proteins and raised antistreptolysin O titre (ASOT). Treatment is with antibiotics to eliminate the organism, NSAIDs for the arthralgia, and steroids for the carditis. Long-term penicillin prophylaxis is required as the syndrome will recur on subsequent group A streptococcal infection.

Various aspects of respiratory disease are covered in other chapters (allergy, vasculitis, and miscellaneous syndromes); Goodpasture's syndrome is covered below.

Idiopathic pulmonary fibrosis (cryptogenic fibrosing alveolitis)

Inflammatory lung fibrosis may occur in association with connective tissue diseases (SLE, Sjögren's syndrome, antisynthetase syndrome), and as a consequence of drug exposure. However, many cases have no obvious trigger or association. Patients present with severe progressive breathlessness; a fulminant presentation, often with fever and cough, is referred to as the Hamman–Rich syndrome. Biopsies show activated macrophages and a neutrophil infiltrate. In the early stages there is a lymphoid infiltrate (before fibrosis develops), and excess local cytokine production can be demonstrated (TNF-α, IL-2, γ-IFN, TGF-β, IL-8). Lung function shows a reduced forced vital capacity (FVC) and diffusion capacity, with desaturation on exercise. BAL may be helpful as part of the diagnostic work-up (see Part 2), particularly where there is a lymphocytosis. Chest X-ray (CxR) and lung CT demonstrate the typical interstitial fibrosis. Most patients show an acute-phase response with a polyclonal hypergammaglobulinaemia. RhF is found in 50 per cent and ANA in 20 per cent. Treatment is with steroids, with either azathioprine or cyclophosphamide, but the response is often poor and the disease is progressive.

Lymphoid interstitial pneumonitis

This may occur alone, but is more usually found in autoimmune diseases such as Sjögren's syndrome, in association with viral infection (particularly HIV, EBV), and in common variable immunodeficiency. It presents with chronic cough, shortness of breath, and chest pain. There is a lymphocytic alveolitis (CD8+ T cells in HIV and CD4+ T cells in Sjögren's). Biopsy and BAL are the most helpful tests. Hypergammaglobulinaemia is usually found, but is anyway associated with the primary disorders (with the exception of CVID).

5 Organ-specific autoimmunity

Chest
Idiopathic pulmonary fibrosis
Lymphoid interstitial pneumonia

Eosinophilic syndromes

The lung is affected by a variety of hypereosinophilic syndromes:
- Löffler's syndrome: ? a hypersensivity reaction to drugs, parasites, or idiopathic;
- chronic eosinophilic pneumonia;
- tropical pulmonary eosinophilia (due to filariasis);
- Churg–Strauss syndrome (eosinophilic vasculitis—often associated with neuropathy);
- eosinophilia–myalgia syndrome (contaminated L-tryptophan);
- bronchopulmonary aspergillosis; and
- eosinophilic granuloma (Langerhans cell histiocytosis).

Investigations that may help distinguish the cause, other than standard respiratory investigations (CxR, RFTs, CT), include:
- BAL, with lymphocyte subpopulation analysis; if Langerhans cell histiocytosis is suspected, then antibodies to the S-100 antigen should be included in the panel;
- biopsy;
- ANCA;
- IgE and specific IgE (*Aspergillus*);
- *Aspergillus* precipitins;
- identification of parasitic infection (direct identification, serology).

The role of serum eosinophil cationic protein (ECP) levels is uncertain, as it is likely to be raised whatever the cause of eosinophil activation. It may, however, have a role in monitoring the response to treatment and be a more sensitive marker of damaging activity than eosinophil number in the peripheral blood.

Treatment is usually with steroids, once an underlying trigger has been excluded; Churg–Strauss syndrome usually requires additional cytotoxic therapy.

RENAL

Glomerulonephritis

The diagnosis of glomerulonephritis is complex and specialized. It relies upon the synthesis of multiple diagnostic strands, including routine histology, immunofluorescence on biopsies, electron microscopy, as well as serological tests. All the histology should be done in the same laboratory and reported by the same person: it is inappropriate for immunology laboratories to do the direct immuno-fluorescence while not seeing the H&E sections, special stains, and EM.

Necrotizing crescentic glomerulonephritis

Necrotizing crescentic glomerulonephritis is associated with systemic vasculitis (Wegener's granulomatosis, microscopic poly-arteritis), or with renal-limited disease. As the presentation is usually fulminant, a rapid ANCA (usually with anti-GBM (glomerular basement membrane) antibody) is justified, although in practice the patient will be biopsied if possible and plasmaphereseed acutely, starting immunosuppressive therapy at the same time. Routine serology for ANA, dsDNA, C3, C4, and acute-phase react-ants should also be taken as a baseline. Positive ANCA by immuno-fluorescence should be titred (so that the reduction by plasmapheresis can be checked) and should be typed as proteinase 3 (Pr3) or myeloperoxidase (MPO) positive. A small number of patients will have both ANCA and GBM antibodies. Monitoring of patients subsequently should include ANCA titre and CRP/ESR—a rising titre of ANCA may herald relapse, but the numeric value has no relation to disease activity.

Treatment is with high-dose steroids with cyclophosphamide. Initial treatment is given as pulsed intravenous therapy: the merits of continuous oral cyclophosphamide therapy versus pulsed intra-venous or oral are still debated. Azathioprine has been suggested as a possible alternative to cyclophosphamide after the initial phase, but personal experience has been that it is less effective in Wegener's granulomatosis.

Immune complex glomerulonephritis

Immune complex glomerulonephritis may be triggered by a host of antigenic stimuli:
- bacteria: nephritogenic streptococci; staphylococci (SBE); treponemes; mycoplasma; salmonella;
- viruses: EBV, CMV, HIV, hepatitis B, hepatitis C;
- fungi: *Candida* (systemic infection);
- parasites: *Plasmodium* species, *Schistosoma*, *Toxoplasma*;
- drugs: xeno-antisera (serum sickness);
- connective tissue diseases: SLE, mixed connective tissue disease (MCTD) (rarer);
- tumours: lymphoma, carcinoma;

Tests for diagnosis	Tests for monitoring
Urinalysis (sediment for casts)	Urinalysis (sediment for casts)
Renal Biopsy	Cr & E
Cr & E	Fbc
Fbc	ESR/CRP
ESR/CRP	ANCA titre
ANCA & titre	
Anti-GBM (quantitate if positive)	
ANA	
dsDNA	
C3, C4	

- complement deficiency: any component; C3-nephritic factor (secondary consumption).

The circumstances under which the glomerulonephritis develops gives useful clues. Activity of the renal disease is marked by the presence of casts (especially red-cell) in the urinary sediment. The type of immune deposits in the biospy also give important clues as to the underlying aetiology

Post-streptococcal glomerulonephritis is accompanied by a reduced C3, normal C4, and elevated C3d. ASOT will be high although the rise may take at least a week. Normally, the C3 level will return to normal within 8 weeks. A persistently low C3 with normal C4 beyond this time, in the presence of renal disease, suggests the presence of a C3-nephritic factor, an autoantibody that stabilizes the alternate pathway C3-convertase. This autoantibody is associated with partial lipodystrophy.

Mixed essential cryoglobulinaemia is now known to be caused by hepatitis C, which explains the high incidence of mixed essential cryoglobulinaemia in northern Italy. There is a type II cryoglobulin with rheumatoid-factor activity; the paraprotein component is usually IgMκ, and the bone marrow often shows a monoclonal expansion of B cells. Features of the disease, other than immune complex glomerulonephritis and hepatitis, include arthralgia, skin rashes, and neuropathy. Treatment of the underlying HCV infection (with α-IFN ± ribavirin) often improves the paraproteinaemia and cryoglobulinaemia. Treatment of the abnormal plasma-cell clone may require cytotoxics; plasmapheresis may be necessary to reduce the cryoglobulin level. Type II or type III cryoglobulins may also be detected in other chronic infections that cause glomerulonephritis, such as SBE.

Both IgA nephropathy and the renal lesion in Henoch–Schönlein purpura are characterized by deposition of IgA immune complexes in the glomerulus. Both diseases may be associated with HLA Bw35. Serum IgA levels are variable but may be significantly elevated. However, this is not a specific test, as liver disease and infections may also lead to persistent elevation of IgA. It has been suggested that some types of IgA nephropathy may be associated with IgA class ANCA, although this is not fully substantiated.

Tests for diagnosis	Tests for monitoring
Urinalysis (for casts)	Urinalysis (for casts)
Cr and E	Cr and E
Fbc	Fbc
CRP/ESR	CRP/ESR
ANA, dsDNA, ENA	Other tests depend on underlying disease
C3, C4, C3d	
C3-nephritic factor if C3 persistenetly low	
Cryoglobulins (low C4, no ANA, DNA; check for HCV)	
RhF	
Serum immunoglobulins and electrophoresis (high IgA Henoch–Schönlein, IgA nephropathy; paraproteins in mixed essential cryoglobulinaemia)	
Infectious serology (ASOT)	

Goodpasture's (anti-GBM) syndrome

Anti-GBM disease is characterized by glomerulonephritis and sometimes pulmonary haemorrhage which may lead to secondary pulmonary haemosiderosis. Lung involvement without renal disease is rare. Onset is usually sudden and may be preceded by flu like symptoms and arthralgia. The disease may be triggered by toxin exposure (hydrocarbon solvents) or infections, and smokers are more likely to develop lung haemorrhage than non-smokers. It may also be caused by penicillamine therapy. It is associated with other autoimmune diseases, including Wegener's granulomatosis, M-PAN, thyroid disease, Behçet's disease, coeliac disease, inflammatory bowel disease, thymoma, lymphoma, and other malignancies.

The disease is characterized by the presence in almost all cases of an autoantibody directed against the non-collagenous region of the α3-chain of type IV collagen. This antigen is missing in patients with Alport's syndrome (hereditary deafness and glomerulo nephritis), and these patients make a nephritogenic antibody if transplanted with a normal kidney. Type IV collagen forms the basement membrane in both the glomerulus and lung, but is also found in the cochlear basement membrane, eye, choroid of the brain, and in liver, adrenal, pituitary, and thyroid (eye and brain disease may occasionally be found in anti-GBM disease). The disease is strongly MHC-associated (DRw15(DR2)/DQw6, DR4/DQw7).

The disease is diagnosed by the typical appearance of basement membrane deposition of IgG (rarely IgA or IgM) and a C3 (linear staining) which is best seen in the glomeruli, but can be seen on good bronchial biopsies as well. Serum invariably contains high levels of circulating anti-GBM antibodies, which should be quantitated, to allow monitoring of therapy. The patient should be screened for coincident ANCA-positive vasculitis. As the disease can occur in a transplanted kidney, if antibodies are still present transplantation should be deferred for a minimum of 6 months and preferably 12 months after the antibody has disappeared from the circulation. Serial monitoring over long periods is therefore justified.

Treatment is with acute plasmapheresis (although the controlled trial data to support this are sparse), or immunoadsorption with protein G columns (experimental) followed by steroids and cyclophosphamide (intravenous pulsed therapy), although the optimal regime has not been defined. Aggressive therapy should be continued until the antibody level drops significantly.

Tests for diagnosis	Tests for monitoring
Urinalysis	Urinalysis
Cr and E	Cr and E
Fbc	Fbc
Renal biopsy with immunofluorescence	ESR/CRP
ESR/CRP	Anti-GBM — quantitative
ANCA	RFTs (diffusing capacity)
Anti-GBM — quantitative	
RFTs (diffusing capacity)	

GASTROINTESTINAL TRACT

Autoantibodies against gut endocrine cells have been described in association with other autoimmune diseases but no specific syndromes have been associated with them.

Achalasia

Achalasia results from damage to the myenteric inhibitory neurones of the lower oesophagus, leading to dysphagia and eventual massive dilatation of the oesophagus. It occurs in early to middle adult life. A similar problem occurs in the trypanosomal disease, Chagas disease. There is a marked increase in the risk of subsequent oesophageal carcinoma. Antibodies have been described that recognize the neurones of Auerbach's plexus in the oesophageal wall in the idiopathic form of the disease, suggesting a possible autoimmune basis. This needs further confirmation.

Crohn's disease

Crohn's disease is an inflammatory disease affecting any part of the bowel, which may also be accompanied by disease distant from the bowel (skin, muscle). It presents with diarrhoea and abdominal pain, or with evidence of the extragastrointestinal complications. The inflammation is transmural and granulomata are present. There is superficial ulceration and crypt abscesses. Skip lesions are common, and the deep penetrating ulceration frequently gives rise to fistulas. The disease is associated a seronegative arthritis, uveitis and sclerosing cholangitis, as well as features of malabsorption (especially of vitamin B_{12}, as the terminal ileum is frequently affected). It has long been suspected that the disease is related to an infection and current attention has focused on *Mycobacterium paratuberculosis*, which causes Jonne's disease in cattle. The MHC association is with HLA-DR2/DQ5. There is evidence of both a cell-mediated response, but also increased B-cell activity with immunoglobulin and complement deposition in damaged bowel. Activated macrophages are present and mast-cell numbers are increased. A range of autoantibodies have been identified in Crohn's disease, as well as in ulcerative colitis, including non-MPO P-ANCA (up to 25 per cent of patients), anticardiolipin, antimycobacterial heat-shock protein, rheumatoid factors, and anti-goblet cell. None of these antibodies has realistic diagnostic value. Monitoring is best done with acute-phase markers ESR/CRP. α1-acid glycoprotein (orosomucoid) was said to be more sensitive as an acute-phase marker for inflammatory bowel disease, but in really adds nothing over CRP. Treatment is with steroids, azathioprine, cyclosporin A, and 5-aminosalicyclic acid derivatives.

238

5 Organ-specific autoimmunity

Gastrointestinal tract
Achalasia
Crohn's disease

Ulcerative colitis

This is an inflammatory disease limited to the colon. Presentation is usually with bloody diarrhoea. There are a number of extra-intestinal manifestations, including seronegative arthritis (sacroilitis), uveitis, pyoderma gangrenosum, erythema nodosum, and sclerosing cholangitis. Pan-colitis may cause a toxic megacolon. There is a significantly increased risk of carcinoma of the colon, so those with pan-colitis will usually have a totally colectomy, which is curative; for milder disease regular surveillance by colonoscopy may be sufficient. Unlike Crohn's disease, the disease is continuous and does not include the presence of granulomata. Otherwise the histology is similar. There is an increase in activated T cells (CD4+ DR+, CD45RO+) and also of inflammatory cells, including neutrophils. Autoantibodies to colonic epithelial cells have been described (which are cytotoxic), and atypical P-ANCA (non-MPO) are also seen; a number of candidate antigens have been suggested as the target for this atypical P-ANCA, including lactoferrin and cathepsin G. None of the antibodies is diagnostically useful because of their occurrence in other diseases. Inflammatory markers (ESR/CRP) are elevated and provide a useful way of monitoring disease. Treatment is with topical or systemic steroids, azathioprine, and 5-aminosalicyclic acid derivatives.

Whipple's disease

This is a rare disease of the bowel now known to be caused by infection with an unusual bacterium called *Tropheryma whippelii*. Presentation is with diarrhoea, weight loss, and abdominal pain; there may be an arthritis, cardiac, respiratory, and CNS involvement. Features of a significant protein-losing enteropathy may occur, with a secondary hypogammaglobulinaemia, and also gut loss of T cells, leading to a secondary combined immunodeficiency. Biopsies show typical Schiff-positive macrophages abundant in the bowel wall. There are no routinely available serological tests, but PCR-based tests are available on an experimental basis.

5 Organ-specific autoimmunity

Ulcerative colitis
Whipple's disease

Coeliac disease

This is a common inflammatory disease of the small intestine, triggered by wheat gliadin (gluten). It is particularly common in western Ireland (prevalence 1 in 300), and in the UK occurs in 1 in 1500 people. It is associated with HLA-B8, DR3, DQ2. Ten per cent of patients will have selective IgA deficiency. The symptoms can come on at any age: in childhood there is failure to thrive, while in adults it often comes to light during the investigation of un-explained anaemia (usually iron-deficient). Malabsorption may be obvious, but many patients do not have significant steatorrhoea, and indeed many adult patients may have a normal or increased weight (due to compensatory hyperphagia). There is a strong association with the blistering skin rash, dermatitis herpetiformis (see below) and with autoimmune diseases particularly diabetes, thyroid disease, Addison's disease, and SLE.

The differential diagnosis for coeliac disease is wide, and includes inflammatory bowel disease, true food allergy (excess eosinophils on biopsy), infections (*Giardia*), and connective tissue diseases (scleroderma). The gold standard for diagnosis is still biopsy of the jejunum, although endoscopic biopsy of the duo-denum usually gives satisfactory and equivalent results. The typical histological features are of total villous atrophy. However, sub-total villous atrophy, and in the early stages an increase in intra-epithelial lymphocytes are also compatible with the diagnosis, indi-cating that total villous atrophy is NOT required to make the diag-nosis. How much gluten is being consumed by the patient at the time will have a significant bearing on the biopsy findings. Serological tests include the detection of R1-reticulin antibodies, IgG and IgA antibodies to gliadin, and IgA endomysial antibodies. The latter are the most sensitive and specific and are therefore the test of choice. Patients must however be checked for IgA defi-ciency, so that an IgG endomysial antibody can be checked (as IgA endomysial antibodies will not be found in a coeliac patient with IgA deficiency!). However, IgA (or IgG) EMA-positive patients should all undergo biopsy as confirmation, as the treatment is life-long gluten avoidance. The endomysial antigen has now been iden-tified as tissue transglutaminase: solid-phase assays do not seem to provide any significant advantage over immunofluorescence or monkey oesophagus. Tests for associated endocrine disease may be relevant.

The abnormal bowel returns to normal when gluten is withdrawn from the diet and the antibodies gradually disappear, allowing the IgA/IgG EMA to be used as a tool to monitor compliance with the diet. Compliance is important, as continued exposure to gluten increases the risk of intestinal lymphoma (T cell). Secondary splenic atrophy is also a problem (Howell–Jolly bodies on blood film) and such patients should be treated in the same way as fully asplenic patients, with prophylactic antibiotics and regular checks on pneumococcal and Hib antibodies, with appropriate booster immunizations as required to maintain antibody levels. Dermatitis herpetiformis usually responds to gluten withdrawal, but may require treatment with dapsone (care in G6PD-deficient patients).

Tests for diagnosis	Tests for monitoring
Fbc	Fbc
Markers of malabsorption (Fe, B_{12}, folate, Ca^{2+}, clotting)	Markers of malabsorption (Fe, B_{12}, folate, Ca^{2+}, clotting)
ESR/CRP (inflammatory bowel disease)	IgA or IgG EMA
Autoantibody screen (reticulin)	Pneumococcal/Hib antibodies (if splenic atrophy)
IgA endomysial antibody (EMA)	β2-microglobulin, serum Igs + electrophoresis (if concerns over lymphoma)
Test for IgA deficiency (do IgG EMA)	
Small bowel biopsy	
Tests for other autoimmune endocrine disease	

LIVER

Primary biliary cirrhosis (PBC)

PBC is a disease of older women (90 per cent of patients are female). The cause is unknown but epidemiological work on clusters of disease suggests a possible infectious aetiology. It is particularly common in the north-east of England. It is not strictly a cirrhotic disease, as the primary pathology is inflammation around the portal triads (intrahepatic bile ducts), leading eventually to fibrosis, although occasional overlap patients occur with features of PBC and also of chronic autoimmune hepatitis. There is increased HLA-DR expression on the biliary epithelium and an infiltrate of CD4+ T cells specific for biliary epithelial antigens. An excess of IgM-producing B cells is also seen around the biliary ducts. The disease is strongly associated with other autoimmune diseases, including Sjögren's syndrome, thyroid disease, cryptogenic fibrosing alveolitis, CREST (calcinosis, Raynaud's, oesophageal dysmotility, sclerodactyly, and telangiectasia), and renal tubular acidosis. Clinical features include profound fatigue in the prodrome, followed by intense itch, arthralgia and, with disease progression, hepatosplenomegaly, xanthelasma, skin pigmentation, and eventually hepatic decompensation with jaundice.

Immunological tests

Liver-function tests show elevated alkaline phosphatase; caeruloplasmin, lipoproteins, and cholesterol are also raised. The typical immunological features are the presence of mitochondrial antibodies, found in 96 per cent of cases. A variety of different mitochondrial antibody patterns are identifiable (with difficulty!) by immunofluorescence. The M2 pattern is most commonly associated with PBC. M2 autoantigens have now been identified as trypsin-sensitive molecules on the inner mitochondrial membrane. The primary antigen is the large multimeric 2-oxo-acid dehydrogenase complex, pyruvate dehydrogenase (PDC). M2a recognizes the E2 subcomponent (dihydrolipoamide acyltransferase) of PDC (95 per cent of PBC). M2c recognizes the E2 antigen of oxoglutarate dehydrogenase (OGDC) (39–88 per cent of PBC) and branch-chain 2-oxo-acid dehydrogenase (BCOADC) (54 per cent), and the protein X component of PDC (95 per cent). M2d and M2e antigens are E1-α and E1-β components of PDC (41–66 per cent and 2–7 per cent, respectively). Solid-phase assays are available for M2 antigen and should be used to confirm the specificity of antibodies identified by immunofluorescence. These antibodies recognize conserved epitopes on related proteins found in fungi and bacteria. The antibodies, which are mainly IgM and IgG3, are known to inhibit enzyme function and may penetrate viable cells. Total IgM levels are polyclonally raised, often significantly (20–30 g/l), although the reason for this is not known.

Other antibodies have been thought to identify subgroups of PBC: M9 antibody (? anti-glycogen phosphorylase) may be marked

Tests for diagnosis	Tests for monitoring
Fbc	Fbc
LFTs (including γ-GT)	LFTs (including γ-GT)
Caeruloplasmin	Caeruloplasmin
Cholesterol and lipoproteins	Cholesterol and lipoproteins
CRP/ESR	CRP/ESR
Anti-mitochondrial antibodies	
M2-antibody	
HEp-2 screen (multiple nuclear dots, ring staining)	
Serum immunoglobulins and electrophoresis	

for early PBC with a benign prognosis (also found in low titres in healthy individuals); M4 antibody may be a marker of aggressive disease (? anti-sulphite oxidase). Non-M2 anti-mitochondrial antibodies (AMAs) are found in myocarditis, SLE, syphilis, and in some drug reactions.

Antinuclear antibodies are also found in PBC: HEp-2 cells may show multiple nuclear dots (MND) and ring-nuclear staining. MND-ANA are found in 10–44 per cent of PBC patients, especially associated with Sjögren's syndrome. The MND antigen is Sp100 which is structurally similar to MHC antigens. It may occur in the absence of AMA, but it is not clear whether this subgroup is clinically different. Ring-nuclear staining is due to autoantibody to the major glycoprotein of nuclear pores (gp210) and laminin B receptor. Both may occur in AMA-negative PBC.

Treatment

Treatment with immunosuppressive drugs is unhelpful. Colchicine and penicillamine have both been tried with limited benefit. Ursodeoxycholic acid may improve symptoms but does not alter the prognosis. Transplantation is used for end-stage disease.

Autoimmune hepatitis

Before a diagnosis of autoimmune hepatitis can be made, it is important to exclude toxic (alcohol, drugs), metabolic diseases (Wilson's disease, haemochromatosis, α1-antitrypsin deficiency), and viral causes, although there is a complex link between autoimmune hepatitis and HCV. It is predominantly a disease of younger women (90 per cent of patients are female). There is a strong association with HLA-B8, DR3, DR4. It may present with acute hepatitis, jaundice, profound malaise and fatigue, and amenorrhoea in women (?autoimmune). There may be marked extrahepatic features: vitiligo and alopecia, thyroid disease, pernicious anaemia, type I diabetes mellitus, autoimmune haemolytic anaemia and ITP, rheumatoid arthritis, ulcerative colitis, glomerulonephritis, cryptogenic fibrosing alveolitis, and coeliac disease.

The major features are piecemeal necrosis of hepatocytes in the periportal region. There is an infiltrate of CD4+ T cells and B cells. Later stages of the disease show typical cirrhosis. Liver-function tests show markedly elevated transaminases. Markers of hepatitis virus infection are absent. There is a polyclonal hypergammaglobulinaemia (mainly IgG and IgA). Autoantibodies to nuclear components, dsDNA, smooth muscle (anti-actin), LKM antibodies, and liver membranes (anti-asialoglycoprotein receptor) can be detected. Low-titre AMA may also be detected. The pattern of antibodies present has led to a classification scheme for autoimmune hepatitis:

Type 1 (lupoid hepatitis)

Mean age onset 35 years; high frequency of extrahepatic symptoms; 90 per cent of cases are female; ANA, smooth-muscle antibodies (SMA), liver membrane antibodies, ds-DNA antibodies.

Type 2a

Onset in childhood in 50 per cent; female predominance; frequent extrahepatic symptoms; hypergammaglobulinaemia is less than in type 1; IgA LOW; LKM-1 antibody positive; anti-thyroid, anti-GPC antibodies frequent.

Type 2b

HCV associated; HCV-RNA positive, antibodies to HCV positive; no female predominance; occurs in over-40s; milder disease; no extrahepatic features; LKM-1 positive (NB HCV antigen cross-reactive with P450 (IID6) cytochrome).

Type 3

Female predominance (90 per cent); onset around 35 years; hypergammaglobulinaemia. Antibodies to SLA (soluble liver antigens = liver cytokeratins 8 and 18); less commonly also SMA and AMA.

Type 4

Overlap syndrome of autoimmune hepatitis and PBC; AMA positive with antibodies to M2 antigen

Other autoantibodies in hepatitis

Liver–kidney microsomal antibodies may be found in autoimmune hepatitis and recognize different hepatic cytochrome enzymes:
- LKM-1: cytochrome P450 (IID6): associated with types 2a and 2b autoimmune hepatitis. Antibodies to LKM-1 may be triggered by HCV and HSV as both have proteins sharing homology with P450 (IID6).
- LKM-2: cytochrome P450 (IIC9). Drug-induced, tienilic acid, in France only.
- LKM-3: glucuronyl transferase. Hepatitis delta infection. These antibodies are specific to human liver.
- Liver microsome antibodies (LM): cytochrome P450IA2. Drug-induced hepatitis, dihydrallazine.

Treatment

The treatment depends on the underlying cause; any viral trigger (HCV) needs direct treatment (α-IFN $\pm$ ribavirin). Immunosuppressive therapy with corticosteroids (high dose) is used and a good initial response defines a good prognosis. Azathioprine is useful for maintaining remission. Cyclosporin A and tacrolimus have also been used. Liver transplantation may be required for end-stage disease in young patients.

Sclerosing cholangitis

This is an inflammatory disease of intra- and extrahepatic bile ducts, leading to fibrosis. It is more common in men than in women and can occur at any age. It may lead to cholangiocarcinoma. It is strongly associated with inflammatory bowel disease. Liver-function tests are similar to those for PBC. Anti-mitochondrial antibodies are absent, the IgM is not raised, and atypical P-ANCA may be found. Immunosuppressive treatment is unhelpful, liver transplantation may be required.

AUTOIMMUNE HAEMATOLOGICAL DISORDERS

Immune thrombocytopenia (ITP)

ITP can occur at any age and is characterized by thrombocytopenia, with increased marrow megakaryocytes, and shortened platelet survival. Presentation is usually with sudden onset of petechiae, particularly around the feet, and bleeding (nose, gums, bowel, urinary tract). It can be triggered by infection (including HIV), by drugs (the list is very long!), or by malignancy (lymphoma, adenocarcinoma), in association with common variable immunodeficiency and in association with other autoimmune diseases (SLE, thyroid disease, autoimmune hepatitis). Neonatal alloimmune thrombocytopenia may occur in mothers who are negative for the platelet antigen PL^{A1}, who become sensitized in prior pregnancies where infants are $PL^{A1}+$, or by blood transfusion; other platelet antigen systems have also been involved.

It appears that antibody-coated platelets are destroyed by the phagocytic cells in the peripheral blood. Many platelet antigens have been shown to be targets for the autoimmune response, including GPIIb/IIIA and GP V (after chickenpox). However, detection of anti-platelet antibodies is difficult and few centres offer this routinely. There is a wide variety of tests. The diagnosis can usually be made clinically and with the assistance of a bone marrow examination. Investigations need to rule out associated autoimmune disease (SLE), immunodeficiency, and malignancy.

Treatment is complex and should be undertaken by a haematologist. Any underlying cause should be treated or removed (drugs). Therapy is determined by the severity of the thrombocytopenia counts of $<20 \times 10^9/l$ usually lead to bleeding problems. First-line therapy is either steroids or hdIVIg. Second-line therapies include cytotoxics, danazol, and splenectomy. If splenectomy is undertaken the usual precautions should be taken (see Chapter 3 and above under Coeliac disease)

Tests for diagnosis	Tests for monitoring
Fbc and platelet count	Platelet count
Viral serology	
Serum immunoglobulins	
Autoantibodies (ANA, dsDNA, ENA, thyroid)	
Anti-platelet antibodies (?)	
Bone marrow	

Immune haemolytic anaemia

Immune haemolytic anaemia is divided into to categories dependent on the temperature at which haemolysis takes place. Warm haemolytic anaemia:

- idiopathic autoimmune (AIHA);
- secondary to other diseases: SLE, CVID, lymphoid malignancy, hepatitis.

Cold haemolytic anaemia:

- idiopathic cold agglutinin disease;
- cold agglutinins secondary to infection (*Mycoplasma pneumoniae*, EBV);
- cold antibody disease (Donath–Landsteiner antibody, occurs in childhood or secondary to syphilis): paroxysmal cold haemoglobinuria;
- cold antibody disease secondary to lymphoma (CHAD).

Other causes of haemolytic anaemia include drug induced (which may be due to bystander immune-complex-mediated damage or due to direct binding of antigen, e.g. penicillin, to the red cell membrane causing the formation of an immunoreactive neo-antigen). Massive haemolysis may occur following mismatched blood transfusion (ABO incompatibility, pre-formed isoagglutinins), and as a result of rhesus incompatibility (rhesus haemolytic disease of the newborn).

The immunological process is identified by the Coombs test which identifies the presence of immunoglobulin and C3 on the red cell membrane. The assays are done at different ranges to identify warm or cold antibodies, and then panels of typed red cells may be used to identify the specificity of the antibody. In the direct test, an anti-human IgG is used to demonstrate pre-bound IgG on the patient's red cells; while in the indirect test, the patient's serum is incubated with normal erythrocytes to demonstrate the presence of anti-red cell antibodies in the serum. Pre-bound antibody can be eluted from the red cell for further studies.

Antigenic specificities vary according to the cause of the anaemia most warm antibodies are against the rhesus system antigens or against the Band 3 anion transporter. Cold antibodies due to *Mycoplasma* recognize the I-antigen, while those induced by EBV recognize i-antigen. Lymphoma-associated cold agglutinin disease is characterized by a monoclonal IgM (usually κ not λ) with anti-I specificity. The Donath–Landsteiner antibody recognizes the P antigen. Three classes of drug-induced antibodies to red cells are recognized:

- antibodies binding to the drug itself on the red cell, where red cell damage is 'accidental': these antibodies are usually warm;
- drugs binding to a complex of drug and red cell membrane antigen (but binding only weakly or not at all to red cells without the drug): these may be cold antibodies;
- antibodies induced by the drug but binding to the red cell in the absence of the drug and recognizing Rh antigens: these antibodies are usually warm.

Tests for diagnosis	Tests for monitoring
Fbc	Fbc
LFTs (bilirubin and LDH)	LFTs (bilirubin and LDH)
Haptoglobin (reduced in haemolysis)	Haptoglobin (reduced in haemolysis)
Direct and Indirect Coombs test	Direct and Indirect Coombs test
Cold agglutinins	Cold agglutinins
Bone marrow	
Viral serology	
Serum immunoglobulins and electrophoresis	
Cryoglobulins	
Autoantibodies (ANA, dsDNA, ENA, thyroid)	

Treatment

Treatment of any underlying disorder is required (lymphoma, infection), and any suspect drug should be stopped. Treatment is similar to that for ITP and splenectomy may be required. hdIVIg is much less effective than in ITP.

Autoimmune neutropenia

This may occur alone or in conjunction with other autoimmune diseases, such as SLE, rheumatoid arthritis (Felty's syndrome), Sjögren's syndrome, PBC, autoimmune hepatitis, or malignancy such as lymphoma or large granular lymphocyte (LGL) leukaemia. It may be triggered by infection (CMV, EBV) or by drug exposure (penicillins and cephalosporins), due to immune mechanisms. Agranulocytosis may occur after exposure to a number of drugs, of which the most important is carbimazole.

All patients will require a bone marrow examination if neutropenia is severe and persistent. Other than testing for associated autoimmune features, attempts to detect anti-neutrophil specific antibodies are hampered by the non-specific binding of immunoglobulins via neutrophil Fc receptors. However, two potential surface antigens (NA1 and NA2, recognizing isoforms of CD16, FcγRIII) have been identified in primary autoimmune neutropenia of childhood; in adults some patients have had antibodies against the complement receptor CD11b/CD18.

Treatment is not usually required until the neutrophil count falls below 0.5×10^9/l. Co-trimoxazole and antifungal prophylaxis may be required. G-CSF may be valuable in shortening the period of agranulocytosis, and may be given as a test in patients who are chronically neutropenic in order to assess the response: responders can then be given treatment if they develop infection. hdIVIg has been used in primary autoimmune neutropenia, but is much less effective that in ITP.

Paroxysmal nocturnal haemoglobinuria

This disease is due to an acquired (clonal) deficiency of complement control proteins on the red-cell surface due to a failure to synthesize glucosylphosphatidylinositol membrane anchors (common to a number of important surface molecules). The affected molecules of red cells include CD55 (decay accelerating factor), CD59 (Homologous restriction factor-20, HRF20), and homologous restriction factor (HRF65, C8-binding protein), all of which prevent accidental lysis of red cells. Red cells tend to lyse at night when the pH of serum drops (hence the name), and the diagnostic test is Ham's acidification test. There is often an associated iron deficiency and leukopenia and an increased risk of haematological malignancy. Androgen therapy may be helpful; steroids are not. Bone marrow transplantation may be required.

5 Organ-specific autoimmunity
Autoimmune neutropenia
Paroxysmal nocturnal haemoglobinuria

Aplastic anaemia

Aplastic anaemia, affecting all bone marrow lineages, may arise following infections (hepatitis B, hepatitis C) or exposure to toxins (drugs (chloramphenicol), solvents (benzene)), or it may be idiopathic. There is evidence in the idiopathic forms of a cellular immune response inhibiting erythropoeisis and about 50 per cent of patients respond to treatment with ATG/ALG. Androgenic steroids may help, but corticosteroids do not. Cyclosporin A may be of benefit. Blood transfusion support is required and bone marrow transplantation is the definitive procedure.

Anti-Factor VIII antibodies (acquired haemophilia)

Acquired Factor VIII inhibitory autoantibodies may occur in association with SLE and other autoimmune diseases, drug therapy (phenytoin, penicillin, chloramphenicol, and sulphonamides) or as an idiopathic autoimmune disease. The antibodies can cause a severe clotting disorder, which can be overcome by very high-dose Factor VIII infusions. Two types of patient are identified: low-titre antibodies with a low response, and high-titre antibodies with a high response to further Factor VIII challenge. Plasmapheresis or specific immunoadsorption with protein A columns (antibodies are usually IgG1 or IgG4) may be required acutely. hdIVIg may also be beneficial. Steroids and cytotoxic agents may also be used in conjunction with other measures. Tolerance induction using regular Factor VIII treatment has been tried with variable success. Desmopressin® (DDAVP) mobilizes Factor VIII from storage and may be a useful adjunct to treatment when inhibitor levels are low. Clotting can be controlled using partially activated complexes that bypass the level of inhibition.

5 Organ-specific autoimmunity

Aplastic anaemia
Anti-Factor VIII antibodies

SKIN

The skin is a very easy organ in which to investigate autoimmune disease, due to its accessibility for biopsy. Very considerable progress has been made in the past few years in identify the target antigens involved in autoimmune skin disease. In clinical practice autoantibodies may be detected either by direct immuno-fluorescence (DIF) of snap-frozen biopsies or by indirect immuno-fluorescence (IIF) using the patient's serum. The use of hypertonic saline prior to staining of biopsies splits the epidermis away from the dermis, between the lamina lucida and the lamina densa, and allows the site of autoantibody binding to be more clearly identi-fied: this is important in distinguishing epidermolysis bullosa acquisita from bullous pemphigoid. Significant disease may be present with little or no circulating antibody and therefore DIF plays a major role in diagnosis. However, this needs to be carried out carefully by an experienced laboratory in order to obtain reliable results.

Tests for diagnosis of blistering skin disease	Tests for monitoring
Skin biopsy (H&E, immunofluorescence, split skin, EM)	IgA EMA (DH only for compliance with gluten-free diet (GFD)
Indirect immunofluorescence (monkey oesophagus)	
IgA endomysial antibody	
Tests for associated autoimmune diseases	

Bullous pemphigoid

This is a disease of the elderly and is characterized by the presence tense, itchy blisters over limbs and trunk. The blistering stage may be preceded by papules or urticaria. Mucous membranes may be involved in up to a third of patients. The blister is subepidermal on histology. DIF and IIF show mainly linear IgG and C3 at the dermo-epidermal junction, binding to the epithelial side of the basement membrane (on a saline-split preparation); on immunoelectron microscopy the IgG is located on the lamina lucida. The rate of positivity in DIF is up to 90 per cent and for IIF up to 70 per cent. Other immunoglobulin classes may be detected. Drug reactions may cause similar bullous lesions but with negative immuno-fluorescence. IgE and eosinophil counts may be raised, although these are not diagnostically useful. Two autoantigens have been identified: BPAg1, 230 kDa (chromosome 6) and BPAg2, 180 kDa (chromosome 10). BPAg1 is similar to desmoplakin I and is likely to form part of the hemi-desmosome, which provides the major site of attachment between the internal cytoskeletal proteins and the external matrix. Antibodies to BPAg1 are only found in bullous pemphigoid, BPAg2 is also a hemi-desmosomal protein, but anti-bodies are also found in herpes gestationis.

Mild disease can be treated with topical steroids, but high-dose oral steroids are usually required; these can be tapered once remission is obtained and the remission may be sustained once steroids are withdrawn. Additional immunosuppressive therapy is rarely required, but azathioprine, cyclophosphamide, cyclosporin A and dapsone have all been proposed. Plasmapheresis has been found not to be of benefit. hdIVIg is now being studied and some reports suggest benefit. Tetracycline and niacinamide have also been proposed as treatment, although this is controversial: the mechanism of action is obscure.

Herpes gestationis

This is a rare itchy and blistering rash associated with pregnancy. The onset is in the second or third trimester or occasionally in the immediate postpartum period. The infant may also be affected due to transplacental passage of the IgG antibody; this usually resolves spontaneously as maternal antibody decays. The umbilicus is involved, in contrast to another rare disease: pruritic urticaria and plaques of pregnancy (PUPP). It may recur in subsequent pregnancies and in response to hormonal changes during the menstrual cycle or in response to the oral contraceptive pill. It is associated with HLA-DR3 and DR4. The pathology shows the presence of eosinophils which may be accompanied by a peripheral blood eosinophilia. The autoantigen is the 180kDa BPAg2 antigen and DIF shows linear deposits of C3 at the dermo-epidermal junction in almost all cases, with IgG in up to 50 per cent. The staining on immuno-EM is localized to the epithelial lamina lucida. IIF is positive in only 30 per cent of patients. Biopsy with DIF is therefore the diagnostic test of choice. Treatment is with steroids (20–60 mg/day) together with antihistamines to control itch. This may pose problems for the pregnancy and careful monitoring is required.

Cicatricial pemphigoid

See autoimmune eye disease, below.

Pemphigus vulgaris

This is a serious blistering disease, which if unrecognized and untreated is invariably fatal. The blisters are flaccid and tend to rupture, with the split occurring in the epidermis itself. This leads to the characteristic sign (Nikolsky's sign), where gentle lateral pressure leads to sloughing of the skin both in affected areas and in apparently normal areas. The blisters typically occur on the head and trunk and in the groins, although no part of the skin is spared. Mucosal lesions are common and the disease often presents with oral involvement. The disease is more common in middle age and particularly in persons of Jewish or Mediterranean extraction. Rarely it may occur as a familial disease. It is associated with HLA-A10 and also HLA-DR4/DQw3 or DR6/DQw1. The histology shows acantholysis or separation of the keratinocytes. DIF on skin biopsies shows the deposition of IgG and C3 in the intercellular spaces of the epidermis, giving a chickenwire appearance, in almost all cases. IIF on monkey oesophagus gives a similar pattern in over 90 per cent of patients. The autoantigen is now known to be a 130 kDa protein identified as cadherin (Dsg3), which is homologous to desmoglein and occurs complexed to plakoglobin. The complex occurs at sites of adherence between neighbouring keratinocytes. Complement plays a key role in the immune process and complement breakdown products can be detected in blister fluid. Local plasmin formation is also important in separation of the cells. Diagnosis requires both DIF on a suitable biopsy, together with IIF on serum. Low titres of serum antibodies giving a similar staining pattern have been reported in SLE, myasthenia gravis with thymoma, burns, and some cutaneous infections (leprosy).

A rare form of pemphigus, with a characteristic neutrophilic infiltrate, has been described in which the antibody is IgA and the autoantigens are desmocollin I and II, components of the desmosome. The DIF shows a chickenwire staining pattern, located in the basal layers only with anti-IgA antiserum.

The treatment is with corticosteroids in high dose (1–2 mg/kg/day); azathioprine is the preferred second-line agent, although cyclophosphamide, cyclosporin A, and methotrexate have all been used successfully. In the neutrophilic variant, dapsone is helpful because of its effects on neutrophil activity. Plasmapheresis appears to be of no benefit., but again hdIVIg is being explored as a possible therapeutic approach.

Pemphigus foliaceus

This is a rare variant of pemphigus vulgaris which rarely involves the mucosal surfaces. The blistering is more superficial than in pemphigus vulgaris and as a result the prognosis is better. Studies in Brazil on the endemic form (fogo selvagem) suggest that it may be triggered by an infectious agent, perhaps transmitted by an insect vector. It may also be seen as a reaction to certain drugs, such as penicillamine, captopril, and other ECA inhibitors. DIF may show that the immunofluorescence is more superficial than in pemphigus vulgaris. The autoantigen is different from that in pemphigus vulgaris (PV) and is a 160kDa component of the desmosome, desmoglein-1. The treatment is the same as for PV.

265

Paraneoplastic pemphigus

A variant of pemphigus, accompanied by erythema multiforme, has been reported in association with lymphomas, chronic lymphocytic leukaemia, and thymoma. The pathology shows acantholysis but there is also necrosis of the keratinocytes and basement membrane damage. There is IgG and C3 deposition, both in the intercellular substance and along the basement membrane. The autoantigens are desmosomal proteins, desmoplakin I and II, although other possible antigens may be involved. The disease tends to be resistant to treatment.

Epidermolysis bullosa acquisita

This is a blistering disease accompanied by marked skin fragility affecting particularly sites of trauma such as hands and feet. There is an association with inflammatory bowel disease, especially Crohn's disease The disease can often be difficult to distinguish from other blistering diseases. There is a linear staining with IgG and C3 of the basement membrane on DIF, but this is not diagnostic; on split-skin preparations the staining is seen to localize to the dermal side. IIF may also be positive. The autoantibody appears to react with type VII procollagen. Treatment is difficult and the response to steroids and cytotoxics is poor. Plasmapheresis and hdIVIg may be more effective.

Dermatitis herpetiformis (DH)

DH is an intensely itchy blistering rash that is associated with gluten intolerance. Typical sites for the rash include the elbows, buttocks, and thighs. DIF on the skin biopsy shows typical granular IgA deposits on the dermal papillae. IgA endomysial antibodies will be positive and jejunal/duodenal biopsies will often show features of coeliac disease even in the absence of clinical symptoms. A gluten-free diet will eventually lead to resolution of the rash, but resistant cases may require treatment with dapsone, having first excluded G6PD deficiency.

Linear IgA disease

There is a group of rare blistering disorders also associated with IgA deposition in the skin on DIF that are not associated with gluten intolerance. However, the rash is often similar to DH. DIF shows linear (rather than granular) IgA deposition along the basement membrane and a 97 kDa antigen (LAD-1) has been identified in most cases. Treatment is with dapsone (with the caveats noted above).

5 Organ-specific autoimmunity

Epidermolysis bullosa acquisita
Dermatitis herpetiformis
Linear IgA disease

AUTOIMMUNE EYE DISEASE

The eye has a number of interesting immunological properties that alter the propensity for immune-mediated disease, including the curious feature that antigen injected into the anterior chamber induces tolerance rather than immunity. In addition, the eye has no true lymphatics, relatively poor vascularity and, as the retina is an extension of the CNS, there is a blood–retinal barrier that limits passage of molecules in either direction. Ocular involvement is a common feature of many connective tissue and vasculitic diseases.

Investigation of uveitis

Uveitis occurs as a consequence of a wide range of systemic diseases; the site of inflammation gives some clues as to the cause:

- Anterior uveitis:
    - seronegative arthritis (ankylosing spondylitis, Reiter's disease, psoriatic arthropathy);
    - infections (herpes simplex, herpes zoster, TB);
    - idiopathic;
    - vasculitis (Behçet's syndrome).
- Posterior uveitis:
    - infections—mainly in immunocompromised (HIV, CMV, candida, other fungi, syphilis, Toxoplasma, TB);
    - vasculitis (Behçet's, polyarteritis);
    - sarcoidosis;
    - rare eye diseases (Eales disease, VKH, birdshot retinopathy).
- Pan-uveitis:
    - connective tissue diseases (polychondritis, SLE);
    - infections (*Brucella, Toxoplasma*, TB, viruses);
    - vasculitis (Behçet's, Wegener's);
    - sympathetic ophthalmitis;
    - sarcoidosis.
- Intermediate uveitis:
    - Fuchs heterochromic iridocyclitis (abnormal pigmentation of the iris);
    - pars planitis (may be associated with MS);
    - juvenile rheumatoid arthritis.

Investigations should therefore be aimed at most likely causes; infection needs to be excluded, as the appropriate treatment for non-infectious uveitis is steroids together with azathioprine and/or cyclosporin A. Aggressive therapy is justified if vision is to be preserved. Patients require regular monitoring of therapy (see Chapter 10).

Tests for diagnosis of uveitis	Tests for monitoring
Fbc	Fbc [azathioprine]
Cr & E	Cr & E [CyA]
Glucose	LFTs [Azathioprine]
LFTs	Glucose [high dose steroids]
CRP/ESR	CRP/ESR
Angiotensin converting enzyme	Cyclosporin levels
Viral/Toxoplasma/Brucella serology (if exposure suspected)	
ANCA	
ANA [+ dsDNA, ENA, C3, C4]	
Chest radiograph	
Mantoux test	
Fluorescein angiogram	

271

Ocular cicatricial pemphigoid

This disease leads to subepithelial fibrosis of conjunctivae and, if untreated, can cause blindness, through damage to the corneal surface. The mouth is also involved, giving a gingivitis and ulceration; this may rarely also spread to involve the larynx and oesophagus. Rarely, there is also skin disease. Autoantibodies to a 120 kDa basement membrane antigen can be detected, and these are found on direct immunofluorescence as continuous linear staining at the epithelial basement membrane, located on immuno-EM to the lamina lucida; IgG, IgA, and complement are deposited. Circulating epithelial antibodies are rarely present: studies claiming to detect them have used neat serum, which is likely to give meaningless results. Putative antigens include epiligrin (a ligand for keratinocyte integrins) and an unidentified 45 kDa protein. Where the skin is involved, antibodies to BPAg1 and BPAg2 have been detected (see Bullous pemphigoid, above) There is an association with HLA-DQ7 (DQB*0301) and B11. Topical therapy is rarely effective and oral steroids, cyclophosphamide or dapsone will be required. Drug-induced pemphigoid has been associated with pilocarpine, ephedrine, and idoxuridine.

Sympathetic ophthalmitis

This syndrome occurs penetrating trauma to one eye, which is then followed by a progressive granulomatous pan-uveitis in the un-injured eye after a variable interval. It is thought that damage to the uveal tract triggers an autoimmune response: autoantibodies to retinal photoreceptors and Müller cells (normally responsible for nutritional support for the photoreceptor) may be detected. One of the major autoantigens is the retinal S-antigen (arrestin). It may also be associated with lens-associated uveitis, although the latter may occur alone and may be cured by lens removal. Vitiligo, alopecia, and whitening of the eyelashes (poliosis) may occur. Early removal of the traumatized eye and aggressive immunosuppressive therapy may be required.

5 Organic-specific autoimmunity

Ocular cicatricial pemphigoid
Sympathetic ophthalmitis

Vogt–Koyanagi–Harada disease (VKH)

This is a rare bilateral granulomatous pan-uveitis occurring in adults and leading to visual failure. It is more common in Japan and South America. It is similar to sympathetic ophthalmitis and is also associated with vitiligo, alopecia, and poliosis. There is a strong HLA association with DR53. High titres of anti-retinal antibodies can be detected, also against the retinal S-antigen. High levels of circulating γ-interferon have been noted. Corticosteroids and cyclosporin A are the recommended treatments.

Cancer-associated retinopathy

This is a very rare paraneoplastic syndrome associated with small cell carcinoma of the lung. It is associated with destruction of the photoreceptors, and autoantibodies against the retina are detectable.

Birdshot retinopathy

This is a rare primary uveitis, with a retinal vasculitis, affecting predominantly middle-aged white females. It is strongly associated with HLA-A29. Treatment is with immunosuppressive agents including steroids, cyclosporin A, azathioprine, and more recently with high-dose IVIg.

5 Organ-specific autoimmunity

6 Connective tissue disease

Rheumatoid arthritis

Aetiology

RhA is often thought of as a joint disease: this is incorrect, it is a multisystem disease in which arthritis is a major component. An infectious trigger has been sought for many years, without success. The best candidate pathogens include EBV, *Mycobacterium tuberculosis*, and *Proteus mirabilis*. A genetic background is required (DR4) although this varies according to the ethnic background of the population. Other genetic factors may include T-cell receptor and immunoglobulin gene polymorphisms.

Clinical features

Morning stiffness and fatigue are early signs. There may be low-grade fever. Joint pain and swelling follow and the arthritis is often deforming. Hand joints are typically affected. Radiographic changes are typical. Non-articular features include Sjögren's syndrome, lymphadenopathy, scleritis, cutaneous vasculitis and ulceration, nodules both of skin and lung, pleurisy, alveolitis, pericarditis, endocarditis (with valvular involvement), splenomegaly (with ulceration and neutropenia = Felty's syndrome), myositis, mononeuritis multiplex, and cord compression from spinal involvement. Amyloid is a long-term complication from chronic inflammation.

Immunopathology

Most of the pathology is located in the joint, with evidence for activation of T cells, macrophages, and endothelial cells. There is increase synovial vascularity. Both CD4+ and CD8+ T cells are found in the joint tissues. 'Memory' T cells (CD45RO+, CD29+) predominate and there is restriction of TcR Vβ usage suggestive of a superantigenic effect. Large quantities of cytokines can be detected in the joint fluids. Endothelial cell activation and the production of chemokines (interleukin -8 (IL-8), RANTES, MCP-1, Gro-α, and ENA-78 (epithelial neutrophil activating peptide)) ensure a major influx of inflammatory cells. Autoantibodies are produced, including rheumatoid factors, anti-nuclear antibodies, and antibodies to keratin and filaggrin. The pathogenic role of these autoantibodies is uncertain. IgG molecules in RhA have been shown to have markedly reduced glycosylation, although the significance of this is uncertain.

Immunological tests

Rheumatoid factors are found in 67–85 per cent of patients, depending on the type of assay used. Most detected rheumatoid factors are IgM class, although it has been suggested that RhF-patients may have RhF of other classes. Rheumatoid factors are not diagnostic tests for RhA (see Part 2). The highest titres of RhF are found in patients with extra-articular disease. There is no correlation of disease activity with antibody titres.

Tests for diagnosis	Tests for monitoring
CRP/ESR	CRP/ESR
Fbc	Fbc
Immunoglobulins	ENA [for development of Sjögren's]
ANA	
ENA	
RhF	

Cryoglobulins may be found and these are usually type II or type III (i.e. with RhF activity), often in association with Felty's syndrome. Hypergammaglobulinaemia is usually present, due to chronic inflammation, and this is invariably polyclonal, although small monoclonal bands may be present. Urine may contain an excess of free polyclonal and sometimes monoclonal light chains. Complement C3/C4 are usually elevated, as are acute-phase proteins, although patients with Felty's may have reduced levels.

Anti-nuclear antibodies may be found, both on rat liver and HEp-2 cells. ANAs are most commonly found in Felty's syndrome. These include antibodies against a nuclear antigen RA-33 a ribonucleoprotein, and rheumatoid-associated nuclear antibodies (RANA), against an antigen which is present in high levels in EBV-transformed cell lines. This antibody is also found in SLE and MCTD patients. Antibodies are also detected against granulocyte nuclei (GS-ANA), which may be difficult to distinguish from P-ANCA when testing is done by fluorescence; these are also associated most strongly with Felty's syndrome. Associated Sjögren's syndrome will be accompanied by the presence of antibodies to Ro and/or La.

Antibodies to keratin and pro-filaggrin have been described and it has been suggested that these are more specific for RhA and may correlate with disease activity.

In active disease, both CRP and ESR will be elevated. CRP is the most sensitive marker of activity, due to its wide dynamic range, and is the most useful marker to monitor response to treatment. Other markers of disease activity that have been studied include cytidine deaminase, calprotectin, and serum hyaluronate. None of these are routinely available yet. Monitoring of cytokines is not used routinely. Anaemia of chronic disease is often present and there may be lymphopenia (both CD4+ and CD8+ cells).

Treatment

Proper supportive care (physiotherapy, occupational therapy) is essential. Drug therapy includes NSAIDs, usually with gastric protection, and analgesics as first line. Low-dose corticosteroids are now back in favour to slow the progression of erosive disease. Disease modifying drugs (DMARDs) include gold, penicillamine, methotrexate (low dose weekly) and hydroxychloroquine: these have complex immunomodulating action (Chapter 10). Gold and hydroxychloroquine both interfere with TNF production. Cyclosporin has been used to reduce the activation of CD4+ T cells. Immunotherapies with anti-CD4 monoclonal antibodies (MAbs), anti-CD52 MAbs, anti-TNF, and IL-1 antagonists have all been tried, with varying degrees of success. Problems with all MAb-based therapies have included high levels of reactions to xenogeneic proteins, even if attempts have been made to humanize the antibodies. Severe and persistent T-cell lymphopenia has been induced in some trials, raising concerns over risks of opportunist infections. Surgical replacement of damaged joints may restore function and relieve pain.

280

Childhood rheumatoid arthritis

Childhood-onset seropositive RhA is rare and usually presents with general malaise a polyarthritis of the small joints of the hands and feet. Because of the frequent appearance of RhF following infection, European guidance suggests that three positive tests over a 3-month period are required to confirm the diagnosis, although bearing in mind the half-life of the antibodies this is probably too short an interval. This disease is associated with DR4. Diagnosis and management are as for the adult disease.

An RhF-negative polyarthritis is also seen in children, this may be severe. It is associated with DR5 and DR8.

6 Connective tissue disease

Rheumatoid arthritis
Childhood rheumatoid arthritis

Juvenile chronic arthritis (JCA)

Clinically this is divided into two types: pauci-articular and systemic forms. The latter is usually referred to as Still's disease.

Aetiology and immunopathology

As with many connective tissue diseases (CTDs), this is not well understood. The immunogenetics of pauci-articular disease is complex: DR8 and DR5 show the strongest correlation with pauci-articular disease. Other genes include DPB1 and A2. Rubella virus has been implicated as a possible trigger.

Systemic disease is also associated most strongly with DR5 and DR8, but also with DR4.

Clinical features

The clinical diagnosis of pauci-articular disease is one of exclusions. Usually age of onset is 1–3 years, with a 4:1 female predominance. Systemic features are an exclusion, and the usual features are those of painful or painless swelling of one or two joints. Uveitis may develop and regular screening is required when ANAs are detected.

Still's disease typically has a high spiking fever, accompanied by malaise and rigors. There is usually a pale, salmon-pink rash which comes and goes, usually in parallel with the spikes of fever. Hepatosplenomegaly and generalized lymphadenopathy are usually present. There is polyarthralgia and polyarthritis. Pericarditis and pleurisy are also common. A rare macrophage-activation syndrome has been described, with encephalopathy, hepatitis, disseminated intravascular coagulation (DIC), and haemophagocytosis. Amyloid may be a long-term complication

Immunological tests

Rheumatoid factor is rare (<5 per cent) in pauci-articular disease and, when present, suggests that the course will be that of juvenile RhA with polyarticular disease. Anti-nuclear antibodies are frequently present, and it is important to ensure that the normal range for significance is appropriately adjusted for the paediatric population. In small children, titres of 1/10 and 1/20 are highly significant, whereas such titres would not be considered important in adults. Detection is important as female patients with arthritis and positive ANA, especially if also Ro antibody positive, have a high incidence of uveitis. Antibodies to histones H1 and H3 are also associated with uveitis. Antibodies to retinal S-antigen may also be found (in 30 per cent). Other antibodies detected include anti-histone antibodies (often in those without uveitis). Detection of anti-dsDNA antibodies should lead to consideration of childhood lupus. There is frequently evidence of complement consumption with raised C3d, even when C3 levels are within the normal range. Acute-phase proteins are minimally elevated. High ESR should prompt a search for other causes, including leukaemia and infection.

Tests for diagnosis	Tests for monitoring
CRP/ESR	CRP/ESR
Fbc	Fbc
RhF	ENA [uveitis risk]
ANA	Histone antibodies
ENA	C3/C4
Histone antibodies	C3d
DNA	
C3/C4	
C3d	
Immunoglobulins	

It is important to realize that the development of diagnostically helpful antibodies often *follows* rather than precedes the development of clinical disease. Repeating antibody measurements at 3-monthly intervals is therefore strongly advised if there is strong clinical suspicion of disease.

In Still's disease, there are no specific tests. ESR and CRP are very high, with anaemia, leucocytosis, and thrombocytosis. There is a polyclonal hypergammaglobulinaemia, although the incidence of IgA deficiency is increased. A small proportion of patients may have RhF and a larger proportion may have ANA (37 per cent). Complement activation may be present. IL-6 and TNF-α levels may be elevated.

Treatment

NSAIDs form the mainstay of therapy for pauci-articular disease, notwithstanding the risks of Reye's syndrome. DMARDs may be required for more severe cases. In Still's disease, NSAIDs are used initially, with steroids reserved for failure of response. Methotrexate is the most effective steroid-sparing agent; gold and sulphasalazine are contraindicated Bone marrow and stem cell transplantation are now being tried for severe cases.

283

Adult Still's disease

The clinical features are very similar to those of childhood Still's, but occurring in young adults. There is the typical fever and rash, often accompanied by sore throat. Hepatosplenomegaly and lymphadenopathy are common. Exclusion of lymphoma may be difficult. There are no diagnostic tests other non-specific inflammatory markers. However, ferritin levels may be exceptionally high and disproportionately elevated when compared to other acute phase markers. NSAIDs, corticosteroids, and DMARDS are all required and the disease may run a chronic course.

Ankylosing spondylitis (AS)

The typical clinical features of this disease include spinal pain and restriction in movement, especially in the lumbar and thoracic regions, accompanied by demonstrable sacroiliitis on radiographs. It is much more common in men than women. It may be associated with inflammatory bowel disease. Anterior uveitis, cardiac lesions involving the proximal aorta and aortic valve, pericarditis and conduction block, and an upper-lobe lung fibrosis occur as complications.

By definition this is a RhF-seronegative arthritis and there are no defining antibodies, although there have been reports of antibodies to proteoglycans and heat-shock proteins, although these are not diagnostically valuable. Acute-phase proteins may be normal or elevated. IL-6 is also elevated. Alkaline phosphatase and creatine kinase (CK) may also be elevated. More than 90 per cent of all cases will be HLA-B27 positive, but as this is a common antigen in the Caucasian population (8 per cent), the diagnostic value of testing for HLA-B27 is of limited value. Of B27-positive persons, 5–10 per cent will develop AS, while 20 per cent go on to develop a reactive arthropathy after infection with agents such as salmonella or chlamydia. DR4 is associated with peripheral joint involvement. Amyloid may develop and there is a recognized association with IgA nephropathy.

287

Psoriatic arthropathy

This usually develops in patients with clinical psoriasis, although if skin lesions are not present, the diagnosis may be difficult. The arthritis is frequently asymmetrical and spinal involvement is common, in contrast to RhA which it most resembles. The disease is associated with HLA-B7 and B27, while DR4 is linked with a peripheral arthritis. A gene has also been identified on chromosome 17. Retroviral-like particles have been described in psoriasis and there is a direct association of guttate psoriasis with streptococcal infections. While the major pathological process is overgrowth of keratinocytes, this now seems to be driven primarily by activated CD4+ T cells and the resultant release of cytokines and growth factors.

There are no specific immunological tests for psoriatic arthropathy, but up 10 per cent of patients will be RhF positive (low titre) and may also have low-titre ANA and autoantibodies against skin antigens. There is polyclonal hypergammaglobulinaemia. Acute-phase proteins are elevated. Anaemia is common and may be both due to chronic disease and also due to folate deficiency from increased cell proliferation. Increased cell turnover may also cause hyperuricaemia and gout. The realization of the central role of T lymphocytes in psoriasis has led to a change in the approach to treatment towards immunomodulation. Care must be taken as some NSAIDs and antimalarials may exacerbate psoriasis. However, gold, penicillamine, hydroxychloroquine, methotrexate, sulphasalazine, azathioprine, cyclosporin, PUVA, and retinoids have all been shown to be useful.

289

Reactive arthritis (including Reiter's syndrome)

This group of diseases presents with a pauci-articular large-joint arthritis, accompanied by back pain (sacroiliitis) and non-articular symptoms, such as balanitis, urethritis, cervicitis, keratoderma blennorrhagicum, pericarditis (with a long PR interval and non-specific T-wave changes), and conjunctivitis. These symptoms can be triggered by a variety of urogenital and intestinal infections, including *Shigella*, *Salmonella*, *Campylobacter*, *Yersinia*, *Klebsiella*, *Proteus*, *Escherichia coli*, *Chlamydia*, *Mycoplasma*, and *Ureaplasma*. It is also associated with inflammatory bowel disease. Fifty-five per cent of cases will be HLA-B27+, but mostly these will be patients with spinal involvement.

ESR/CRP will be elevated and there is anaemia and leucocytosis. RhF and ANA will be absent. Atypical P-ANCA may be seen where there is inflammatory bowel disease.

Treatment is with NSAIDs, together with treatment of the underlying infection or bowel disease.

Other bowel diseases that are associated with arthritis include: coeliac disease (check IgA endomysial antibodies), which responds promptly to a gluten-free diet; intestinal bypass surgery/ bacterial overgrowth (cryoglobulins may be present, and there may be cutaneous vasculitic lesions); Whipple's disease due to infection with *Tropheryma whippelii* (malabsorption with migratory arthritis; no specific tests but hypogammaglobulinaemia may occur).

Systemic lupus erythematosus (SLE) and variants

SLE has taken over from syphilis as being the great mimic. Clinical criteria have been defined: 4 out of 11 criteria are sufficient to confirm the diagnosis (within a window of observation, not necessarily); however, many patients clearly have the disease even though they do not fit the criteria. SLE is strongly associated with other autoimmune diseases, through a shared immunogenetic background.

Aetiology and immunopathology

There is a strong genetic background to SLE: the main contributing factors being: complement deficiency (especially C2, C4 deficiency), HLA-A1, B8, DR3, other HLA genes associated with specific features and/or autoantibodies (DQw1, DQw2 with anti-Ro; DR2, anti-Sm; DQw6, 7, 8 with anti-phospholipid), possibly Tcr and immunoglobulin genes, racial background (especially West Indian), and female sex (M:F = 1:10–20). Men with Klinefelter's syndrome are at increased risk. There is a familial link between SLE and chronic granulomatous disease. The precise cause of lupus is unknown, although a mouse model is known to be deficient of mechanisms for controlling lymphocyte apoptosis (*fas*). Drugs may also trigger lupus, although the association for some of these is weak. The likelihood of a drug causing problems is associated with acetylator status (slow acetylator status increasing the risk).

The disease itself is a prototype immune complex disease, with evidence for incorrectly sized immune complexes being formed that are cleared inefficiently, in part due to an acquired reduction in the CR1 receptor on erythrocytes. Many antibodies thought to be non-pathogenic are now known to be able to penetrate viable cells and interfere with an intracellular target enzyme: these include anti-DNA, anti-RNP, and anti-ribosomal P antibodies. This process is trypsin sensitive. Surface DNA-binding proteins and proteins with a similar structure to DNA will also bind anti-DNA antibodies and this may lead to alterations in cell function. There is evidence of complement consumption, the level of which corresponds to disease activity.

Clinical features

There is no typical presentation and the disease may present to any organ specialist (see table). Any age group may be affected, but younger women are most commonly affected. Fatigue, malaise, and weight loss are often marked in the prodrome. Lymphadenopathy and splenomegaly are common. Presentations with skin disease alone are of a more limited disease (which may progress), discoid lupus, and subacute cutaneous lupus. C2-deficient lupus tends to give a very florid disease with marked cutaneous vasculitic symptoms and is invariably anti-Ro positive. Arthritis with recurrent pleurisy is a common presentation. A high index of suspicion is required. Severe difficulties in diagnosis may occur as ANAs may

6 Connective tissue disease

Systemic lupus erythematosus (SLE) and variants

Clinical features	Associated antibodies
Arthritis (non-deforming)	
Serositis (pleurisy, pericarditis, peritonitis)	
Rashes (including photosensitivity); malar rash	Anti-Ro, anti-La
Urticaria	
Alopecia (including scarring), vitiligo	Anti-melanocyte
Mouth ulcers	
Sicca syndrome	Anti-Ro, anti-La
Glomerulonephritis, nephrotic syndrome	
Neurological disease (psychosis, seizures)	Anti-ribosomal P, anti-neuronal
Peripheral neuropathy, mononeuritis	
Transverse myelitis, optic neuritis	
Myasthenia gravis	AChRAb
Haemolytic anaemia	Positive direct Coombs test (DCT)
Thrombocytopenia	Anti-platelet antibodies, anti-phospholipid
Lymphopenia	Lymphocytotoxic antibodies
Venous thrombosis, pulmonary emboli	anti-phospholipid
Recurrent miscarriage	anti-phospholipid
Endocarditis	anti-phospholipid
Livedo reticularis	anti-phospholipid
Raynaud's phenomenon	cryoglobulins [Type II or III]
Shrinking lung	
Hepatitis	anti-smooth muscle, anti-ds-DNA
Mesenteric vasculitis	
Organ-specific endocrine disease	organ-specific antibodies [thyroid etc.]
Neonatal lupus/congenital complete heart block	anti-Ro, anti-La
Drug-induced	anti-histone, anti-ssDNA
Angioedema	anti-C1-inhibitor, anti-C1q

frequently be found in chronic infection, including bacterial endocarditis and particularly infection with enteric organisms.

The disease may be triggered by stress and by UV light (in patients who are photosensitive). The latter not only causes worsening of skin disease but also sets off systemic manifestations. Infection may also trigger flares, but the role of immunization is more controversial.

As the disease often affects young women, pregnancy is a frequent problem. The effect of SLE on pregnancy is unpredictable. Conception is unlikely with severe active disease. Disease may flare or remit during pregnancy, but frequently flares postpartum (due to sudden hormonal changes). As autoantibodies are invariably IgG, they cross the placenta: anti-Ro and possibly anti-La have been associated with congenital complete heart block due to damage to the fetal conducting system, and also with neonatal lupus that disappears as maternal antibody is removed from the circulation. Complete heart block occurs in the children of 1 in 20 women positive for the antibodies, but if there has been a previously affected baby, the risk rises to 1 in 4.

Systemic lupus erythematosus (SLE) and variants *(cont.)*

Immunological testing

Detection of autoantibodies and complement abnormalities form the mainstay of diagnosis. A full diagnostic screen must include ANA, dsDNA, ENA, HEp-2 cells (for proliferating cell nuclear antigen (PCNA)), anti-cardiolipin ± anti-β2GP-I, lupus anticoagulant, organ-specific autoantibodies (thyroid, gastric parietal cells, DCT, others as clinically indicated), C3/C4, C3d or equivalent, serum immunoglobulins and electrophoresis, and cryoglobulins if Raynaud's is present. Antibodies to histones may be useful in suspected drug-induced lupus erythematosus. Other antibodies may be sought, depending on clinical features (see table).

294

The pattern of ANAs detected may give a clue as to other antibodies present (e.g. coarse speckled = anti-RNP), and should always be reported. Homogeneous ANAs are usually associated with antibodies to dsDNA and histones. Multiple specificities may be present in a single patient. A proportion of SLE patients have always been noted to be ANA-negative: these patients are usually anti-Ro positive. Rodent liver, widely used as a substrate for detecting ANA, has low levels of Ro antigen which may be leached out during the test procedure; HEp-2 cells have much higher levels, so the proportion of ANA-negative lupus falls when this substrate is used for screening. HEp-2 cells also allow the detection of PCNA (see Part 2), another SLE-specific antibody. Antibodies to dsDNA should be checked regardless of the ANA result if SLE is suspected.

Additional antibodies detected on ENA screening give further useful information: anti-Sm is a rare antibody which is highly specific for SLE, but is found mostly in West Indians; anti-RNP may be found in SLE, but always with dsDNA (if anti-RNP is the only specificity, then MCTD is more likely; see below). Anti-Ro and anti-La are associated with features of secondary sicca syndrome, as well as with congenital complete heart block, neonatal lupus, and photosensitivity. Ribosomal antibodies will be detected when a multiblock section is used. ANCA may also be found in SLE, although it is difficult to identify these accurately in the presence of high-titre ANA: solid-phase assays with specific antigens (PR3 and MPO) help here. Rheumatoid factors are usually present but contribute little to the diagnostic process.

Complement studies are essential. C4 reductions are common and do not reliably relate to disease activity, as C4 null alleles are common. When disease is quiescent, the following rule of thumb applies: complete C4 deficiency, no detectable C4; one functioning allele, C4 is half the lower limit of normal; two functioning alleles, C4 is at or just below the lower limit of normal; three functioning alleles, C4 is midway into the normal range. C3 levels are reduced in active disease, although because of an acute-phase response with increased synthesis, the level may not drop below the lower end of the normal range. A measure of C3 breakdown is required (C3d). Measuring haemolytic complement as a monitor of disease activity is too crude and not recommended. It is, however, essential when

SLE is thought to be due to a complete deficiency, and this testing should always be followed up with measurement of individual components. Assays of immune complexes are difficult (impossible?) to standardize and add little to the management. Rare patients with angioedema may have antibodies to C1q or C1 inhibitor.

Skin biopsies show typical deposits of IgG and C3/C4 along the dermo-epidermal junction in a 'lumpy-bumpy' distribution. There may also be deposits around cutaneous blood vessels. Both normal and affected skin show similar findings (this is used to form the so-called lupus band test).

For investigation of anti-phospholipid antibodies, see below.

Serum immunoglobulins are normally increased polyclonally; small monoclonal bands on a polyclonal background may be seen on electrophoresis; reduction in C3 may reduce the β-region and there may also be features of nephrotic syndrome visible on electrophoresis (reduced albumin and raised α2-band). IgA deficiency is common in SLE, and rare patients may be pan-hypogamma-globulinaemic (distinct for hypogammaglobulinaemia secondary to aggressive immunotherapy). Cryoglobulins, if present, will be type II or type III.

ESR is raised in active disease but, paradoxically, CRP is either normal or only trivially raised. High CRPs in patients with SLE suggest intercurrent infection (which may be hard to distinguish from a flare).

Fbc should be scanned for evidence of haemolysis (reduced Hb, increased MCV, confirmed by low/absent haptoglobin and positive DCT), thrombocytopenia, and other cytopenias. Regular monitoring of creatinine and electrolytes, liver and thyroid function tests, and urine (casts, red cells, protein) are all essential. Imaging is essential

Tests for diagnosis	Tests for monitoring
Fbc	Fbc
Cr&E	Cr&E
LFTs	LFTs
TFTs	TFTs
Urine [rbcs, casts, protein, creatinine, clearance]	Urine [rbcs, casts, protein, creatinine, clearance]
ANA	dsDNA
dsDNA	C3/C4
ENA	C3d
HEp-2 screen	ESR/CRP
Histone antibodies [drug-induced only]	
Ribosomal antibodies [CNS]	
Organ-specific autoantibodies	
Anti-phospholipid antibodies	
DCT	
C3/C4	
C3d	
Haemolytic complement [CH100/APCH100]	
Immunoglobulins	
Cryoglobulins [Raynaud's]	
ESR/CRP	

to confirm organ-specific problems and MRI is particularly valuable. Renal biopsy may be helpful in view of the wide range of histopathological abnormalities that may be identified.

Monitoring of lupus patients must include regular Fbc, Cr&E, LFTs, TFTs, urine, CRP/ESR, and C3/C4/C3d plus dsDNA. A rising titre of dsDNA often heralds relapse; complement studies and acute-phase markers give an indicator of current activity, although this must always be interpreted in the light of clinical symptoms. There is no value in monitoring ANA titres. Frequency of monitoring is dependent on disease activity and the type of drugs being used (i.e. more frequent when cytotoxics are being used). It is worth rechecking full serology every so often (every 6–12 months), as antibodies may come and go and the disease pattern may evolve or change in parallel. As the half-life of antibodies is about 3 weeks, measurements of autoantibodies are rarely of value more frequently than monthly (unless a patient is being plasmapheresed).

Treatment

Mild disease can usually be managed with NSAIDs, although there are reports that patients with SLE are more prone to develop hepatic abnormalities and aseptic meningitis. Rashes can be treated with topical steroids, and sunblocks are essential in sunny climes. Fatigue, arthralgia, and skin disease respond well to antimalarials: hydroxychloroquine is the safest. Systemic disease usually responds to low-dose steroids (20–30 mg/day); azathioprine can be used as a steroid-sparing agent. More serious organ involvement, e.g. glomerulonephritis, haemolytic anaemia, requires aggressive therapy with pulsed intravenous steroid with intravenous or oral cyclophosphamide. Neurological involvement is difficult to treat and there is no consensus: high-dose steroids can be tried but may be more likely to trigger a steroid psychosis; the role of cytotoxics is uncertain. Plasmapheresis may be an adjunct in severe disease while waiting for a clinical effect from cytotoxics, but should not be used alone because of potential rebound worsening of the disease. Patients on any form of immunosuppressive therapy need to have their humoral and cellular immune status monitored, and preventive measures, such as low-dose co-trimoxazole and antifungals, may be required. IVIg should be used only with care as it may make the immune complex component of the disease worse (contraindicated if there is a high-titre RhF, renal impairment (high dose)). The aim should always be for the lowest dose of treatment compatible with maintaining remission. Chronic steroid therapy should be accompanied by bone protection therapy. Oral contraceptives are not contraindicated, but low-oestrogen or progesterone-only pills should be used. Splenectomy may be required for thrombocytopenia where this is antibody mediated and resistant to immunosuppressive therapy: great care needs to be taken with these patients in view of the increased infective risk.

6 Connective tissue disease
Systemic lupus erythematosus (SLE) and variants
Paediatric SLE

Paediatric SLE

The disease in children is very similar to that in adults. Difficulties arise because the marker antibodies are frequently not present until the child has been ill for some time, making diagnosis difficult. There is often also overlap of symptoms with childhood connective tissue diseases. Before puberty, the male to female ratio is increased compared to that in adults (1:5).

The use of diagnostic tests should be applied just as in adult disease; however, where there is a high suspicion of disease, but no antibodies, tests should be repeated at regular intervals (every 2–3 months), as antibodies may appear later. Remember that significant titres of autoantibodies will be lower in children.

Management follows the same lines as adults, although greater care needs to be taken over the use of steroids, to avoid stunting growth.

Sjögren's syndrome

Sjögren's syndrome may occur as both a primary disorder in its own right, or it may accompany other connective tissue diseases. There is a strong association with other autoimmune diseases, particularly thyroid disease and primary biliary cirrhosis (PBC). The primary pathology is a lymphocytic infiltrate into the exocrine glands, affecting salivary and lacrimal glands, but also glands of the genital and respiratory tracts.

Aetiology and immunopathology

The cause is unknown, although there is some evidence to suggest that viral infections may contribute substantially, including EBV, HCV, and retroviruses. There is an immunogenetic background, shared with other autoimmune diseases, including B8 and DR3. Proto-oncogenes are also expressed and the disease is frequently accompanied by monoclonal expansion of B cells within the glands, accompanied by IgMκ paraprotein production and the development of type II cryoglobulins. The disease may terminate in frank lymphoma.

Clinical features

Clinical features include dry gritty eyes, dry mouth, difficulty swallowing, recurrent parotitis and gingivitis, recurrent chest infections, and dyspareunia. There may be subclinical pancreatitis. Fatigue and malaise are marked and early features. Arthralgia and arthritis are common. Interstitial lung disease may be found on CT scanning. A Fanconi syndrome may occur. Both CNS and peripheral nerve involvement have been reported. Features of other autoimmune diseases will be present. Raynaud's may be present if there is a cryoglobulin. Salivary glands may be enlarged; lymphadenopathy should always be taken seriously if it does not settle once local infection has been dealt with (risk of lymphoma). Secondary Sjögren's appears to be more limited (sicca symptoms).

Clinical diagnosis may be made by Schirmer's test (normal >15 mm wetting in 5 minutes; <5 mm is abnormal); Rose bengal staining of the cornea may demonstrate corneal loss.

Immunological testing

Diagnostic testing should include ANA, dsDNA, ENA, RhF, thyroid and mitochondrial antibodies, C3/C4, serum immunoglobulins and electrophoresis, cryoglobulins, β2-microglobulin, CRP/ESR, and IgG subclasses. If the ANA is negative and primary Sjögren's is suspected, then salivary gland antibodies may be helpful. HEp-2 screening may also pick up other specificities known to be associated, such as antibodies to the Golgi body and the nuclear mitotic apparatus.

RhF will be found in 90 per cent of patients developing arthritis; 70 per cent will be positive for anti-Ro, and 40 per cent for anti-La. ANA will usually show a fine speckled appearance. dsDNA will be negative. Thyroid antibodies are common (30 per cent) and mito-chondrial antibodies will be found in those going onto develop PBC.

Complements will usually be normal or elevated (this is not a complement-consuming disorder); low levels should raise questions about the primary underlying diagnosis.

There is invariably a marked restricted-clonality hypergamma-globulinaemia, often with IgMκ paraproteins on immunofixation. The increase in IgG is restricted to IgG1, with reductions seen in IgG2, IgG3 and IgG4, hence the electrophoretic appearances. Measurement of IgG subclasses is therefore a helpful adjunctive test, as no other conditions give this pattern, other than myeloma. Cryoglobulins should always be sought, particularly if there is any cutaneous involvement. β2-Microglobulin should be monitored as a marker of lymphoproliferation.

ESR and CRP are high, with an anaemia of chronic disease. Raised alkaline phosphatase of liver origin may indicate PBC. Thyroid function must be checked at baseline and regularly thereafter.

Long-term monitoring of patients should be undertaken at the clinical level; regular checks for paraproteins and evidence of lymphoproliferation are essential. Clinical checks should include thyroid and liver, in view of the strong association with Sjögren's syndrome. There is no value in monitoring the autoantibodies.

Tests for diagnosis	Tests for monitoring
Fbc	Fbc
Cr&E	Cr&E
LFTs	LFTs
TFTs	TFTs
Urine (glucose, amino acids – Fanconi)	Urine (glucose, amino acids – Fanconi)
ANA	Immunoglobulins, electrophoresis
dsDNA	β_2MG
ENA	ESR/CRP
HEp-2 screen	
Organ-specific autoantibodies	
C3/C4	
Immunoglobulins & electrophoresis	
β_2MG	
Cryoglobulins [Raynaud's]	
ESR/CRP	

Sjögren's syndrome *(cont.)*

Treatment

Symptomatic treatment with lubricants forms the mainstay of treatment; spectacles help reduce the drying effect of the air. Meticulous attention to oral hygiene reduces the oral infective problems. Hydroxychloroquine is valuable for the arthralgia and fatigue. The role of steroids and cytotoxics is less clear and it has been suggested that these may increase the rate of progression to lymphoma; however, they are necessary if there is extraglandular involvement and/or vasculitis. Long-term follow-up needs to be instituted for early identification of malignancy.

Undifferentiated connective tissue disease

This usually comprises a clinical syndrome which does not fulfil the criteria for any one connective tissue disease, either clinically or serologically. Typical features include Raynaud's, polyarthritis, rash, and myalgia. Such patients need to be treated symptomatically while being followed clinically and serologically (testing as for lupus, see above). Some will resolve spontaneously and others will progress to a more clearly defined disease.

6 Connective tissue disease

Sjögren's syndrome
Undifferentiated connective tissue disease

Mixed connective tissue disease (MCTD)

Whether MCTD is truly a distinct entity has been questioned by some experts, on the basis that it may evolve into SLE or other typical connective tissue disease, or that these diseases may evolve into MCTD. Even if it forms part of the spectrum of SLE, it is distinct enough to be considered separately. It is associated with DR4 and DQ3. Clinical features include: arthralgia (96 per cent), swollen hands (88 per cent), Raynaud's (84 per cent), abnormal oesophageal motility (77 per cent), myositis (72 per cent), and lymphadenopathy (68 per cent). Other clinical features that may occur include serositis, leucopenia, thrombocytopenia, sclerodactyly, pulmonary fibrosis (with reduced gas transfer, 70 per cent), pulmonary hypertension, and aseptic meningitis. Trigeminal neuropathy may occur in 10 per cent. Fatigue and malaise are common in the prodrome. Early reports suggested that nephritis was rare, but this is now known not to be true, with up to 50 per cent of patients suffering this complication.

There is polyclonal hypergammaglobulinaemia, with cryoglobulins; C3/C4 may be reduced and C3d elevated. Autoantibodies show a coarse speckled ANA, absent or low level of anti-dsDNA antibodies, and strongly positive anti-U1 RNP (90–100 per cent of true MCTD patients); the presence of high levels of anti-dsDNA suggests SLE not MCTD. RhF is positive in 40–60 per cent. Antiphospholipid antibodies may be associated with pulmonary hypertension. ESR/CRP are elevated and there is an anaemia of chronic disease; thrombocytopenia may be due to anti-platelet antibodies or the presence of anti-phospholipid antibodies. CK may be elevated from muscle involvement but also in aseptic meningitis and trigeminal neuropathy.

Treatment is with NSAIDs and/or hydroxychloroquine for fatigue, myalgia, and polyarthritis. Steroids plus cytotoxic agents (azathioprine, cyclophosphamide) are used for severe organ involvement; methotrexate is used where there is evidence of erosive joint disease. Anticoagulation is used for the anti-phospholipid antibodies. Raynaud's phenomenon requires treatment with vasodilators, calcium-channel blockers, ACE inhibitors, ketanserin, prostacyclin infusions, fish oil, and topical nitrates.

Mixed connective tissue disease (MCTD)

Tests for diagnosis	Tests for monitoring
Fbc	Fbc
Cr&E	Cr&E
LFTs	LFTs
CK	CK
TFTs	Urine (rbcs, casts, creatinine clearance)
Urine (rbcs, casts, creatinine clearance)	C3/C4
ANA	C3d
dsDNA	Diffusing capacity and lung function
ENA (Ul RNP)	
RhF	
Anti-phospholipid antibodies	
Immunoglobulins	
Cryoglobulins	
C3/C4	
C3d	
ESR/CRP	
Diffusing capacity and lung function	

Polymyositis/dermatomyositis (PM/DM)

Polymyositis and dermatomyositis may be idiopathic (no known accompanying disease) or they may be associated with malignancy. Juvenile forms also exist. Rare forms of myositis include inclusion-body myositis, eosinophilic myositis, granulomatous myositis, and orbital myositis (orbital pseudotumour).

Aetiology and immunopathology

These disease tend to be common in patients of African origin and also in females. Older patients tend to be more affected, but the diseases can occur at any age. In adult patients there is a strong association with underlying malignancy, both carcinoma and, more rarely, lymphoma: the muscle disease often appears at a time when the tumour is still occult and it is debated how intensively one should investigate to identify the tumour. The muscle disease will often remit when the tumour is treated. Seasonal variations have been noted in onset, with anti-Jo-1 disease occurring in the spring and anti-SRP myositis in the autumn, possibly suggesting an association with an infectious agent, as yet unidentified.

T cells are involved, both CD4+ and CD8+ T cells infiltrating affected muscle, and restriction Vβ gene usage suggests that the recruitment is specific to muscle antigens. Muscle fibres express MHC class II antigens and there is an increase in local expression of adhesion molecules (ICAM-1). B cells seem to play little role, and the pathogenicity of the autoantibodies known to occur is uncertain. There is evidence for significant involvement of complement in the muscle-fibre destruction and it has been hypothesized that the role of high-dose IVIg in PM/DM is to interfere with complement activation.

A very wide range of autoantibodies have been identified, although many are not routinely available through diagnostic laboratories. The PM/DM-associated antibodies comprise one of the most complex of any autoimmune disease. The most important subgroup of PM/DM is associated with transfer-RNA synthetases, which accounts for about 30 per cent of cases. The most important antibody is anti-Jo-1. This antibody, together with the rarer antibodies (see table), identifies the anti-synthetase syndrome, characterized by an aggressive myositis, prone to relapse, accompanied by a high incidence of interstitial lung disease, mechanic's hands, Raynaud's syndrome, inflammatory polyarthritis, sclerodactyly, and sicca syndrome. The response of this subgroup to treatment is much poorer, but it is less likely to be associated with malignancy. Anti-Jo-1 antibodies frequently rise before the onset of overt muscle damage, indicating a possible pathogenic role, especially as it is now known that autoantibodies may enter selected viable cells.

Other antibodies, recognizing other nuclear antigens, have been identified: anti-signal recognition particle (SRP) in adult PM (lung disease uncommon); anti-Mi-2 in dermatomyositis; anti-KJ in PM with Raynaud's and lung disease. Polymyositis may occur as part of overlap syndromes, such as MCTD (anti-U1 RNP),

Anti-synthetase syndrome antibodies	Target antigen
Anti-Jo-1 (25%)	histidyl-t-RNA synthetase
Anti-PL-7 (rare)	threonyl-t-RNA synthetase
Anti-PL12 (rare)	alanyl-t-RNA synthetase
Anti-OJ (rare)	isoleucyl-t-RNA synthetase
Anti-EJ (rare)	glycyl-t-RNA synthetase

polymyositis–scleroderma overlap (anti-PM–Scl), SLE–myositis overlap (anti-Ku).

Clinical features

The major clinical feature is proximal muscle weakness with pain. Onset may be acute with fever. Distal muscle involvement is rare, and should raise other diagnostic possibilities (infection (viral, bacterial, parasitic), inclusion-body myositis and metabolic problems). Gottren's papules are often seen on the knuckles, and the typical heliotrope rash around the eyes and a generalized erythematous rash (may be photosensitive) mark out DM. There may be signs of inflammatory arthritis and scleroderma; mechanic's hands (thickened, cracked skin) identify the anti-synthetase syndrome. There may be dyspnoea from lung involvement; with accompanying pain pulmonary embolus may be suspected. Although the heart is rarely involved, presentations with atypical chest pain may be diagnostically difficult due to raised CK, unless the CK-MB fraction is rapidly available. Diaphragmatic involvement typically leads to dyspnoea when lying flat. Gastrointestinal disease may occur (slowed transit, reflux). Renal disease is rare, but high serum myoglobin levels may trigger renal impairment if there is very active myositis.

Investigation

As well as immunological investigations, muscle biopsy and electromyogram (EMG) should be considered. MRI is excellent at identifying affected muscles non-invasively. Biopsy may not be necessary in a typical presentation associated with typical autoantibodies. Lung function, including gas transfer, mouth pressures, and CT of lungs are essential. As the disease may be patchy within a muscle, a normal biopsy does not categorically exclude disease. Anti-Jo-1 recognizes primarily a cytoplasmic antigen: this will not be recognized on rodent liver. If PM/DM are suspected, then screening on HEp-2 cells is most revealing as many of the cytoplasmic and nuclear antigens associated with myositis can be identified from the patterns of staining; antibodies to Jo-1 should be specifically requested. Nucleolar ANA may also be seen, although these may also be found in patients with scleroderma. Antibodies to PM–Scl and other synthetases may be available from certain specialist centres.

Polymyositis/dermatomyositis (PM/DM)
(cont.)

Management

Management is with high-dose steroids. Failure to control disease with acceptable levels of steroids is an indication for second-line therapy: weekly methotrexate (where there is no lung disease), azathioprine or cyclophosphamide, or possibly cyclosporin. Both steroids and cyclophosphamide can be given as intravenous pulse therapy, particularly if there is progressive lung disease. Intolerance of, contraindications to, or failure of first- and second-line agents should lead to consideration of the use of high-dose IVIg. Patients with malignancy-associated PM/DM respond poorly to immuno-suppressive therapy, as do those with the anti-synthetase syndrome.

Polymyositis/dermatomyositis (PM/DM)

Tests for diagnosis	Tests for monitoring
Fbc	Fbc
Cr & E	Cr & E
Urinalysis	CK
CK	CRP/ESR
Serum myoglobin	Lung function
HEp-2 screen	
Anti-Jo-1	
Anti-PM–Scl	
Anti-RNP	
CRP/ESR	
Lung function	

Overlap syndromes

Patients often exhibit features of more than one connective tissue disease. Moreover, clinical features may change over a period of time, and this may be accompanied by changes in the serological profile. It is therefore wise not to be too dogmatic in pigeon-holing patients.

Recognized overlap syndromes include the following:

- Mixed connective tissue disease: see above. Marker antibody profile is anti-U1 RNP in the absence of anti-dsDNA.
- 'Rhupus': a form of lupus with more aggressive destructive arthritis more typical of rheumatoid arthritis, but with other typical lupus features. There are no specific serological markers, as many patients with SLE have rheumatoid factors anyway, without developing overt features of RhA. Whether this is a true overlap syndrome is debatable.
- Polymyositis–scleroderma overlap: features of polymyositis and scleroderma, although the myositis may be mild. Serologically defined by detection of anti-PM–Scl.
- SLE–myositis overlap: features of SLE with prominent myositis. Serologically defined by detection of anti-Ku.

309

Systemic sclerosis: CREST and limited variants

There are many variants of scleroderma, including localized and systemic forms. There is also considerable overlap with other connective tissue diseases (SLE, MCTD, PM/DM). The pathological process is very similar to that of chronic graft-versus-host disease. The CREST syndrome (calcinosis, Raynaud's, oesophageal dysmotility, sclerodactyly, and telangiectasia) forms an entirely clinically and serologically distinct subgroup.

Aetiology and immunopathogenesis

There is a female preponderance (M:F = 1:4). Childhood onset is rare. A wide range of MHC antigens have been associated with scleroderma variants, including DR1, DR3, DRw52, DR5, although there is significant racial variation. There is a strong association of scleroderma-like conditions with environmental factors (dust exposures, organic solvents such as vinyl chloride, resins, toxic oil drugs such as cocaine, bleomycin, fenfluramine). The contribution of silicone breast implants to scleroderma is uncertain. The precise immunological involvement is unclear, but targets include endothelial cells and fibroblasts, with cytokine production leading to increased collagen synthesis. There are obvious vascular changes such as vasomotor instability (Raynaud's) but also direct damage to blood vessels, such as can be seen in nailfold capillaries. Unlike other connective tissue diseases, there is very little in the way of a systemic inflammatory response, and CRP/ESR may be low or normal.

A variety of autoantibodies have been identified, although the significance of some of them has not been fully elucidated (see Part 2). Anti-centromere antibodies and anti-Scl-70 antibodies are mutually exclusive: only two cases of the presence of both antibodies together have ever been reported.

Clinical

Localized forms include linear morphoea ('coup de sabre') and limited scleroderma where the changes are limited to the extremities, without systemic manifestations. Raynaud's phenomenon is severe. The CREST syndrome has a more generalized involvement and may give rise to late pulmonary hypertension, but less often to renal involvement. Systemic sclerosis, on the other hand, leads to major renal and lung involvement. Involvement of the kidney may lead to rapid onset of severe hypertension and renal failure, due to obliteration of the glomeruli (scleroderma kidney). Lung disease includes interstitial fibrosis, an increased risk of carcinoma, bronchiectasis, and pulmonary hypertension. Gastrointestinal involvement leads to severe oesophageal reflux, malabsorption due to poor small bowel motility, and bacterial overgrowth; secondary problems may arise from a deficiency of key vitamins and minerals. Poor colonic motility may lead to pseudo-obstruction. There is an association with thyroid disease, primary biliary cirrhosis, and rare

Nuclear antigens targeted	Nucleolar antigens targeted
Centromere (CENP-A, CENP-B, CENP-C) 80% CREST patients	RNA polymerases I, II, III: 23% systemic disease (speckled nucleolar)
Scl-70 (topisomerase I): 30% systemic, 10% limited	Fibrillarin (clumpy)
	PM–Scl: scleroderma–myositis overlap (homogeneous)
	To: rare, limited scleroderma (homogeneous)

neurological involvement (neuropathy). The vascular disturbance may lead to ischaemia of the ends of digits which, if not treated rapidly, will lead to dry gangrene and progressive reabsorption of the terminal phalanges. Systemic forms are often accompanied by a prodrome of malaise and fatigue. Rarely, there may be renal and lung involvement without cutaneous involvement.

Immunological testing

Screening for anti-nuclear antibodies may reveal the presence of nucleolar staining patterns, or speckled patterns due to the presence of anti-centromere antibodies. HEp-2 cells give the best differentiation of the staining patterns and these should be followed up by specific tests for Scl-70. Assays for individual nucleolar antigens are not routinely available. No immunological tests are useful for monitoring. In the CREST syndrome there may also be antibodies to the M2 antigen (25 per cent); 30 per cent will be positive for rheumatoid factor. ESR/CRP will be low. All patients should be screened for thyroid disease. All patients with Raynaud's should also be checked for cryoglobulins. Baseline lung function, including gas transfer, chest radiograph ± CT scanning should be carried out for all systemic forms. Likewise, renal function needs to be assessed. Both organs should then be monitored regularly.

Management

Many drugs have been tried in scleroderma but few have stood the test of proper double-blind, placebo-controlled trials. Penicillamine and colchicine have been used, with some evidence that they slow progression. Steroids only help with active inflammatory problems such as myositis or arthritis. Cytotoxics such as azathioprine and cyclophosphamide may have some benefit. Cyclosporin may be of benefit (but watch renal function!). Raynaud's may be difficult to control. Avoidance of cold, wearing warm clothing and heated gloves may help. Other treatments to be tried include high-dose fish oil or evening primrose oil, slow-release or long-acting calcium-channel blockers (nicardipine, felodipine, amlodipine, nimodipine), ACE inhibitors, topical GTN (glyceryl trinitrate) ointment or 5-HT antagonist (ketanserin, not a licensed drug). Acute ischaemia should

Systemic sclerosis: CREST and limited variants *(cont.)*

be treated with prostacyclin infusion: although the half-life is only seconds, the clinical effect may last for months (reasons unknown). Infection in sclerodermatous skin needs aggressive treatment, often with intravenous antibiotics. Malabsorption should be sought and treated. Omeprazole, low dose erythromycin, or cisapride may help with reflux and improve motility. Octreotide may also help (unlicensed indication). Continuous oxytetracycline may reduce bacterial overgrowth.

Tests for diagnosis	Tests for monitoring
Fbc	Fbc
Cr&E	Cr&E
Creatinine clearance/isotopic clearance	Creatinine clearance/isotopic clearance
Tests for malabsorption	Tests for malabsorption
Thyroid function	Thyroid function
Liver function	Liver function
Lung function (gas transfer)	Lung function (gas transfer)
Chest imaging (X-ray, CT)	Chest imaging (X-ray, CT)
Anti-nuclear antibodies	
HEp-2 screen	
Anti-Scl-70	
Mitochondrial antibodies	
Cryoglobulins	
CRP/ESR	

Anti-phospholipid syndromes

This set of syndromes (now sometimes referred to as Hughes' syndrome) is associated with antibodies against a range of biologically relevant phospholipids.

Aetiology and immunopathology

Both sexes may be affected, although it appears to be more common in females. MHC association has been reported (DR4, DR7, among others). Why the antibodies arise is not known, although non-pathogenic antibodies may be induced by infection.

The antibodies appear to recognize a variety of different phospholipids, but pathogenic antibodies seem to require the presence of a co-factor, β2-glycoprotein-I (apolipoprotein H). Antiphospholipid antibodies may also arise secondary to infection (such as syphilis, EBV infection) but these antibodies do not require the presence of β2-glycoprotein-I, and do not seem to cause a clotting disorder.

The spectrum of antibodies include both anti-cardiolipin antibodies and lupus anticoagulants. Either may be found in the absence of the other, but the clinical significance is identical. The activity of the antibodies *in vivo* is complex, but includes activation of platelets, interference with endothelial cell function (reduced prostacyclin production, reduced thrombomodulin function), complement activation, and reduced levels of proteins C and S, leading to a pro-coagulant effect.

Clinical

Anti-phospholipid antibodies can occur either as an isolated finding or in association with other connective tissue disease, usually SLE. Major clinical features are arterial and venous thromboses, with pulmonary emboli, recurrent miscarriage, and thrombocytopenia. As the arterial system can be affected; strokes in young people should always be investigated. Recurrent minor cerebrovascular occlusions may lead to a multi-infarct dementia. Other clinical syndromes associated include the Budd–Chiari syndrome, chorea, transverse myelitis, pulmonary hypertension (recurrent asymptomatic PEs), and cardiac valve lesions. Livedo reticularis is a useful cutaneous marker, and may be associated with Sneddon's syndrome (hypertension, cerebrovascular disease, and livedo).

Immunological tests

Clinical suspicion should lead to testing for IgG and IgM anti-cardiolipin antibodies (ACAs) and clotting studies, which should include APTT (prolonged) and a dilute Russell's viper venom test (dRVVT; prolonged). Fbc should be scanned for thrombocytopenia. The significance of IgM anti-cardiolipin antibodies alone is uncertain, but if associated with clinical features of recurrent thrombosis should be treated seriously. IgA ACAs have been described: the significance is unknown. A false-positive VDRL test may be noted but this is not diagnostically helpful. Assays for β2-glycoprotein-are available and may help to distinguish between antibodies of no significance triggered by infection and those of pathogenic significance. At present it is not clear that they are necessary for routine management. There is no correlation between the numerical value of ACAs detected by ELISA and the severity of symptoms, although there has been a suggestion that levels may correlate with neurological disease in SLE. To determine whether there is a primary or secondary anti-phospholipid syndrome, a full search should be done for other markers of connective tissue diseases. There is no indication that routine monitoring of levels is helpful.

Tests for diagnosis	Tests for monitoring
Fbc	Fbc
IgG and IgM ACA	
APTT	INR (if on warfarin)
dRVVT	
Anti-β_2-glycoprotein-1	
ANA	
dsDNA	
ENA	
C3/C4	
Other clotting studies (thrombophilia screen)	
exclude homocysteinuria	

Management

Asymptomatic patients require no treatment, or just low-dose aspirin. Symptomatic patients should be warfarinized for life with an INR of 3–4; if thrombotic events continue, low-dose aspirin should be added. The role of steroids ± cytotoxics is controversial, but may be tried where there are continuing catastrophic thrombotic events: do not expect there to be much change in antibody levels. Plasmapheresis may be tried, but beware of rebound rises in antibody. For management of pregnancy, no treatment or low-dose aspirin is recommended for those with either no history or a history only of first-trimester loss. Where there is a history of second/third-trimester loss the treatment is low-dose aspirin ± subcutaneous heparin. If there is a previous history of thrombosis, then low-dose aspirin and heparin are suggested, even for first pregnancies. Intravenous immunoglobulin may also be valuable Thrombocytopenia is rarely severe, but if it is, high-dose IVIg and steroids may help. Splenectomy may increase the thrombotic tendency if the platelet count rebound is very high, and so needs to be considered carefully. Danazol may also be of benefit.

7 Vasculitic syndromes

Causes of vasculitis

The term vasculitis implies inflammation affecting predominantly the blood vessels. The effects of the process depend on the location of the inflammatory change and the size and type of the vessel involved. It is unclear why there is selectivity for vessels of a certain type, size, or location. Although at present vasculitis is divided into primary and secondary, it is likely that, with the passage of time, we shall identify environmental triggers for most the so-called 'primary vasculitides'.

Primary

Many classifications have been proposed for primary vasculitis, but the most satisfactory is that based on the size of the vessel involved and on the presence or absence of granulomata. However, there is considerable overlap in the size of vessels involved.

Secondary

318

There are many causes of secondary vasculitis and the following is not an exhaustive list:
- infections: bacterial (streptococci), spirochetes (syphilis, Borrelia), fungal, mycobacterial, rickettsial, viral (VZV, CMV, hepatitis A, B, and C, influenza), with and without cryoglobulins;
- malignancy: hairy-cell leukaemia, lymphoma, acute myeloid leukaemia, with and without cryofibrinogens;
- drugs: biologicals (serum sickness), oral contraceptive, sulphonamides, penicillins, thiazides, aspirin, illicit drugs (cocaine, amphetamines, LSD);
- secondary to other autoimmune diseases: primary biliary cirrhosis, Goodpasture's syndrome, SLE, RhA, systemic sclerosis, Sjögren's syndrome, polymyositis/dermatomyositis, hypocomplementaemic urticaria, relapsing polychondritis;
- secondary to inflammatory bowel disease: ulcerative colitis, Crohn's disease;
- mimics of vasculitis: cholesterol embolus, myxoma embolus, ergotism.

	Small artery	Medium artery	Large artery	Veins
No granuloma	Buerger's disease	Buerger's disease	Takayasu's disease	Buerger's disease
	Henoch–Schonlein purpura	Kawasaki syndrome		Behçet's disease
	Microscopic polyarteritis	Polyarteritis nodosa		
	Primary angiitis of the CNS	Churg–Strauss syndrome		
	Behçet's disease	Cogan's syndrome		
	Hypergammaglobulinaemic purpura of Waldenström			
With granuloma		Wegener's granulomatosis	Takayasu's disease	
		Lymphomatoid granulomatosis	Giant cell arteritis	

Diagnostic tests

The most important diagnostic test is often biopsy of the affected organ, which is particularly convenient if the skin is involved. Some vasculitides may mimic neoplasia, e.g. Wegener's and lymphomatoid granulomatosis, and may therefore be difficult to distinguish on imaging. Imaging is an essential source of diagnostic information in cranial vasculitis (MRI is better than CT), unless invasive biopsy is considered justified. Angiography is particularly helpful in identifying large and medium-vessel disease. Where there is suspected involvement of the coronary arteries, ECG, echocardiography, and coronary angiography will be required.

Immunoglobulin measurements contribute very little to diagnosis, being on the whole non-specific. Electrophoresis is necessary to identify paraproteins but it is important to consider the possibility of cryoglobulinaemia and cryofibrinogenaemia. Complement measurements (including complement breakdown products or other tests of complement turnover) are essential, particularly in secondary vasculitis. Autoantibody testing should include antinuclear, ENA, dsDNA, and ANCA. The role of anti-endothelial cell antibodies (AECA) is not determined as these antibodies do not seem to be disease specific. The acute-phase response is mostly high (except in the case of SLE (although the ESR is high) and scleroderma). In some vasculitides the caeruloplasmin is significantly elevated: this accounts for the greenish colour of the serum from patients with active vasculitis. Regular monitoring of the acute-phase response provides useful information on the response of the disease to treatment.

The full blood count will often show the anaemia of chronic disease, together with a thrombocytosis. There is often a lymphopenia.

321

SMALL-VESSEL PRIMARY DISEASE

Henoch–Schönlein purpura (HSP)

HSP is mainly disease of small children, with a peak age of onset around 3 years, although it can occur at any age and does occur in adults, in whom it is possibly more chronic. There is a male predominance. There is often a history of a preceding upper respiratory tract infection. The typical clinical feature is palpable purpura especially at sites of pressure (socks). These occur in crops, often with an urticarial component, and may become confluent. There is gastrointestinal involvement, often with GI haemorrhage and associated with colic, vomiting, and intussusception (3 per cent). Renal disease with nephritis occurs in 50 per cent, although in most cases this recovers spontaneously and does not lead to long-term renal damage. It may recur in transplanted kidneys in the small proportion who do have progressive renal damage (4–14 per cent). Testicular involvement, pulmonary haemorrhage, pancreatitis, and CNS involvement are all very rare complications. There is fever in 45–75 per cent and often a migratory arthralgia. Attacks may recur every few weeks to months and are thought to be triggered by β-haemolytic streptococci.

Immunology

IgA-containing immune complexes can be detected in affected tissues, including glomeruli. These involve both IgA1 and IgA2 but contain mostly polymeric IgA. IgA rheumatoid factors are also detectable and the levels are highest in the acute phase of the disease. Total IgA may be increased polyclonally; complement C3 and C4 are normal but C3d is increased, indicating an increase in complement turnover. Properdin levels are decreased while C1q levels are normal, suggesting alternate pathway activation. Properdin and C3 deposits can be detected in affected kidneys. In practice, only complement C3, C4, and total immunoglobulins will be measured, as the diagnosis is usually made clinically. Assays for IgA immune complexes and IgA rheumatoid factors are not routinely available. Acutely, the CRP will be elevated.

Treatment

Treatment is most often not required as HSP is a self-limiting disease; aspirin should be avoided as it will exacerbate the bowel bleeding. Steroids reduce symptoms but do not shorten the illness. Factor XIII, which is required for healing of the bowel wall, has been used experimentally by infusion to reduce GI haemorrhage. There is no conclusive evidence to support the use of plasmapheresis or cytotoxics, although the latter would be used if there was major glomerular involvement with significant proteinuria.

Tests for diagnosis	Tests for monitoring
Urinalysis	Urinalysis
Fbc	Fbc
Cr&E	Cr&E
CRP/ESR	CRP/ESR
C3, C4, C3d	C3, C4, C3d
Serum immunoglobulins and electrophoresis	
(Renal or skin biopsy)	

IgA nephropathy

IgA nephropathy (Berger's disease) is probably closely related to HSP, and may be HSP with renal disease but no rash. Again there is a male preponderance and often a history of a preceding upper respiratory tract infection. Unlike HSP, it may be familial. There may be bowel involvement and arthralgia. It is also associated with IgA immune complexes and IgA RhF. *Haemophilus parainfluenzae* membrane antigens have been detected in the kidney and it is thought that this may be the candidate triggering antigen. There is usually progressive disease, with a persistent polyclonal elevation of IgA.

Buerger's disease (thromboangiitis obliterans)

This disease affects predominantly small and medium-sized arteries and veins. It occurs mainly in male smokers above 30 years of age (less than 5 per cent of patients are non-smokers). It presents as a migratory thrombophlebitis with claudication in the lower limbs, and less commonly in the upper limbs; Raynaud's phenomenon is common. Ischaemic features will arise with peripheral gangrene. Systemic features are usually absent and there is no acute-phase response. The histology shows infiltration of blood vessels by neutrophils early, then mononuclear cells later. Eventually fibrosis of the vessel supervenes. Active inflammatory lesions improve when smoking ceases, suggesting a direct toxic effect, although fibrotic lesions will not improve. Diagnosis is on the history backed up by angiography. The most important therapeutic intervention is cessation of smoking. Aspirin, vasodilators, and anticoagulants are of no proven value, although infusions of prostacyclin may help. Amputations may be required.

Hypersensitivity ('allergic') vasculitis

This is a generic term for small-vessel cutaneous vasculitis, which is less used now. It is not a discrete disease and may be caused by drugs, infections, SLE/SS, cryoglobulins, inflammatory bowel disease, HSP. The typical features include purpura, urticaria, ulceration, bullae, and systemic features (fever, arthralgia, myalgia).

7 Vasculitic syndromes

IgA nephropathy
Buerger's disease (thromboangiitis obliterans)
Hypersensitivity ('allergic') vasculitis

Microscopic polyarteritis

MPA is an aggressive small-vessel vasculitis, which is distinct from polyarteritis nodosa. It may occur in families, suggesting either a transmissible agent or a genetic background. The illness is often of relatively sudden onset with a short prodrome of fever, malaise, and myalgia/arthralgia, followed by onset of glomerulonephritis with hypertension and renal insufficiency. There may be pulmonary haemorrhage mimicking Goodpasture's syndrome: this has a high (75 per cent) mortality. Extrarenal complications include weight loss, episcleritis, and rarely coronary artery involvement. Renal biopsies show a necrotizing glomerulonephritis without evidence of granulomata. The renal lesions are similar to those found in Wegener's granulomatosis. Angiography of the mesenteric vessels does not show microaneurysms, thus distinguishing MPA from polyarteritis nodosa (PAN). P-ANCA, with anti-myeloperoxidase specificity on ELISA, can be detected in the serum of 45 per cent of patients and 45 per cent have C-ANCA with proteinase 3 specificity. The treatment is with high-dose (usually pulsed intravenous) steroids and cyclophosphamide. There may be an acute role for plasmapheresis in preserving renal function.

Tests for diagnosis	Tests for monitoring
Urinalysis	Urinalysis
Creatinine clearance (or isotopic equivalent)	Creatinine clearance (or isotopic equivalent)
Fbc	Fbc
Cr&E	Cr&E
C3, C4, C3d	C3, C4, C3d
ANCA (anti-Pr3 and anti-MPO)	ANCA (anti-Pr3 and anti-MPO)
Anti-GBM	Anti-GBM
ANA [dsDNA]	
Renal biopsy	

Primary angiitis of the CNS (PACNS)

Primary cerebral vasculitis is very difficult to diagnose antemortem without recourse to biopsy which, of course, has significant hazards. The disease is a rare one, primarily of small arteries of the cortex and meninges, and presents in older patients with headache, disturbance of higher mental function, and strokes. A more benign variant has also been described. Systemic symptoms are absent (if they are present then it is likely that there is a systemic vasculitis with cerebral involvement). Histology show that most cases have a granulomatous infiltrate around the blood vessels. CSF may be normal or show elevated protein and cell count. MRI scanning and angiography may be required to establish the extent of the disease. No specific immunological tests are helpful. Similar features have been found following the use of cocaine, amphetamines, and phenylpropanolamine, in ergotism and with phaeochromocytomas, suggesting a vasospastic origin. An association with viral (herpesviruses) and mycoplasma infections has also been postulated: turkeys infected with *Mycoplasma gallisepticum* develop a very similar illness. Treatment is with steroids and cyclophosphamide, as for Wegener's granulomatosis. The use of cerebral vasodilators (nimodipine, nicardipine) has also been advocated to relieve vasospasm.

Behçet's disease

This disease is characterized by recurrent orogenital ulceration, similar to aphthous ulceration but deeper and which may heal with scarring. Eye disease is often present, including anterior and posterior uveitis, retinal vasculitis, and optic atrophy. Vascular features include thrombophlebitis, deep vein thrombosis (DVT), and arteritis. There is arthralgia/arthritis which is often asymmetric and typically affects large joints, especially the knees. CNS disease is due to vasculitis and typically causes pontine lesions. Other CNS complications include pseudotumour cerebri, myelitis, meningitis, and organic brain syndromes. CNS disease is rare but a poor prognostic marker. Pulmonary haemorrhage (with diffuse infiltrates), nephritis (rare), and amyloid may all occur. Venous thrombosis may lead to a Budd–Chiari syndrome and vena caval obstruction. The histology shows transmural vascular inflammation with arterial and venous involvement.

The disease is common in eastern Mediterranean countries where there is a strong association with HLA-B5 (B51) and also an increase in DR2, DR7, and DR52. However, sporadic cases occur and these do not have the same MHC associations. The cause of the disease is unknown. Immunological features include an excessive response of polymorphs to fMLP, IgA antibodies to the 65 kDa heat-shock protein of bacteria, and detectable anti-endothelial cell antibodies (these are non-specific).

Immunology

There are no routine diagnostic markers. There is a significant acute-phase response, complement C9 is often increased, and there are high circulating levels of von Willebrand factor (vWF). Anti-cardiolipin antibodies may be raised in some cases. Twenty-five per cent of patients may have cryoglobulins, and immunoglobulins are polyclonally increased. The MHC-associated cases, but less often sporadic cases, show the phenomenon of pathergy, the development of sterile skin pustules at the site of minor trauma (e.g. venepuncture sites).

Treatment

Treatment is difficult and is mainly aimed at symptom control. The arthritis is usually treated with NSAIDs, while the ulceration may be helped with colchicine or thalidomide; the latter drug should not be used in women of child-bearing age without discussion of the teratogenic risks, and it is advisable to obtain a detailed consent, together with baseline nerve conduction studies, before embarking on therapy. Corticosteroids have a beneficial short-term effect, but there is little evidence for long-term benefit. Systemic vasculitis may warrant the use of cyclophosphamide, azathioprine, chlorambucil, or low-dose weekly oral methotrexate, although the evidence for benefit is small. Eye and CNS involvement carry a poor prognosis and cyclosporin A or tacrolimus (FK506) have been shown to be of significant benefit, although the disease usually relapses when

Tests for diagnosis	Tests for monitoring
Fbc	Fbc
Cr & E	Cr & E
ESR/CRP	ESR/CRP
Anti-cardiolipin antibodies	[cyclosporin A levels]
Lupus anticoagulant [dRVVT]	
Exclusion antibodies [ANCA, ANA]	

the drugs are withdrawn. Unfortunately few controlled trials of therapy have been undertaken. Other drugs that have been used include dapsone and clofazimine. Anticoagulants need to be used with care and are probably contraindicated if there is retinal disease.

331

MEDIUM-SIZED BLOOD VESSELS

Polyarteritis nodosa (PAN)

The main clinical features of PAN include fever, weight loss, painful nodular skin lesions (which need to be distinguished from erythema nodosum), hypertension (often with a tachycardia), abdominal pain (cholecystitis may be a feature), myalgia, arthralgia, mononeuritis multiplex, peripheral neuropathy, and orchitis. There is a very strong association with hepatitis B infection, and a very high incidence in areas where HBV is endemic. About 20 per cent of cases are associated with HBV, although this figure is higher in endemic areas. Recent data suggest that the incidence is declining with the increasing use of HBV vaccines. It has also been associated with tuberculosis and HIV infections. There is a very strong link with hairy-cell leukaemia, and a PAN-like vasculitis may be the first feature of the leukaemic process. It is not an uncommon disease, with a prevalence of 63 per million.

The major diagnostic features are the presence of micro-aneurysms on mesenteric and renal angiography and the absence of ANCA. The latter is a relatively new definition as older studies claimed that ANCA was present in a proportion of cases of PAN. The inflammatory change is limited to medium-sized arteries and there is no evidence of small-artery involvement, which if present would indicate a diagnosis of MPA. There is a profound acute-phase response and usually a leucocytosis. Poor prognosis is indicated by proteinuria above 3 g/24 hours, renal insufficiency, pancreatitis, and cardiomyopathy.

Treatment is with corticosteroids and cytotoxics, either cyclophosphamide or azathioprine. It has been suggested that vidarabine, an antiviral agent, be used for HBV-associated disease in conjunction with plasmapheresis to reduce the antigenic load: this is still experimental.

Churg–Strauss (CSS) variant

CSS is thought to be a subset of PAN in atopic individuals. There is usually an allergic prodrome which lasts several years, typically causing asthma. It has also been recorded in asthmatics treated with leukotriene-antagonists although this may be due to steroid withdrawal in undiagnosed CSS patients. The onset of the vasculitis is heralded by fever, malaise, and weight loss. Mononeuritis multiplex is common (up to 80 per cent) and there may be other systemic features, such as GI involvement with bleeding, inflammatory bowel-like symptoms, cholecystitis, cardiac involvement with an eosinophilic myocardial fibrosis or pericarditis, and cutaneous vasculitic lesions. The sinuses and upper airways are often involved. The coincidence of upper and lower airway disease suggests that an inhaled antigen is the trigger, although none has been identified so far. The histology shows that small–medium arteries are involved and there is intimal inflammation with eosinophilic infiltrate.

Tests for diagnosis	Tests for monitoring
Urinalysis	Urinalysis
Creatinine clearance (or isotopic equivalent)	Creatinine clearance (or isotopic equivalent)
Fbc	Fbc
Absolute eosinophil count	Absolute eosinophil count
Cr&E	Cr&E
ESR/CRP	ESR/CRP
ANCA (anti-Pr3 and anti-MPO)	ANCA (anti-Pr3 and anti-MPO)
IgE	Eosinophil cationic protein
Eosinophil cationic protein	
Exclusion antibodies (ANA, dsDNA)	
Renal or nerve biopsy	

The diagnosis is mainly one of clinical suspicion, backed up by biopsies. The chest radiograph may show infiltrates. There is a marked peripheral blood eosinophilia ($>1.5 \times 10^9$/litre), and levels of eosinophil cationic protein (ECP) are raised in active disease. This protein is known to be neurotoxic and therefore may account for some of the neurological sequelae. Measurement of ECP may be helpful in monitoring the disease, although it is not a specific marker for CSS. The IgE is also often raised, although this is less helpful as a diagnostic or monitoring tool. There is a significant acute-phase response. It has been suggested that autoantibodies to eosinophil peroxidase may be present, which may give an atypical fluorescent staining pattern on neutrophil cytospins. The diagnostic value of this remains to be evaluated. Otherwise 60 per cent have anti-myeloperoxidase antibodies (P-ANCA) and 10 per cent anti-proteinase 3 antibodies (C-ANCA).

Treatment is with steroids and cytotoxics, usually cyclophosphamide, as for other types of vasculitis.

Cogan's syndrome

This is a rare syndrome of deafness and keratitis, accompanied in up to 72 per cent of cases by a systemic necrotizing vasculitis indistinguishable from PAN, and affecting particularly large blood vessels, especially the aorta and coronary vessels The vasculitis may be florid. Although the trigger is not known, the syndrome has been linked to infections, including *Chlamydia* and *Borrelia*. There are no specific diagnostic tests, but paraproteins may be detected in the serum. It is usually treated as for Wegener's granulomatosis, with high-dose steroids and cyclophosphamide; cyclosporin A has also been used.

Kawasaki syndrome (mucocutaneous lymph node syndrome)

Kawasaki syndrome was first described in Japan, although it is now known to occur throughout the world. It is sometimes also referred to as infantile PAN. It is characterized by a high spiking fever for more than 5 days, accompanied by bilateral conjunctivitis, mucosal damage (lips, tongue), a rash on the hands and feet with desquamation, a diffuse macular exanthem, and cervical lymphadenopathy. Other infectious causes must have been excluded. The feared complication is the development of coronary artery aneurysms, which have a mortality of 1–2 per cent (higher if not recognized). Aneurysms may also occur elsewhere. The histological features of the vascular lesions are identical to those of PAN. The aetiology is obscure but the clustering of cases strongly suggests an infectious agent and there have been reports of an association with Parvovirus B19. It has also been suggested, on the basis of T-cell receptor gene usage, that the disease may be due to superantigenic stimulation, possibly due to staphylococcal or streptococcal superantigenic toxins.

Investigations

There is currently no specific diagnostic test. Both ANCA and AECA are detectable but these may also be found in other febrile childhood illnesses. High levels of circulating soluble TNF receptor have been noted, but this is not a routinely available test. There is often a thrombocytosis and a significant acute-phase response. Echocardiography and occasional angiography are required to evaluate the coronary arteries for evidence of aneurysms.

Treatment

The treatment of choice, shown now in several large studies, is high-dose IVIg (1 g/kg/day for 2 days) together with aspirin (80–100 mg/kg/day for 14 days with monitoring of blood levels), which should be begun immediately the diagnosis is suspected. This regime prevents the development of coronary artery aneurysms if begun early, but has no effect once they are established. If aneurysms are documented, then low-dose aspirin ± anticoagulants should be continued. Although, mostly, the disease does not recur, it has been suggested (although not proven) that treatment with IVIg increases the risk of recurrence (about 3 per cent get recurrent disease).

Kawasaki syndrome (mucocutaneous lymph node syndrome)

Wegener's granulomatosis (WG)

Wegener's granulomatosis occurs in two forms: a systemic disease, which always includes a necrotizing glomerulonephritis, and a limited form in which the disease tends to be localized and in which renal involvement does not occur. It seems to be rare for there to be any progression of the limited form to the systemic form. In both forms there is often a prolonged prodrome of malaise, arthralgia, and myalgia. The cause is unknown, but reports that co-trimoxazole may influence the course of the disease have raised the possibility that it is triggered by an infection.

The limited form presents typically with involvement of the upper and lower respiratory tracts. Sinusitis and otitis are common, and nasal crusting, ulceration, and bleeding occur; the nasal cartilage is often eroded, leading to gradual collapse of the bridge of the nose. Subglottic stenosis is very typical and leads to acute presentation with stridor. There may be haemoptysis and the chest radiograph may show multiple 'cannon-ball' lesions, often with cavitation. Endobronchial disease may also occur, causing lower respiratory obstruction. More central involvement of the head may lead to proptosis and obstruction to the draining veins. Erosion into arteries may also occur. Skin involvement may include a leucocytoclastic vasculitis. Other complications include parotid enlargement, endocarditis (similar to Libman–Sacks endocarditis), transverse myelitis, peripheral neuropathy, and granulomatous bowel disease. Episcleritis and uveitis may occur. The systemic form tends to present as fulminant renal failure, often with pulmonary involvement, high fever arthralgia, and malaise. The lung lesions may be mistaken for tumours.

Investigations

The diagnosis has been revolutionized by the discovery of the association with anti-neutrophil cytoplasmic antibodies (C-ANCA). The major target antigen is proteinase 3, and the autoantibodies are known to penetrate intact cells and to inhibit the function of the enzyme by binding near its catalytic site, as well as by interfering with its inactivation by α1-antitrypsin. The antibody also potentiates neutrophil chemotaxis in response to fMLP, adhesion to endothelium, and nitric oxide production. Pr3 may also be expressed by endothelial cells, although this is controversial, and the C-ANCA may increase adhesive and activation molecules (E-selectin, VCAM-1, ICAM-1) as well as IL-8 production. All of these effects will enhance the inflammatory interaction between neutrophils and endothelium. Ninety-five per cent of patients with WG will have detectable ANCA, of whom 85 per cent will have C-ANCA (anti-proteinase 3) and 10 per cent P-ANCA (antimyeloperoxidase). Anti-neutrophil elastase antibodies have also been detected (P-ANCA pattern on immunofluorescence). Approximately 5 per cent of cases are seronegative. Biopsy is also important and will show the granulomatous vasculitis, often with fibrinoid necrosis.

Other features include a normochromic, normocytic anaemia, with a thrombocytosis, leucocytosis (occasional leukaemoid reactions), and slight eosinophilia. Acute-phase responses are marked. Rheumatoid factors are detectable in about 50 per cent. Immunoglobulins are usually normal. Monitoring of the disease is best carried out with acute-phase markers (CRP/ESR) and serial ANCA measurements. While the antibody titre does not correlate with the degree of disease activity, a rising titre may herald relapse. This is not affected by secondary infection, which will elevate the CRP. Disease activity is also marked by an increase in soluble CD25 (IL-2 receptor), vWF, soluble ICAM-1, and thrombomodulin, but none of these additional markers have been critically evaluated. Renal function must be checked, and the urine sediment inspected for evidence of glomerular damage. It has been suggested that indium-labelled leucocyte scanning is useful for defining sites of disease activity.

Tests for diagnosis	Tests for monitoring
Urinalysis	Urinalysis
Creatinine clearance (or isotopic equivalent)	Creatinine clearance (or isotopic equivalent)
Fbc	Fbc
Cr&E	Cr&E
ESR/CRP	ESR/CRP
ANCA (anti-Pr3 and anti-MPO)	ANCA (anti-Pr3 and anti-MPO)
Renal biopsy (+ other tissues)	Indium-labelled leucocyte scanning
Indium-labelled leucocyte scanning	

Treatment

The mainstays of treatment are steroids, given either orally or as intravenous pulses, and cyclophosphamide, which is given either as continuous oral therapy or as pulsed intravenous/oral therapy: a complex regime has been proposed by the Birmingham group for managing these two agents, which it is claimed has a better efficacy than traditional regimes. The role of azathioprine is uncertain, but it is probably less effective. Low-dose weekly methotrexate (20–30 mg/week) has also been shown to be successful. As noted above, co-trimoxazole may have a disease-modifying effect, although this is still uncertain; however, all patients should receive low-dose treatment with this agent as prophylaxis against *Pneumocystis carinii* pneumonia secondary to immunosuppression. Cyclosporin A (up to 5 mg/kg/day, with monitoring of blood levels) may be effective in combination with steroids. High-dose IVIg (0.4 g/kg/day for 5 days, repeated monthly) has been suggested as an alternative in small uncontrolled trials, and one small controlled trial. Other experimental therapies include the use of anti-CD52 (Campath 1H) ± anti-CD4 monoclonal antibodies or hu-IgG–CD4 chimeric molecules.

Lymphomatoid granulomatosis

This is an unusual condition in which there is a lymphocytic proliferation accompanied a systemic vasculitis affecting mainly small arteries and veins. It is possible that the condition is triggered by infection, possibly EBV. It occurs in patients with autoimmune diseases and in association with HIV. It may be difficult to distinguish from angiocentric lymphoma, and indeed is thought possibly to be an unusual lymphoma variant. Key clinical features include lung involvement with breathlessness and cough, and radiographic evidence of multiple nodules. Upper airways involvement, including sinuses, is common and may mimic lethal midline granuloma. Skin lesions, including nodules and ulcers, are present in over 50 per cent of patients. There may be renal involvement with proteinuria and haematuria. CNS involvement is either due to mass lesions or as a more diffuse process due to vasculitis. Lymph node and splenic enlargement are very rare and the lack of these helps distinguish the condition from true lymphoma. Myalgia and arthralgia occur.

There is no specific diagnostic test other than biopsy, and treatment comprises steroids plus cyclophosphamide, although the difficulty in distinguishing the disease from lymphoma has meant that aggressive lymphoma protocols have also been used. Irradiation may be useful for localized disease.

LARGE-VESSEL DISEASE

Giant-cell arteritis (GCA) and polymyalgia rheumatica (PMR)

These two diseases are closely associated and predominantly affect the elderly, with a peak incidence in the over-70s, although they may occur in younger patients where the diagnosis may not be considered. They are almost exclusively Caucasian diseases and have a female predominance of 3:1; the incidence is >170 per million, making them common diseases. The typical presentation of GCA is with headache, fever, and an anaemia of chronic disease. The temporal arteries are often swollen, red, and tender. Other features include jaw/tongue claudication, sudden blindness (occurs in 10 per cent through retinal artery occlusion or cortical blindness, although the figure is falling with increasing recognition), extraocular muscle palsies, ischaemic symptoms in arms and legs, stroke, and myocardial infarction. It may also be a cause of inflammatory aneurysms of the aorta. It is a cause of pyrexia of unknown origin (PUO) in the elderly. It is incorrect to think of the disease as purely one of the temporal arteries as it is a systemic vasculitis. PMR causes limb girdle pain and there is marked morning stiffness and a mild synovitis without erosive disease. There is an association with HLA-DR4. However, the cause is unknown, although it may occur in association with acute myeloid leukaemia and with HTLV-1 infection.

There are no specific immunological tests at present and the diagnosis is made by temporal artery biopsy. A reasonable length should be removed as the disease process is often patchy. There is an infiltrate of T cells, predominantly CD4+ T cells, and macrophages, with giant cells. Pretreatment for up to a week with steroids will not abolish the typical appearances. Angiography may be required to delineate the extent of disease in major vessels. There is a marked acute-phase response (CRP/ESR), although occasional patients lack this, despite evidence of disease on biopsy. Immunoglobulins and complement are normal.

The treatment is with high-dose steroids (60–100 mg/day may be required initially), which are reduced rapidly to maintenance levels and continued for 18–24 months. The minimum required to keep the disease suppressed is used, as determined by suppression of the acute-phase response (CRP is more useful for monitoring that the ESR) and lack of clinical symptoms. Failure to control the disease with high-dose steroids may require the use of cytotoxic agents such as azathioprine or cyclophosphamide. Treatment of PMR in the absence of GCA requires lower-dose steroids, usually not more than 20 mg/day. The diseases usually burn out over several years and treatment can be withdrawn, although some cases grumble on for even longer periods.

7 Vasculitic syndromes

Giant-cell arteritis and polymyalgia rheumatica

Takayasu's disease

This is predominantly a disease of Oriental patients. There is a strong association with HLA-B52 and 85 per cent of cases are women. The age of onset is usually below 40 years. There is a pre-pulseless phase with exertional dyspnoea, cough, and tachycardia, which is followed after a variable interval by a subacute presentation with fever, malaise, night sweats, nausea, and upper/lower limb claudication. Examination will reveal widespread arterial bruits. Erythema nodosum may occur and there is often an arthralgia with a synovitis; the disease may be associated with adult or juvenile rheumatoid arthritis or spondylitis. It may involve the coronary arteries, and cause interstitial lung disease, pulmonary hypertension, and glomerulonephritis. The aorta and/or pulmonary arteries are involve in 50 per cent of patients. The histology shows a granulomatous infiltrate of multinucleate giant cells with a patchy distribution; the disease begins in media. In the late phase (pulseless) there is transmural sclerosis. The disease may burn out after 5 years, leaving vascular scarring with multiple bruits. Five types are recognized, dependent on arterial involvement:

- type IA: ascending aorta, aortic arch, and arch vessels without aneurysms;
- type IB: as for IA but with aneurysms;
- type II: thoraco-abdominal aorta;
- type III: aortic arch and thoraco-abdominal aorta;
- type IV pulmonary arteries.

The acute-phase response, ESR/CRP, is high in the acute inflammatory phase of the disease but there is no specific test. Immunoglobulins are elevated in some cases. Anaemia and leucocytosis are present on full blood count. Confirmation of the diagnosis requires angiography and biopsy if a suitable accessible artery is affected.

In the inflammatory stage, the disease responds to high-dose steroids. The value of cytotoxic agents is uncertain. Surgery may be required to bypass sclerotic narrowed arteries in the end stage of the disease.

SECONDARY VASCULITIS

Hypocomplementaemic vasculitis

This discrete syndrome is characterized by urticaria with hypo-complementaemia; angioedema may also occur. Skin lesions may leave residual staining of the skin. Unlike allergic disease, the urticaria may be prolonged, lasting up to 72 hours. Forty per cent of patients have renal involvement, with granular IgG along the glomerular basement membrane, and obstructive lung disease has also been documented. There is an acute-phase response. There is a low CH100, and low C1q, C2 and C4. An autoantibody to the collagenous region of C1q has been found and apparently activates the classical pathway of complement. A similar syndrome may also occur with C3-nephritic factor (see Part 2). It is treated with steroids or dapsone (impairs chemotaxis and lysosomal activity of neutrophils and neutrophil adherence).

Erythema elevatum diutinum

This is an exceptionally rare disease, mainly in the elderly (although it may occur in girls in childhood) with cutaneous purpuric lesions accompanied by persistent red/orange plaques (like xanthomata) and violaceous nodules over extensor surfaces. The histology of fresh lesions shows a leucocytoclastic vasculitis, while older lesions show evidence of lipid deposition, with histiocytes. Immunoglobulins are increased. It has been reported in HIV and also in association with myeloma (especially IgA), hairy-cell leukaemia, and cryoglobulinaemia, and it is though to be due to an aberrant immune response to a pathogen (undefined). The first-line treatment is dapsone, also sulphapyridine and corticosteroids.

Erythema nodosum

This is form of small-vessel vasculitis particularly affecting the fat of the subcutaneous tissue. It is invariably secondary to an infective or toxic insult. The characteristic features are of red, hot, painful swellings on the shins, and less commonly on the arms. These resolve slowly, often with desquamation of the skin, and leave a brown pigmented area. They may recur if the underlying disease is not identified. There is often fever, malaise, and arthralgia. The causes are multitudinous, but worldwide the largest cause is mycobacterial infection (TB and leprosy). In the UK the most common causes are streptococcal infection and sarcoidosis. It may also be caused by other infections: viral (EBV); fungal (histoplasma, blastomycosis); bacterial (Yersinia, tularaemia, cat scratch disease, lymphogranuloma venereum). It is also associated with inflammatory bowel disease, leukaemia and lymphoma, pregnancy, the oral contraceptive pill, and sulphonamides.

The most important investigation is the patient's history, including drugs and travel, followed by a chest radiograph. Other investigations will be determined by the type of precipitant suspected. The acute-phase response will be markedly elevated. Treatment is primarily for the underlying disease, but NSAIDs relieve the discomfort. Corticosteroids also relieve the pain but do not speed resolution.

7 Vasculitic syndromes

Erythema elevatum diutinum
Erythema nodosum

Relapsing polychondritis

This is a rare autoimmune disease affecting cartilage. It is a disease of middle age and older, occurring in males and females equally. It typically affects the cartilage of the nose and the pinna of the ear, which become red and exceedingly painful. More rarely, it is associated with damage to the cartilage of the trachea (causing respiratory failure), larynx (causing hoarseness), cardiac valve rings (causing aortic incompetence), and costochondral junctions. There is often a non-deforming arthritis, hearing loss, fever, and malaise; it is a rare cause of PUO. There is a necrotizing vasculitis of small/medium-sized blood vessels, accompanied by a cutaneous vasculitis. Eye involvement includes episcleritis, iritis, and conjunctivitis. There is a mononuclear cell infiltrate of cartilage. A focal chondritis may be seen in SLE. The course may be fluctuating and it is important to distinguish it from Wegener's granulomatosis, Cogan's syndrome, infectious causes, and chondrodermatitis nodularis chronica helicis which is limited to ear.

While it is associated with antibodies to type II collagen, these occur in only 20 per cent of patients, and have little diagnostic or predictive value. IgG and complement are deposited at sites of inflammation. HLA-DR4 is present in 56 per cent of patients compared to 25 per cent of controls, but there is no association with particular HLA-DRB1 alleles and no association with HLA-B27, despite the similarities to ankylosing spondylitis. The acute-phase response is marked (ESR and CRP and complement). The full blood count shows the anaemia of chronic disease.

It is treated with NSAIDs where the disease is mild, and with steroids ± cyclophosphamide or cyclosporin A where the disease is more widespread.

Cystic fibrosis

Patients with CF may develop a vasculitis and this has been associated with the presence of ANCA. Recently the specificity of these ANCAs has been shown to be against the bactericidal/permeability increasing protein of neutrophil granules. This disorder is likely to be triggered by the chronic infection present in CF patients, although the precise relationship remains to be determined. Vasculitis is a poor prognostic marker.

7 Vasculitic syndromes

Relapsing polychondritis
Cystic fibrosis

Infection

Many of the vasculitides discussed above are suspected, or known, to be triggered by infection. Causes include direct microbial invasion of the vascular tree: cryptococcal aortitis, Aspergillus, Salmonella, Pseudomonas; septic emboli. There may be replication of the pathogen in the endothelial cells: rickettsial vasculitis (rickettsia are found in endothelial cells of gangrenous limbs); varicella zoster virus in immunosuppressed patients with lymphoma (cutaneous vasculitis with VZV in endothelial cells). HIV is recognized to cause a wide range of vasculitis responses, including PAN and HSP-like small-vessel vasculitis (leucocytoclastic and neutrophilic), and may include cerebral vasculitis. Tuberculosis not infrequently causes a PAN-like disease. CMV vasculitis accounts for gastrointestinal ulceration, pneumonitis, and skin lesions (ulcers). Syphilis (now rare in the UK) causes an endarteritis, while Borrelia is associated with a vasculitis, particularly accounting for the CNS features (Lyme disease); Bartonella is also associated with a vasculitis.

The mechanisms may include:
- immune complex deposition and complement activation, with secondary recruitment of inflammatory cells;
- type IV hypersensitivity with granuloma formation and activation of T cells, with either direct tissue damage or cytokine release;
- cross-reactive antibodies against pathogens may directly damage host components: this may involve the generation of cryoglobulins (e.g. in HBV).

Malignancy

Vasculitis may occur as a paraneoplastic phenomena, e.g. the association of PAN with hairy-cell leukaemia (strong association). Here the vasculitis resolves with HCL treatment, which includes α-IFN. Leucocytoclastic vasculitis has been associated with myelomonocytic leukaemia, T-cell lymphoma, Wilm's tumour, and renal cell carcinoma (all case reports). Vasculitis is strongly associated with chronic natural killer cell lymphocytosis (urticarial vasculitis, PAN, and acute glomerulonephritis (GN)).

Neoplasms may also present as 'vasculitis': myxoma (diagnose by demonstration of myxomatous material on biopsy). Angiocentric T-cell lymphoma (cutaneous lesions, mainly in the elderly) mimics PAN, WG, and LG.

Vasculitis may present as a neoplasm: Wegener's and lymphomatoid granulomatosis are the best examples. A testicular presentation of PAN is often confused with testicular tumours: biopsy will distinguish between the two and prevent unnecessary orchidectomy.

353

Drugs

Drug-related vasculitis accounts for 10–20 per cent of all dermatological vasculitis. It may present any time after the drug has been started, including after many years of therapy. It is often accompanied by fever, arthralgia, hepatitis, and lymphadenopathy. Systemic vascular involvement is variable and may include lung, heart, CNS, and kidney. There may be typical features of serum sickness.

Any drug is potentially capable of triggering a vasculitic reaction. More common causes include aspirin, penicillin, thiazides, and sulphonamides, AZT and cytokines (α-IFN, which may actually be used to treat vasculitis associated with HBV and HCV), and colony stimulating factors such as G-CSF (the vasculitis is related to the increasing neutrophil count).

Rare cases have been reported with illicit drugs (amphetamines, cocaine, heroin, LSD) but in many of the reports the role of hepatitis viruses has not been excluded.

355

Secondary to connective tissue diseases and other autoimmune diseases

Vasculitis is a well-recognized feature of all of the connective tissue diseases. Rheumatoid vasculitis is a small-vessel vasculitis and is marked by very high levels of rheumatoid factor; atypical ANCA against elastase and lactoferrin (P-ANCA) have been described but do not seems to be specific for rheumatoid vasculitis.

Sjögren's syndrome is associated with vasculitis in 5–10 per cent of cases. This is characterized by purpura, recurrent urticaria, skin ulceration, and mononeuritis multiplex. Raynaud's is common. Systemic vasculitis may lead to involvement of the gut (with bowel infarction); glomerulonephritis is rare. There is hypergamma-globulinaemia, high-titre RhF, anti-Ro antibodies (especially with purpuric lesions), and cryoglobulins are usual (mixed, type II with IgMκ paraprotein). Treatment is with steroids ± cyclophosphamide.

SLE, systemic sclerosis, dermatomyositis/polymyositis, inflam-matory bowel disease, PBC, and Goodpasture's syndrome are all associated with a medium- to small-vessel vasculitis.

Sneddon's syndrome is a complex of livedo reticularis and endarteritis obliterans, especially of medium-sized cerebral arteries, leading to strokes. It is often associated with anti-phospholipid anti-bodies (LAC or ACA).

Cryoglobulinaemia

Essential mixed cryoglobulinaemia (type II, see Part 2) is associated with purpura (leucocytoclastic vasculitis), Raynaud's phenomenon, arthralgia, peripheral neuropathy, Sjögren's syndrome, glomeru-lonephritis, and liver disease. There is usually an IgMκ paraprotein with RhF activity and evidence for a low-grade lymphoproliferative disease. The disease is very common in northern Italy, where there is a major association with chronic HCV infection. It is less commonly found in HBV and EBV infections. Other chronic bacteraemic infections, such as shunt nephritis and low-grade endo-carditis, may also lead to cryoglobulin formation. Complement studies show low C1, C2, and C4. Plasma viscosity is increased. Some patients with glomerulonephritis have an antibody to a 50 kDa renal antigen, although the nature of the antigen is unknown. Plasmapheresis may be required and α-IFN may be tried in order to eliminate HCV.

Cryofibrinogenaemia

This behaves in a very similar manner to cryoglobulinaemia, with cold-related purpura, haemorrhagic ulcers, and thrombosis of superficial blood vessels in exposed extremities. It may be idiopathic or associated with malignancy (see Part 2).

Hypergammaglobulinaemic purpura of Waldenström

A benign disease characterized by purpuric lesions and a polyclonal increase in immunoglobulins. High levels of immune complexes can be detected and there is a cutaneous necrotizing vasculitis. The cause is unknown. Treatment is not required.

Cholesterol emboli

These may mimic vasculitis, with a PAN-like pattern of skin lesions, accompanied by fever, myalgia, high ESR, hypertension, and eosinophilia. The skin biopsy demonstrates the presence of cholesterol clefts. It may arise following invasive vascular investigations as well as spontaneously.

Atrial myxoma

Atrial myxomas mimic vasculitis when emboli are shed: these appear in distal small blood vessels and give the typical appearances of small cutaneous vasculitic lesions, with multiple splinter haemorrhages. More major embolic lesions are the major complication (strokes). The appearances are very similar to those of SBE. There may be a tumour 'plop' associated with prolapse of the tumour through the mitral valve. The tumours may secrete high levels of IL-6 and are therefore accompanied by malaise, an elevated CRP/ESR, and a polyclonal increase in immunoglobulins. The diagnostic test is echocardiography. Treatment is surgical removal. As the tumours are benign, removal is curative and recurrence unlikely.

7 Vasculitic syndromes

Hypergammaglobulinaemic purpura of Waldenström
Cholesterol emboli
Atrial myxoma

8 Miscellaneous conditions

361

Sarcoidosis

Sarcoidosis is an enigmatic disease characterized by the presence of non-caseating granulomata. Common presentations include asymptomatic bihilar lymphadenopathy, uveo-parotid fever (von Heerfordt's syndrome), primary cerebral involvement, and a multi-system presentation, which can affect all organs in the body. Other clinical features include erythema nodosum, arthralgias, and symptoms and signs of hypercalcaemia.

Immunology

The formation of non-caseating granulomata is typical, but not by itself diagnostic, as many other diseases can cause granulomata (infections, lymphoma, carcinoma, beryllium, vasculitic and connective tissue diseases, Crohn's disease). The granuloma comprises a central area of macrophages, epithelioid cells, and Langerhans' giant cells surrounded by lymphocytes (mainly CD4+ cells and plasma cells), monocytes, and fibroblasts. The macrophages are activated and release enzymes and 1,25-dihydroxycholecalciferol hence the tendency to hypercalcaemia. There is peripheral blood lymphopenia (T and B cells), cutaneous anergy, and poor *in vitro* tests of lymphocyte proliferation. T cells have an 'activated' phenotype and T-cell receptor studies show skewing of the V_β chain usage and this might be compatible with a response to a single, as yet unidentified, pathogen. There have been numerous candidate pathogens but none have stood the test of time. Serum immunoglobulins are elevated and, as a result, low-level autoantibodies may be present. Bronchoalveolar lavage specimens show a lymphocytosis (predominantly CD4+ T cells with high levels of activation and adhesion markers) and monocytes/macrophages (also activated with elevated MHC class II). Soluble activation markers, such as sIL-2R, are raised.

Laboratory tests

No specific diagnostic tests are available for sarcoidosis. There are raised ACE levels in about 60 per cent of patients (released by epithelioid cells in the granulomata). Hypercalcaemia may be present. Serum immunoglobulins show a polyclonal elevation of all classes, but predominantly IgG. Low-titre rheumatoid factors and anti-nuclear antibodies may be present. Peripheral blood lymphocyte analysis will show a generalized lymphopenia, with a proportional reduction in all cell types. DTH testing will show anergy. There is no clinical need to assess lymphocyte proliferation *in vitro*, although it will be reduced. Measurement of sIL-2R also adds little to management. Biopsy with appropriate immunohistochemical staining is helpful. The Kveim test, in which an extract of sarcoid spleen is injected under the skin and biopsied 4–6 weeks later, is helpful: a granuloma forms at the site of injection. This test, which uses human material, is less popular now. BAL studies are helpful where there is interstitial lung disease, although the changes are no specific. In cases of cerebral disease, CSF oligoclonal bands may be present (again not specific). Lung function testing and appropriate radiological studies are essential.

Treatment

Cases of asymptomatic disease picked up by chance on chest radiography require no specific treatment. For symptomatic disease low- to moderate-dose steroids are used. Occasionally patients require other immunosuppressive drugs as steroid-sparing agents (cyclophosphamide, methotrexate, and azathioprine). Cyclosporin A and hydroxychloroquine may be helpful through their effects on T-lymphocyte activation. Patients with uveitis may require aggressive treatment to preserve vision.

Amyloidosis

This group of conditions that cause multisystem disease is often overlooked clinically. The diseases are characterized by the deposition of polymerized proteins in an insoluble β-pleated sheet form either generally or in a single organ, depending on the type of polymerizing protein. Once established, it is virtually impossible to eliminate the deposits.

AL amyloid

In this type of amyloid the deposited protein is derived from immunoglobulin light chains (λ:κ = 2:1—the opposite of that found in myeloma), and is often associated with evidence of lymphoproliferative disease. Typical clinical features include hepatosplenomegaly, cardiac failure due to infiltration, malabsorption, nephrotic syndrome, and peripheral neuropathy (especially carpal tunnel syndrome); macroglossia may be present. Deposits may occur in the skin and there may be a bleeding tendency due to selective absorption of clotting factors. It is a disease predominantly of older people. Serum and urine should be checked for the presence of monoclonal immunoglobulins and free light chains: sensitive techniques may be required to demonstrate the paraproteins, which are present in up to 80 per cent of cases; paraprotein levels are often low. Some paraproteins may not be detected as the light chain is highly abnormal or polymerized in circulation, such that it does not react with the usual antisera, or the band overlaps on electrophoresis with other protein bands. Biopsy of an affected organ and Congo red staining, which gives apple-green birefringence, is helpful; more specific immunostaining with anti-light chain antisera may give reactions, although the distorted protein structure may prevent reactivity. Bone marrow examination is essential. There is no curative treatment, but steroids, melphalan, and colchicine may slow down the rate of progression; symptomatic organ-specific treatment will be required.

AA amyloid

This form of amyloid is due to the polymerization of serum amyloid A protein (SAA), an acute-phase protein, whose levels rise in response to IL-1 and IL-6. It is a complication of chronic infection or inflammation (TB, bronchiectasis, rheumatoid arthritis, ankylosing spondylitis, etc.) and presents predominantly with hepatosplenomegaly, nephrotic syndrome, and malabsorption; cardiac and nerve involvement is rare. Biopsies will confirm the presence of the amyloid deposits, and the serum will contain high levels of acute-phase proteins (e.g. CRP); SAA is not normally measured routinely. The treatment is aimed at the underlying disease to eliminate the drive to high levels of SAA.

Two inherited disorders also give rise to AA amyloid: familial Mediterranean fever (FMF, see below) is also complicated by AA amyloid, which may be prevented by colchicine treatment. AA amyloid is also associated with the Muckle–Wells syndrome of urticaria associated with fever and deafness.

Other acquired amyloids

Another acquired amyloid is dialysis amyloid, related to the polymerization of β2-microglobulin (Aβ2MG): this is related to failure of certain older (cuprophane) haemodialysis membranes to clear β2MG and also to the duration of haemodialysis. Current membranes do not have this problem to the same extent. Widespread deposition of β2MG occurs but these deposits may resolve slowly with a successful transplant or on switching to dialysis with more permeable membranes. Serum β2MG levels will rise to very high levels (>20 mg/l).

Amyloid deposition has been associated with prions in Creutzfeldt–Jakob disease, where the prion protein, PrP, is mutated and becomes amyloidogenic. A β-amyloid protein has also been identified in certain cases of Alzheimer's disease and is associated with the typical neurofibrillary tangles. This protein is derived from a larger precursor amyloid β-precursor protein (AβPP), and in Alzheimer's it appears that the processing is defective, leading to an abnormal β-amyloid.

Amyloid deposits are found in patients with type II maturity-onset diabetes, where the amyloidogenic protein seems to be islet amyloid polypeptide, which is normally co-secreted with insulin. The latter may also account for the occurrence of this type of amyloid in association with insulinomas.

Senile cardiac amyloid is very common in the elderly and is due to deposition of polymerized atrial natriuretic factor.

Medullary thyroid carcinoma may be associated with a form of amyloid derived from pro-calcitonin and calcitonin.

Inherited amyloids

There are a number of rare inherited amyloid deposition diseases related to rare mutations in proteins: these include transthyretin, apolipoprotein A-I, gelsolin, fibrinogen, cystatin C, and lysozyme. Clinical features are variable but renal and neurological involvement, both central and peripheral, are common.

Investigations

The most important aspect of diagnosis is biopsy, with an appropriate request to the histopathologist to check for amyloid. Ideally an affected organ should be biopsied, but rectal biopsy may be positive. Urine and serum should be electrophoresed and preferably immunofixed to detect low-level paraproteins, which should, of course, be quantitated. CRP should be measured as a marker of elevated acute-phase proteins. SAA measurement is available in some laboratories. If an AL amyloid is suspected, bone marrow examination is advisable.

365

Familial Mediterranean fever (recurrent polyserositis)

This is an inherited disease, most common in Jews, Arabs, Turks, and Armenians, especially those living around the Mediterranean basin. It is inherited as an autosomal recessive. In some ethnic groups the disease has been associated with a gene on the short arm of chromosome 16. Clinical features include attacks of abdominal pain with high fever, mimicking acute peritonitis but settling over 24–48 hours. Pleuritic chest pain, arthritis, which may be destructive and mimic RhA, and skin rashes also occur. Pericarditis may occur rarely. As noted above, AA amyloid may be a long-term complication of repeated attacks, especially in Jews. The involved serosal surfaces have an inflammatory infiltrate, mainly neutrophils; joint fluid also shows a high neutrophil count during an acute attack.

Investigations

The biggest clue is the periodic fever lasting 103 days. There is a peripheral blood leucocytosis, mild anaemia, and the ESR rises during attacks. Fibrinogen levels are high (>5 g/l); serum immunoglobulins are non-specifically polyclonally elevated. Autoantibodies are not found. Biopsies need to be considered if AA amyloid is suspected.

Treatment

Colchicine in a daily dose of 1–1.5 mg will reduce the frequency and severity of attacks markedly and reduce the risk of developing amyloid.

Hyper-IgD syndrome

This rare syndrome comprises bouts of fever, lymphadenitis, and occasionally arthritis. Severe immunization reactions are a particular feature. Humoral immune responses may be poor, with reduced IgM, raised IgG_3 and very high IgD levels. IgD can be measured with commercial RID assays.

8 Miscellaneous conditions

Familial Mediterranean fever (recurrent polyserositis)
Hyper-IgD syndrome

Chronic fatigue syndromes

This is a diagnosis of exclusion, but fatigue is a major feature of many medical problems so careful history taking, examination, and investigation are required to eliminate treatable causes. Although patients use the term ME, this is a misnomer and should not be used. Patients are often sent to an immunologist because of the reports of immunological abnormalities: however, none of the findings are either diagnostically or therapeutically helpful. Fatigue is extremely common, and is the most common reason for visiting a GP. Significant fatigue is that lasting beyond 6 months. Other symptoms include non-specific arthralgia, without arthritis, myalgia, headaches, sore throats, difficulty concentrating, as well as debilitating fatigue. Weight loss is *not* a feature and should always prompt a detailed search for an underlying medical or surgical cause. Patients often slow the diagnostic process down by self-diagnosing ME, which tends to switch off doctor's critical faculties. Often patients come with beliefs, fostered by lay publications or by visits to alternative practitioners, that they have multiple allergies, are reacting to mercury amalgam fillings, have chronic *Candida* overgrowth: the evidence to support these aetiologies is scant.

The chronic fatigue syndrome is a hotch-potch of miscellaneous syndromes, dependent on the speciality of the 'expert'! Included within the spectrum are:

- irritable bowel syndrome
- food allergy
- fibromyalgia
- somatization disorder
- effort syndrome
- overtraining syndrome (see Sports immunology, below)
- patients with otherwise unexplained persistent fatigue and or atypical pain
- patients with significant medical disorders.

It is not a new syndrome and has been well described from Victorian times onwards (neurasthenia).

What CFS is not:

- 'ME'—there is no pathological evidence for myalgic encephalomyelitis!
- This is now accepted by the major patient support groups.
- No satisfactory operational definition of 'ME' exists, or is likely to be described.

Differential diagnosis

In hospital practice, up to 25 per cent of patients may turn out to have other medical or surgical problems: the differential diagnosis is long but includes:

- chronic infections: EBV, (HIV), coxsackievirus, *Toxoplasma*, *Brucella*, *Yersinia*, *Borrelia*;
- connective tissue diseases: SLE, Sjögren's syndrome, rheumatoid arthritis, polymyositis often have a long prodrome of fatigue;
- other autoimmune diseases: especially thyroid disease, Addison's disease, diabetes mellitus, pituitary disease;

- gastrointestinal disease: PBC, autoimmune hepatitis, coeliac disease;
- neurological disease: MS, degenerative disease (including CJD);
- cardiac disease: cardiomyopathy (alcohol, thiamine deficiency);
- poisonings: carbon monoxide, heavy metals, prescription drugs (e.g. β-blockers, minor opiate analgesics);
- malignancy;
- primary psychiatric disorders: depression (but a secondary depression is common), somatization disorder, stress;
- malingering (rare but usually perpetuated by obvious financial benefit from maintenance of sick role).

UK case definition for CFS

The UK criteria have evolved out of the need to identify homogeneous groups of patients for research trials. They provide a useful basis for clinical work, although not all patients will always fit into the criteria.
- Severe disabling fatigue affecting physical and mental functioning
- Minimum duration of symptoms = 6 months
- Functional impairment = disabling
- Mental fatigue required
- No other symptoms required

The Americans have a similar but slightly different case definition.
- Physical causes of fatigue excluded
- Psychiatric disorder excluded
  - psychosis
  - bipolar disorder
  - eating disorder
  - organic brain disease

Epidemiology

- Institutional epidemic outbreaks (Royal Free disease): these differ substantially from sporadic disease
- 'Chronic fatigue', loosely defined, is very common in the community:
  - prevalence of 20–30 per cent
    - 10–20 per cent of attenders in primary care complain of chronic fatigue (loosely defined)
    - for 5–10 per cent this will be the primary reason for consultation
    - only a minority fulfil the case definition for CFS (see above)
  - female-to-male ratio = 2 : 1
- The prevalence of CFS is much lower, but similar figures have been obtained from the USA and UK (using the different criteria):
  - point prevalence, 0.08–1 per cent range using restrictive criteria

Chronic fatigue syndromes *(cont.)*

- point prevalence of up to 2.6 per cent using UK (Oxford) criteria
- there are no reliable data on incidence
- It has been estimated that there may be as many as 150 000 cases in the UK

Virology

Definable fatigue syndromes are well documented after:
- Epstein–Barr virus
  - persistent EBV IgM positive (chronic EBV)
    - only occurs in 10 per cent of EBV-infected individuals;
- *Toxoplasma*;
- cytomegalovirus;
- other infectious agents (non-specific response).

The history of viral infection preceding the onset of fatigue may be unreliable, as ill health may precede viral infection on close questioning (reverse causality) and many patients have no history of antecedent illness. There appears to be no difference in likelihood of viral infections in case-control studies of CFS.

CFS and enteroviruses

There is no convincing evidence for chronic enteroviral infection of muscles in CFS patients as the original studies purporting to show this have not been repeatable. Likewise, the utility of the 'VP1' (for a common enteroviral antigen) test has not been confirmed in subsequent studies and therefore cannot be used as a test for 'CFS/ME'. Coxsackievirus and echovirus infections are very common in the community, making it difficult to prove the link.

Immunology

So far, there is no evidence for a primary immunological abnormality underlying CFS, although many immunological abnormalities have been described in patients suffering from CFS. The abnormalities described are likely to be secondary and are inconsistent, although this may be due to poor matching of patients.

Abnormalities described are:
- minor abnormalities of IgG subclasses;
- increased CD5+ CD19+ B cells;
- poor B-cell function;
- low levels of autoantibodies (RhF);
- reduced CD4+ T cells; increased CD8+ T cells;
- increased markers of T-cell activation;
- abnormalities of NK cells and monocytes;
- no clear changes in cytokine production (NB difficulties in measuring cytokines in biological fluids).

Significant immunological abnormalities should raise doubts about a diagnosis of CFS.

New research has shown similarities with the fatigue found in primary biliary cirrhosis and Sjögren's syndrome. Antibodies against nuclear pore antigens may be found in 60–70 per cent of CFS patients in one study.

Muscle abnormalities

There are no characteristic abnormalities:
- CK may be mildly elevated;
- NMR studies demonstrate abnormal metabolism.

Neurological abnormalities

There are no diagnostic abnormalities; however, a range of abnormalities has been documented, the significance of which are uncertain at present:
- MRI scanning may show white matter abnormalities;
- single-photon emission tomography (SPET) reflects abnormalities of regional cerebral perfusion;
- SPET abnormalities identified in brain stem; lesser abnormalities are reported in patients with depression (these results need further confirmation);
- dynamic tests of the hypothalamic–pituitary–adrenal axis demonstrate abnormal responses;
- subgroup of CFS patients may have low cortisols (usually high in depression).

Psychiatric changes

There is no convincing evidence to show that CFS is purely a psychiatric disorder. Depression may be present but is usually secondary. Other psychological factors may be present. There is an increased risk of developing psychiatric disorder in CFS patients (two- to 7.5-fold compared to chronic disease controls). There is overlap with somatization disorders. It has been accepted by the Royal Colleges' Report that CFS is *not* simply a psychiatric disorder, even though we do not understand fully what CFS really is. Recognition and treatment of coexistent depressive illness is essential to good management of CFS.

Assessment

This is usually a lengthy procedure. Take care to assess the patient objectively (and try to ignore the long-standing patient's interpretation of events).

Are criteria for CFS met?

What is the degree of disability?

What are the patient's beliefs about his or her illness?

Are there any symptoms/signs of other medical problems?

Low-grade fever, muscle wasting, orthostatic hypotension, pallor, breathlessness, tremor allowable (deconditioning due to prolonged rest).

Chronic fatigue syndromes *(cont.)*

- Marked weight loss, lymphadenopathy, and fever >38 °C require further investigation and should not be accepted as part of CFS.
    Look specifically for evidence of neurological disease (MS, motor neurone disease) and endocrine disease (goitre, abnormal pigmentation, visual fields) and connective tissue diseases (fatigue may be an very early feature of CTD).

Investigations

Investigation should be guided by the history and examination. There are no diagnostic tests. The basic screen includes:
- Fbc, differential white count;
- acute-phase response (evidence for inflammatory disease—ESR/CRP);
- LFTs, Cr&E, TFTs, CK, blood sugar;
- autoantibody screen (ANA, AMA, HEp-2 screen for nuclear pore antibodies);
- urine (protein/sugar);
- viral serology (EBV, *Toxoplasma*, *Brucella*, Lyme disease, coxsackie), dependent on risk factors.

Other tests to consider include cortisol, Synacthen® test, glucose tolerance test (prolonged to pick up reactive hypoglycaemia), endomysial antibodies, all dependent on specific clues from the history and examination.

Management

An holistic approach is required:
- evaluate the contribution of life events and psychological background;
- identify significant secondary depression and deal with this;
- deal with bizarre beliefs;
- reassurance early that no serious medical condition has been identified;
- detailed explanation of current theories of CFS;
- expected prognosis;
- limit investigation (and control multiple referrals!);
- management by the smallest possible team;
- physical re-conditioning
  - graded exercise;
- drug therapy is symptomatic (not curative)
  - NSAIDs for muscle ache
  - antidepressants (for reactive depression)
  - (there is no indication that newer drugs are any better than older drugs);
- psychological support
  - cognitive behaviour therapy (often resisted by patients);
- general support from a sympathetic medical team.

Management is usually difficult and time consuming for those where no identifiable medical condition is identified. There is no place in management for immunoglobulin therapy, either intravenous or intramuscular; trials of cytokine therapy have been uniformly disappointing. A full and sympathetic explanation of the symptoms is required. Emphasizing the need for a graded return to activity early is essential, as prolonged periods of rest lead to rapid deconditioning of muscles and delay recovery. Antidepressants may be necessary for dealing with secondary depressive symptoms but do not fundamentally alter the speed of recovery; cognitive behaviour therapy is said to help, although it is time consuming and not always widely available. Education about avoiding the more extreme forms of dietary manipulation is essential. Limitation of investigation and multiple medical referral is appropriate as allowing these perpetuates illness behaviour and delays recovery.

Outcome

The prognosis is variable:
- most patients show significant improvement over 2 years;
- 'cure' rate is probably 6–13 per cent (several different series);
- it is important to discuss adaptation of the patient's life style to his or her illness early on;
- there are no laboratory markers that predict outcome.
  A poor outcome associated with:
- late presentation;
- unaddressed psychosocial factors;
- poor management ('there is nothing wrong with you—it's all in your mind');
- inadequate rehabilitation (failure to encourage exercise perpetuates deconditioning);
- secondary gain;
- perpetuation of bizarre beliefs (*Candida* syndrome, total allergy syndrome).

373

Bizarre beliefs and treatments

There is no convincing evidence that CFS is caused by:
- *Candida* hypersensitivity or overgrowth;
- total allergy syndrome;
- mercury amalgam dental fillings;
- magnesium deficiency.

There is no convincing evidence at present to support the use of the following treatments in CFS:
- immunoglobulin (intravenous or intramuscular);
- antihistamines;
- interferons (usually make the symptoms worse);
- antivirals (except where there is a proven persistent EBV infection);
- antifungals;
- magnesium;
- colonic irrigation;
- anti-*Candida* diets;

Chronic fatigue syndromes *(cont.)*

- low-allergen diets;
- enzyme-potentiated desensitization.

Children with CFS

The syndrome is *rare* in children. Beware of 'Munchausen syndrome by proxy'. Management is more complicated and must address family issues. Depression is common (60–80 per cent of childhood CFS cases). The therapeutic management proceeds as in adults with a proper history and examination to exclude other organic medical or psychiatric disease. Investigation should be kept to the minimum, mainly to provide reassurance to the family of the normality of tests. Psychosocial factors (bullying) and psychiatric problems must be dealt with, as must peer-relationship problems and school avoidance (avoid home tuition as this encourages social isolation). Aim for a recovery programme including graded physical and intellectual exercise, with identification of recovery goals.

An excellent report on the causes, diagnosis, and management of chronic fatigue has been produced by the Royal Colleges of Physicians, Psychiatrists and General Practitioners (Chronic Fatigue Syndrome: Report of a joint working party of the Royal Colleges of Physicians, Psychiatrists and General Practitioners; Royal College of Physicians, London 1996)

8 Miscellaneous conditions
Chronic fatigue syndromes

Sports immunology

Considerable attention has been paid to the immunology of sport, the interest being generated by perceptions of changes in susceptibility to infection which may be attributable to alterations in immune function as a result of exercise. It is important to distinguish between the immediate effects of exercise, which may depend on the intensity and duration, and longer-term effects arising as a result of the training process. Studies of immunological function in the resting state, even of trained athletes, rarely shows much deviation from normal, indicating that many of the effects are short-term changes related to the acute bout of exercise. Chronic changes only become apparent during very hard training. Many of the effects on the immune system are mediated fully or in part by the pathways linking the neurohumoral axis and the immune system. Clinicians should not forget that illicit drugs taken to boost performance may also have effects on immune function.

Acute phase response

Exercise has been demonstrated to increase acute-phase proteins (CRP, fibrinogen, haptoglobin), although considerable amounts of exercise (>2 hours) are required. This corresponds with the demonstration (with all the usual caveats about measuring cytokines) of increased levels of IL-1 (although this is contentious), IL-6, α- and γ-interferon, and TNF-α in serum. LPS-stimulated release of cytokines by monocytes is also increased by adrenaline, present in high levels during exercise. IL-2 levels are reduced.

Innate immune response

There is a significant increase in C3a following exercise, and the greater the duration of exercise, the greater the rise. It is thought that damage to muscle fibres may be the trigger for alternate pathway activation. A leucocytosis is noticeable after quite short bursts of exercise, which is likely to be due to increased mobilization, while after marathons, a persistent marked neutrophil leucocytosis is apparent. A monocytosis may also be found. Adrenaline may play a role in the mobilization, although it may still occur in the presence of β-blockade. The neutrophils are also activated, and granule components may be detected in the circulation.

NK cell numbers are increased in absolute and percentage terms and NK activity is increased, except in high-intensity exercise (such as a marathon), when it is reduced.

Specific immunity

Many effects on the specific immune system have been described, although the relationship to clinical status is often obscure.

B-cell function

The following changes have been documented during and immediately after acute exercise:

- no significant change in B-cell numbers;
- reduced salivary IgA after long-duration exercise;
- reduction of circulating antibody-producing cells;
- monocyte-induced suppression (indomethacin inhibitable, suggesting role for prostaglandins).

T-cell function

The following changes have been documented during and immediately after acute exercise:
- increase in T cells (CD8+ > CD4+);
- altered CD4:CD8 ratio;
- increased CD4+ CD45RO+ T cells (? activation or altered trafficking);
- reduced proliferative response to PHA and ConA;
- increased proliferative responses to IL-2, LPS, PWM;
- increased soluble activation markers after long-duration exercise (sIL-2R, sCD8, sICAM-1, sCD23, sTNF-R, neopterin).

It has been suggested that many of the effects on the immune system are mediated by the combination of changes in circulating and local hormones, including catecholamines, growth hormone, endorphins, and cortisol (which may be responsible for late effects). Hypoxia and hyperthermia may also contribute. A fashionable theory suggests that increased muscle demand for glutamine as an energy source starves the immune system of an essential metabolic precursor, leading to impaired function.

377

Adaptive changes during training

The resting immunology of athletes during training does not normally show very dramatic changes. During low-intensity training there is a reduction of total lymphocyte count, with a reduction of CD4:CD8 ratio. More intense training tends to have less effect. NK cells numbers increase slightly. Most trained athletes show slightly higher neutrophil counts, although some long-distance runners may have a neutropenia. Neutrophil (and monocyte) function is normal. The acute changes in immunological parameters seen in trained athletes tend to be less than in sedentary individuals undertaking a similar workload.

Exercise and infection

Many athletes believe that they have increased susceptibility to infection (usually upper respiratory tract infections) immediately after bouts of intense exercise, either during training or after competitions. The acute changes noted above may give a window of opportunity to pathogens that accounts for this observation. This window may last up to 2 weeks. The risks seems to be mainly in the longest distance (marathon) runners.

Overtraining

There appears to be a J-shaped curve relating overall immune function to exercise, so that low and moderate levels of exercise improve immunological function, while high levels lead to immunological impairment. However, it is difficult to ascertain for any given individual what level of exercise will be compromising immune function. The overtraining syndrome has many feature in common with the chronic fatigue syndrome (CFS; see above).

Short-term fatigue is a normal consequence of exercise; however, prolonged fatigue is usually a marker for overtraining. This can usually be attributed to inappropriate training and/or competitive programmes that do not allow adequate recovery periods. This can often be laid at the door of the athletes themselves, striving to improve their performance.

The precise nature of the overtraining syndrome is uncertain, but might relate to chronic overproduction of acute-phase cytokines (e.g. TNF), hormones (cortisol and thyroid hormones are increased while testosterone is decreased). Interference with the neuro-humoral axis may occur, and patients may have features of anxiety and depression. Chronic glutamine deficiency has also been invoked, although it is unlikely that this is the sole cause, or even the primary cause. The situation may be confused if illicit performance-enhancing drugs have been taken, and information on this should always be sought directly.

Beware that high-intensity exercise may be a surrogate form of anorexia in young females particularly: such athletes are at high risk of serious complications of exercise due to inadequate nutrition and over-exercising: stress fractures, premature osteoporosis, and iron-deficiency anaemia.

Immunology

The immunological changes of optimum training are difficult to analyse, but include increased NK cell numbers and activity, minor changes in T- and B-cell numbers and little change in serum immunoglobulins. Levels of soluble markers such as IL-2R, sCD8, sICAM-1, sCD23, and sTNF-R are all increased. Very heavy training and/or competition tend to lead to a reduction in cell numbers and function and reductions in antibody levels. Exercise itself tends to mobilize cells from storage pools (spleen, marginated cells) but this effect is transient. In the overtraining syndrome, lymphocyte numbers and NK cells are reduced and there is evidence of *in vivo* activation on the basis of expression of activation markers CD25, CD69, and HLA-DR (on T cells). *In vitro* mitogen responses are reduced (a common finding where there is evidence of increased *in vivo* activation). Phagocytic cell function is impaired.

Laboratory tests

Investigation should be geared towards excluding other contributors to fatigue:
• full blood count including differential white count;

- acute phase (ESR/CRP);
- thyroid and liver function tests;
- serological tests for chronic infection (EBV, *Toxoplasma*);
- vitamin and mineral status (iron, especially in women, folate, B12);
- serum immunoglobulins and lymphocyte surface markers if there is a history of significant infections.

Routine diagnostic use of *in vitro* tests of NK and T-cell function are not normally required for management.

Treatment

A firm explanation is required as to the cause of the problem and a period of reduction of training to basal levels for a period of several months may be required, followed by a gradual increase. Emphasizing the need to have peaks and recovery troughs in the training programme is essential. Attention to diet and vitamin and mineral supplementation may be required. There is no good scientific evidence that high-dose vitamin C helps, but many sportsmen have empirically found that it reduces the susceptibility to infection: it may, however, cause renal stones as it is metabolized to oxalate. This may be a particular problem in athletes who are prone to dehydration during competition so it is important to emphasize the need for adequate hydration.

379

Depression and immune function

There is now a reasonable body of evidence that there is a close link between mental state and immune function. Lymphocytes have receptors for certain neurotransmitters (catecholamines) as well as neurohormones (endorphins), and cytokines such as IL-1 affect cerebral function (fever, hormone release). Chronic or severe acute stress may both be immunosuppressive and lead to an increased risk of infection through multiple neurohumoral pathways. The same changes are seen in prolonged depressive illness.

Findings may include minor lymphopenia and reduced NK cells, as well as poor NK function and reduced immunization responses. However, routine investigation of the immune system is not warranted unless there is evidence of a major susceptibility to bacterial or viral infection.

Immunology of infection

Dealing with infection is the primary function of the immune system and the reader is referred to the standard immunology text-books for details of this. There are, however, certain clinically important points that need to be borne in mind when interpreting immunological tests taken in patients with active infection.

Neutrophils

A neutrophilia, often with a left shift (i.e. immature cells newly emigrating from the marrow) and toxic granulation is a major early feature of bacterial infection. However, severe neutropenia may also result from overwhelming sepsis due to consumption exceeding the marrow capacity for production: this obviously has to be distinguished from a primary neutropenia *causing* the infection. Bone marrow examination may help. If severe, G-CSF may speed recovery.

Monocytes

Monocytosis is often seen in viral infections and a compensatory monocytosis is also seen during infective episodes in neutropenic patients.

Eosinophils

Marked eosinophilia is a feature of parasitic infections. However, in the UK marked eosinophilia with fever is more likely to be due to a hyper-eosinophilic syndrome with or without vasculitis, rather than an infection. Levels of eosinophil cationic protein (ECP) may be significantly raised and are important in diseases like Churg–Strauss vasculitis, as high levels of ECP are neurotoxic.

Lymphocytes

Acute viral and bacterial infections often lead to a generalized pro-portional lymphopenia. In viral infections this will be followed by a rise in the CD8+ cytotoxic T cells, leading to a marked reversal of the CD4:CD8 ratio. There is usually an increase in activation markers (CD25, HLA-DR). This is *not* a finding limited to HIV infection and therefore lymphocyte marker analysis will not act as a surrogate HIV test. EBV infection often leads to a marked lymphocytosis, with B cells followed by CD8+ T cells. Very high B-cell counts may occur following EBV infection in bone marrow transplant patients where there are insufficient T cells to control the EBV-driven B-cell proliferation (B-lymphoproliferative disease).

Serum immunoglobulins

Acute bacterial infection may lead to severe pan-hypogamma-globulinaemia; this may lead to erroneous diagnosis of a primary antibody deficiency. It is therefore essential that the tests are repeated when the infection has been treated. Starting IVIg under such circumstances is not only dangerous and unnecessary but will also prevent a proper diagnosis being reached. More commonly, there will be an initial rise in IgM followed by a polyclonal rise in IgG which then returns to normal.

Chronic infection will lead to significant polyclonal increases in immunoglobulins and may be accompanied by the appearance of monoclonal bands in the serum. These represent the overexpansion of clones of B cells producing antibody against the persisting pathogen. These bands are often multiple and set on a polyclonally increased background. Excess free light chains may also be found in the urine. The bands will disappear within a few months of satisfactory treatment. Persistently raised IgM or IgA may be found in tuberculosis.

Complement

Viral infection tends to have little effect on complement, but acute bacterial infection will often lead to reductions of C3 and C4 (as well as Factor B if measured) although as complement components are under acute-phase control, there may be normal levels despite significant consumption. Complement breakdown products will be increased and haemolytic complement assays may show reduced activity related to critical reductions in one or more component (usually in the terminal lytic sequence). Patients with bacterial endocarditis often show marked reductions of C3 and C4. In patients with suspected post-streptococcal nephritis, persistence of a low C3 beyond 6 weeks should prompt a check for a C3-nephritic factor, an autoantibody that stabilizes the alternative pathway C3-convertase and leads to unregulated C3 cleavage. In patients with meningococcal disease, assay of haemolytic complement to look for complement deficiency should be deferred at least 4 weeks: doing the tests early often leads to confusing results.

CRP

The highest levels of CRP (>300 mg/l) are seen in bacterial infection, and often the very highest levels are seen in *Legionella* infection. Beware of elevated CRP in infection with herpes viruses, especially EBV (levels up to 100 mg/l). High levels may also be seen in certain malignancies, including lymphoma and hypernephroma. The latter is worth remembering as it often presents as a PUO.

Reproductive immunology

Pregnancy

Pregnancy is a form of allograft and non-rejection is a complex multifactorial process. Implantation is the first part of the process and the immune system plays a part in this. Uterine macrophages are activated and produce high levels of cytokines which increase PGE2 levels, thought to be essential for implantation. Decidual cytokine production modifies the blastocyst; key cytokines appear to be leukaemia inhibitory factor (LIF) and colony-stimulating factor 1 (CSF-1). Tubal cytokines (TNF-α, TGF-β, and epidermal growth factor (EGF)) all enhance blastocyst maturation while it is in transit. Blastocysts themselves are active, producing adhesion molecules (increased by cytokines) and high levels of progesterone.

The trophoblast is the key to prevention of fetal rejection. Cytokine production by the trophoblast enhances a maternal Th1 to Th2 switch (IL-10, PGE2), and it expresses a non-polymorphic MHC antigen, HLA-G (similar to class I), without class I or II molecules. The trophoblast is also resistant to complement-mediated lysis, through the expression of CD55 (decay accelerating factor (DAF)) and CD59 (HRF20).

Immunological changes can be documented during pregnancy, with a reduction in T cells (mainly CD4+) which reaches a nadir around the seventh month. NK cell numbers also fall but B-cell numbers and function remain static. Antibody synthesis and serum immunoglobulin levels are essentially unchanged. Despite the change from Th1 to Th2, there is no evidence for increased susceptibility to infection, with the exception of *Listeria* which has a tropism for the placenta and requires macrophages and T cells for clearance (these are locally suppressed). There are no changes in solid organ allograft tolerance during pregnancy but autoimmune diseases may behave unpredictably. Lupus may get worse or better during pregnancy, but may relapse immediately after delivery due to the sudden hormonal changes. Vaccine responses are normal.

Pre-eclampsia

Pre-eclampsia has some immunological features, in that there is evidence of complement consumption, with reduced C4, and it is also associated with high-titre anti-thyroid antibodies.

Recurrent miscarriages

There are many immunological theories for recurrent miscarriages, but many have little in the way of supportive evidence.
- Antibody mediated
  - anti-phospholipid antibodies—well substantiated
    - anti-sperm antibodies—not substantiated
    - anti-trophoblast antibodies—not substantiated
    - blocking antibody deficiency (anti-paternal antibodies): these antibodies are well documented but appear

to be irrelevant to pregnancy outcome (agammaglobu-
linaemic women and mice have normal pregnancies)
- absence of complement regulatory proteins CD55 and
CD59 on trophoblast—no evidence so far.
- Cell mediated
  - excessive Th1 response: some evidence of increased Th1
  cytokines (γ-IFN and TNF-α, both of which are aborti-
  facient in mice) and Th1 responses to trophoblast antigens
  in recurrent aborters—this is a strong possibility
    - deficiency of Th2 cells/cytokines: no human evidence
    yet
    - deficiency of decidual 'suppressor' cells: uncertain
    whether this is cause or effect
    - inappropriate MHC class I and II expression: evidence
    in mice only, none from humans
  - HLA homozygosity: no convincing evidence as inbred
  mouse strains reproduce normally.

Laboratory investigation

The most important well-defined cause is the presence of anti-
phospholipid antibodies, and this should always form part of the
screen for causes of recurrent miscarriages. These autoantibodies
have a pro-coagulant effect and seem to lead to microthrombosis in
the placenta, leading to placental failure. Investigation should
include tests for IgG and IgM cardiolipin antibodies as well as for
the presence of a lupus anticoagulant. The latter will cause the
APTT to be prolonged, and the prolongation will not be reversible
by normal serum. The dilute Russell viper venom test (dRVVT) is
more specific. Often patients will have a moderate thrombocytopenia ($80-120 \times 10^9$/l). The significance of the detection of IgM
cardiolipin antibodies alone is debated: these may be found during
and after infections. Rare patients with the clinical feature of the
anti-phospholipid syndrome may be found who only have high-titre
IgM anti-cardiolipin antibodies over prolonged periods.

Other autoantibodies should be sought, including anti-thyroid
peroxidase (microsomal) antibodies, anti-nuclear antibodies, antibodies to ENA (especially Ro and La). C3 and C4 should be
measured. These tests should identify otherwise 'silent' cases of
SLE.

Management

Joint obstetric and medical management is required for such
patients: low-dose aspirin or heparin may be required. Those with
antibodies but no previous history of thrombosis or pregnancy loss
should be tried on low-dose aspirin first. Those with a prior history
of thrombosis should go onto heparin, and those with recurrent miscarriages and a previous history of thrombosis should go onto
aspirin plus heparin. Heparin is associated with occasional severe
osteoporosis in pregnancy. It is not yet clear whether this effect is

385

also seen with low molecular weight heparins. Obviously the risks of these therapies must be fully discussed with the patient. If these treatments are unsuccessful, then consideration may be given to using high dose IVIg as an immunoregulatory agent, which has been shown to be helpful in small controlled trials. Full counselling concerning potential infective risks (hepatitis, spongiform encephalopathies) must be given and recorded in the notes.

For recurrent miscarriages not associated with anti-phospholipid antibodies, the optimal treatment is unknown. Many manipulations have been tried but there are few good clinical trials. In 58 per cent of untreated patients successful pregnancy may ensue, and this figure rises to 85 per cent with good supportive psychotherapy. There is no convincing evidence that leucocyte transfusions, steroids, cyclosporin A, progesterone (immunosuppressive in high doses), or other drugs make a significant difference.

Immunological diseases of pregnancy

Blood group incompatibility

See Chapter 5

Alloimmune thrombocytopenia

See Chapter 5

Autoimmune diseases

Autoimmune diseases in the pregnant mother that are accompanied by IgG autoantibodies may occur in the fetus/neonate due to placental transmission of the antibody. This also confirms the pathogenicity of some antibodies. Myasthenia gravis and thyroid disease may both occur following placental transmission of antibody.

Mothers with SLE who are anti-Ro or anti-La antibody positive are at increased risk of having babies affected with either neonatal lupus, characterized by a photosensitive rash (made worse if the baby is given photo therapy for jaundice) or more seriously with the development of *in utero* complete heart block. The former is a self-limiting problem that disappears over the first 6 months of life as maternal antibody is catabolized. The latter is a serious and life-threatening problem. The antibodies appear to react with the developing neonatal cardiac conducting system, causing inflammation followed by fibrosis and then conduction failure: this begins around the eighth–twelfth week of pregnancy (i.e. earlier than books traditionally say that antibody crosses the placenta). Cardiac failure may develop *in utero*, leading to a hydropic fetus and death. Dexamethasone has been used experimentally with variable success to reduce the inflammatory response as it crosses the placenta (prednisolone is metabolized by the placenta). Immediate insertion of a pacemaker is required on delivery. Only a proportion of anti-Ro+ mothers (1 in 20) will be affected, but if one pregnancy has been affected the risks in subsequent pregnancies are much higher (1 in 4). Although less common, anti-La has also been associated with congenital complete heart block.

There is some evidence to suggest that children with either neonatal lupus or congenital complete heart block are more likely to develop lupus in their own right in later life.

Immunodeficiency

Primary antibody deficiency occasional comes to light during pregnancy when routine testing fails to identify isohaemagglutinins in the pregnant mother. Replacement therapy should be started at once to ensure approximately normal levels of placental transfer. Failure to do so means that the neonate will be at significant infective risk during the first 6–9 months of life, and if no maternal replacement has been undertaken, then the infant should be given at least 6 months of IVIg in normal replacement doses, while continuing to receive the normal childhood immunizations.

Maternal infection (including rubella and the herpesviruses; see Chapter 3) during pregnancy, particularly peripartum, may also lead to neonatal immunodeficiency due to *in utero* or neonatal infection. HIV infection poses particular risks of vertical transmission. Because of maternally transmitted antibody, direct tests for virus are required. Schedules of prophylactic treatment with anti-retroviral drugs are now used to reduce the risk of transmission. Congenital HIV infection is more prone to cause hypogammaglobulinaemia and unsuspected cases may therefore present with recurrent bacterial infections rather than the opportunist infections seen in adults.

9 Transplantation

390

Bone marrow transplantation

Bone marrow transplantation is used for the following conditions:
- severe combined immunodeficiency:
  - all types
  - Omenn's syndrome;
- combined immunodeficiency where there is reason to suspect progression, including:
  - Wiskott–Aldrich syndrome
  - hyper-IgM syndrome
  - activation defects (ZAP70 kinase deficiency, etc.)
  - MHC antigen deficiency
  - X-linked lymphoproliferative disease
  - purine nucleoside phosphorylase deficiency
  - cartilage hair hypoplasia;
- neutrophil disorders:
  - chronic granulomatous disease
  - leucocyte adhesion molecule deficiency (LFA-1 deficiency)
  - Chediak–Higashi syndrome;
- lymphomas and acute leukaemias, usually when in remission;
- solid tumours (Ewing sarcoma, neuroblastoma, germ cell tumours, breast and ovarian cancer);
- inherited metabolic diseases:
  - osteopetrosis
  - Gaucher's disease
  - adrenoleucodystrophy
  - metachromatic leucodystrophy
  - mucopolysaccharidoses;
- juvenile chronic arthritis (experimental).

Conditioning

In the treatment of leukaemia and lymphoma, BMT may be autologous, but in all other conditions allogeneic bone marrow will be used. In any case, conditioning will be required to generate space in the marrow cavity for the incoming marrow to develop. This will involve high-dose cytoreductive therapy, including busulphan and cyclophosphamide, and will lead to a severe aplastic phase during which laminar flow isolation is required. Complications of this phase include veno-occlusive disease of the liver, which is due to hepatic endothelial damage, alopecia, and severe mucositis. Rarer problems include acute myocarditis, and late problems include secondary malignancy, infertility, and leucoencephalopathy. Presence of infection during this phase poses particular problems. IVIg may used prophylactically and antifungal, antiviral, and anti-*Pneumocystis* drugs are usually administered.

Matching

For all allogeneic transplants, MHC matching is required, as the success of the transplant is dependent on the match. Identical sibling matches are the preferred donors, followed by matched unrelated donors. If neither are available, then haplo-identical parental bone marrow can be used or less well-matched unrelated donors. Where a SCID baby requires a haplo-identical marrow, paternal marrow is preferred, to eliminate any residual materno-fetal engraftment. Fully matched marrow from an identical sibling can be used whole, but where there are mismatches, *in vitro* T-cell depletion is used to remove mature T cells that are capable of producing GvHD.

Confirmation of suitability of the chosen donor is usually checked pretransplant, using mixed lymphocyte reactions (MLR) or CTLP or HTLP frequency (Chapter 15). High levels of reactivity in these tests are good predictors of the development of graft-versus-host disease. Cyclosporin A, either alone or with low-dose steroids, is administered to reduce the risks of development of GvHD.

Donors are assessed medically and screened for transmissible infections, including EBV, HIV, CMV, Parvovirus. If there is a mismatch, then prophylactic antivirals should be used. The donor will have to undergo a general anaesthetic for harvest, so cardiorespiratory fitness is essential. Marrow is now tested routinely for stem-cell numbers, with a view to maximizing stem-cell numbers.

For those with no good match, stem-cell harvesting from cord blood for banking is now being set up. Peripheral stem-cell harvesting is also being used for patients with marrow that would be unsuitable for harvesting (i.e. infiltrated with tumour). Experimental systems for enriching bone marrow by selective *in vitro* culture are also being attempted.

The use of growth factors (G-CSF, GM-CSF) is being assessed to speed up the reconstitution process and shorten the aplastic phase in the recipient. Donors may also, under some circumstances, be treated with CSFs to increase stem-cell activity and also to increase peripheral counts of mature neutrophils, which are then cytopheresed for infusion into the recipient during the aplastic phase.

All recipients must receive irradiated cellular blood products, to prevent accidental engraftment of viable donor lymphocytes, until there is evidence of satisfactory immunological recovery, and this should be CMV negative unless the recipient is known to be CMV positive.

Post-transplant monitoring

Many units use very little in the way of post-transplant immunological monitoring. A full blood count and differential indicates the need for red cell and platelet support, and the rise of the neutrophil count gives a good indication of when adequate protective innate immunity has returned. Immunological monitoring does, however, have a role to play in optimizing management and, in particular, in developing strategies for assessing the return of adaptive immunity.

- Serial lymphocyte profiles on peripheral blood demonstrate when safe levels of CD4 T and B cells have returned. Rising NK counts often precede infection and GvHD. Very rapid rises in B cells in the absence of T cells usually indicate B-lympho-proliferative disease secondary to EBV. These should be done at least weekly, or more often if there are problems. An appropriate panel will include CD4, CD8, CD3, CD16/56, CD25, HLA-DR, CD19, or CD20. Other markers may be useful under special circumstances.

- Acute-phase proteins (CRP)—early warning of infection.
- β2-Microglobulin—possibly useful for monitoring GvHD.
- Trough immunoglobulins—to assess adequacy of IVIg replacement (patients may be hyper-catabolic and require increased doses).
- Lymphocyte proliferation assays: the optimum panel of mitogens has yet to be determined. PHA responses are the last to return. ConA responses return earlier, followed by anti-CD3 responses. Flow cytometric assays involving CD69 expression do not correlate well with formal proliferation assays. These assays should only be requested when T cells can be detected in the peripheral blood and then done at monthly intervals.
- Chimerism studies: genetic techniques now allow analysis of the origin of separated cell lineages (using monoclonal antibody coupled to magnetic beads). B-cell recovery is often host even when T cells are donor. Despite this, there is usually full immunological recovery of B-cell function, even if there is an MHC mismatch between T and B cells.
- Long-term monitoring of humoral immune function and cellular reconstitution is required, as the very long-term outlook is as yet unknown.
- The use of specific tests may determine the return of function known to be defective pretransplant and confirm the success of the transplant, e.g. flow cytometric analysis of oxidative metabolism of neutrophils in CGD transplants, where autologous reconstitution may be a concern, and CD40L expression in transplants for hyper-IgM syndrome (although this assay is inhibited by prophylactic cyclosporin A).
- Once prophylactic IVIg has been stopped, the development of IgG subclasses and specific antibodies can be followed. Clues to satisfactory B-cell function include the return of IgM isoagglutinins, and rising IgA and IgM levels, as well as satisfactory B-cell numbers in peripheral blood.

Immunological development

The rate of development is dependent on the conditioning regime, stem-cell dose, use of T-cell depletion, matching of MHC, development of graft-versus-host disease, and intercurrent infection (which may lead to a furious response from the incoming graft). Under optimum conditions, evidence of lymphocyte engraftment is usually present within 28 days, but may be delayed up to 90 days. T-cell reconstitution usually precedes B-cell engraftment. B-cell numbers and function return only very slowly and may take 2 years to return to 'normal'. Occasionally B cells fail to engraft and autologous B-cell reconstitution does not take place: such patients need to remain on IVIg. Return of isohaemagglutinins and a rising IgA and IgM are early signs that can be readily detected despite IVIg. IVIg is usually continued for at least a year (longer if there have been complications such as GvHD) and then stopped. Killed vaccines are usually administered at the time IVIg is stopped and responses checked when the IVIg has disappeared from circulation. A full course of 'childhood' immunizations is required, but live viral vaccines and BCG should not be given until there is evidence of good responses to killed or subunit vaccines and good *in vitro* T-cell function. IgG2 subclass levels rise only very slowly after transplantation, mirroring normal ontogeny.

Some patients with autologous transplants and apparently 'cured' lymphoma may have long-term evidence of continuing immunodeficiency with recurrent bacterial infections, low serum immunoglobulins, and poor specific anti-bacterial responses and lymphopenia. These patients require long-term IVIg therapy replacement.

Results

Bone marrow transplantation for acute leukaemia and lymphomas gives a 50–60 per cent disease-free survival in first complete remission, falling to 30 per cent in second remission and 15 per cent in refractory disease. For SCID, the figures for long-term survival are dependent on the closeness of the match, age at transplant, and the presence or absence of infection at the time of transplant. In the best centres, 90 per cent survival is now regularly achieved for early matched sibling transplants, falling to 30 per cent survival for late transplants in infected recipients with poor matches.

Graft-versus-host disease (GvHD)

Development of graft-versus-host disease is largely dependent on the presence of MHC differences between donor and recipient. It is more likely to occur in unrelated donor transplants, even if well-matched for MHC, because of other antigenic differences coded outside the MHC. The presence of mature T cells in the graft has a major effect. Curiously, a disease resembling GvHD may be seen in autologous transplants, possibly due to the development of autoreactive T cells.

Acute GvHD causes damage mainly to rapidly dividing tissues, such as skin (causing rashes) and gut (where there is profuse diarrhoea). The liver is frequently involved, with rapidly rising bilirubin. GvHD is immunosuppressive, so there is an increased risk of infections. Diagnosis is usually obviously clinically but can be confirmed on biopsy of bowel or skin, where infiltrates of mature T cells can be seen with evidence of MHC class II antigen induction on surrounding tissues. Acute GvHD is graded in severity from I to IV. Damage to tissues is caused by both direct cellular toxicity and also by high levels of released cytokines (IL-1, TNF-α, γ-IFN). Where there is strong evidence that GvHD may be expected, prophylactic treatment with cyclosporin A or methotrexate has been shown to reduce the incidence and/or severity of GvHD. The problem with these regimes is that they add to the immunosuppression and increase the risk of infection in the post-transplant period.

Acute GvHD is treated with pulsed high-dose intravenous steroids, anti-thymocyte globulin (ATG), and monoclonal antibodies directed against mature T-cell antigens (anti-CD52). Tacrolimus may be used instead of cyclosporin A.

In the context of BMT for haematological malignancy, a degree of GvHD is often felt desirable because of a graft-versus-leukaemia (GvL) effect, leading to better elimination of minimal residual leukaemic cells. At present, however, there is no reliable way of developing a specific GvL without a damaging GvHD.

Chronic GvHD has many features in common with systemic sclerosis and related collagen–vascular diseases. The skin becomes thickened and waxy, with increased collagen deposition and pigmentation. There is severe malabsorption due to damage to the intestinal mucosa. There is a sicca syndrome, with dry eyes and mouth. The liver and lungs (interstitial pneumonitis) are frequently involved. Immunosuppression is profound and 25 per cent of patients will die from infection; the dysregulation of the immune system leads to the development of multiple autoantibodies and both hypo- and hypergammaglobulinaemia may occur. Those who have had acute GvHD are more likely to develop chronic GvHD. There is usually a marked increase in peripheral blood CD8+ T cells. The outlook is grim. Treatment is with corticosteroids plus cyclosporin A; thalidomide is being tried (it has an anti-TNF activity).

Solid organ transplantation

Routine solid organ transplantation now includes kidney, liver, heart, lung and, more recently, the small bowel. The shortage of donor organs places a significant constraint on the use of solid organ transplantation. Frequently organs are less than optimal in terms of matching and infection status of the donor. For cardiac transplantation and liver transplantation, MHC matching is rarely carried out, partly due to the need to press ahead quickly with the transplant procedure. Pancreatic transplants are matched for MHC and ABO status. For renal transplants more extensive matching is performed, including testing for pre-formed antibodies, as reasonable preservation fluids have been developed; even so, eventual outcome is dependent on keeping the ischaemic time as short as possible. Screening and matching for CMV status, although recognized to be desirable, is not always possible. Anti-rejection therapy is usually commenced with three drugs (prednisolone, azathioprine, and either cyclosporin A, tacrolimus (FK506), or mycophenolate mofetil), going down to two drugs after an initial period of up to 6 months (depending on progress). It has been observed for many years that both random and donor-specific pre-transplant blood transfusions improve the outcome, although the precise mechanism for this is unclear.

Immunology of rejection

Solid organ rejection is divided into four phases, and these are applicable to all types of organ:

- Hyperacute rejection (<24 hours)—mediated by pre-formed complement-fixing antibodies, usually anti-MHC class I or anti-ABO, recruitment of neutrophils, and vessel thrombosis through platelet activation. There is fever and rapid loss of organ function. Often the organ is affected immediately, as soon as the clamps are removed and the organ is revascularized. There is no treatment and the organ must be removed.
- Accelerated rejection (3–5 days)—mediated by non-complement-fixing antibodies, and recruitment of FcR-bearing cells. There is fever, swelling of the graft, and loss of function. Immunosuppressive therapy is only partially effective and repeated attacks occur, eventually leading to the need for graft removal.
- Acute rejection (6–90 days)—mediated by T cells (both CD4+ and CD8+ T cells are involved), with recruitment of phagocytic cells. Antibody may play a role and the endothelium of the graft is a major target, along with interstitial elements such as tubules. There is loss of function and graft swelling and tenderness, but less fever. Early recognition and aggressive immunosuppressive treatment with pulsed steroids, ATG, ALG, or monoclonal anti-CD3 is often effective, but bouts may recur and progress to chronic rejection. Other monoclonal antibodies, directed against T cells, are under investigation as alternative immunosuppressive agents.

- Chronic rejection (>60 days)—the precise mechanism is unknown but there is usually evidence of progressive fibrotic lesions, with vascular damage, glomerular obliteration, 'vanishing bile ducts', bronchiolitis obliterans, or accelerated coronary artery occlusion, depending on the organ grafted. Treatment is relatively ineffective and function will be lost progressively.

Immunosuppression and infection

The fact that matches are not always good means that solid organ grafts often have to be supported with high levels of continuing immunosuppression over many years. This increases significantly the risk of opportunist infections, and also increases the risks of EBV-driven lymphoid malignancy and cutaneous malignancy in the long term. Grafting organs from CMV-positive donors into CMV-negative recipients also means that acute CMV infection is likely in the post-transplant period. Acyclovir prophylaxis may help to reduce the incidence and severity of such episodes, even though it is relatively inactive against this herpesvirus. However, severe CMV infection may be very difficult to treat while patients remain on high-dose immunosuppression, and the difficult decision must be made to reduce immunosuppression and risk losing the graft. Similar constraints apply to EBV and lymphoproliferation. Azathioprine, in particular, is capable of producing a persistent humoral immunodeficiency when used in high doses over long periods: patients may then start to develop recurrent bacterial infections and should be treated with replacement IVIg.

Transplantation in early childhood (for example heart transplants) followed by immunosuppression may also lead to problems of interfering with normal immunological maturation, particularly with regard to the development of anti-polysaccharide antibody responses. This appears to be a problem mainly in those transplanted under the age of 2, when these responses have not developed.

Laboratory tests

In the immediate post-transplant period the major clinical question always revolves round the presence or absence of rejection or infection. Biopsy with immunostaining is the mainstay of diagnosis; markers such as β2-microglobulin, sICAM-1, and sCD25 (IL-2R) may have a certain predictive value, but also tend to rise in infection so there is no really clear distinction.

When high-dose immunosuppression is used, it is useful to monitor peripheral T-cell numbers to ensure that drugs such as anti-CD3 and ATG have been effective in eliminating T cells. ATG, in particular, suffers from batch to batch variation. Failure of therapy may also be due to the development of anti-mouse or anti-rabbit antibodies in the recipient. Some laboratories can measure these, as part of the monitoring process.

Solid organ transplantation *(cont.)*

Full investigation of T- and B-cell function may be necessary when there are problems of recurrent infections in those on chronic immunosuppression (see Chapter 3). This is particularly important in children receiving transplants (usually cardiac) followed by immunosuppression early in life (under 2 years of age), as the immunosuppression may lead to long-term failure of development of immune responsiveness to polysaccharide antigens.

10 Immunotherapy

Introduction

The aim of this chapter is to giver an overview of the very complex
but exciting area of immunotherapy. Despite great advances in the
basic science, the results of clinical immunotherapy have not been
as good as had been hoped. None the less, the advances in basic
immunology continue to provide new avenues to explore.

Major mechanisms of immunomodulation

- Immunization:
    - active
    - passive
- Replacement therapy:
    - immunoglobulin (IM, SC, IV)
    - C1-esterase inhibitor
    - α1-antitrypsin
    - plasma
- Immune stimulants:
    - drugs
    - cytokines
- Immune suppressants:
    - drugs
    - monoclonal antibodies
    - cytokines and antagonists
    - IVIg
    - antibody removal (plasmapheresis)
- Desensitization:
    - bees and wasps
    - other allergens
- Anti-inflammatory agents:
    - NSAID
    - anti-cytokines (anti-TNF); IL-1ra
    - anti-endotoxin MAb
    - anti-CD4 MAb
- Adoptive immunotherapy:
    - bone marrow transplantation
    - stem-cell transplantation
    - thymic transplants?

405

Passive immunization

Protection is provided by transfer of specific, high-titre antibody from donor to recipient. The effect is transient (maximum protection 6 months). Protection is immediate (unlike active immunization).

- Problems:
  - risk of transmission of viruses
  - serum sickness (including demyelination); acute reactions
  - development of antibodies against infused antibodies reduce effectiveness
  - identification of suitable donors (Lassa fever; rabies).
- Types:
  - pooled specific human immunoglobulin
  - animal sera (antitoxins, antivenins)
  - ?monoclonal antibodies (anti-endotoxin).
- Uses:
  - hepatitis A prophylaxis (but new vaccine provides active immunization and longer prophylaxis)
  - hepatitis B (for needlestick injuries), tetanus, rabies, Lassa fever
  - botulism, VZV (especially during pregnancy and the immunocompromised), diphtheria, snake bites (post-exposure)
  - rhesus incompatibility (post-delivery anti-D).

Active immunization

The purposes of active immunization are to:
- stimulate the production of protective antibody (opsonization, complement fixation, enhanced phagocytosis, blocking uptake (virus neutralization));
- stimulate antigen-specific T cells: whether these are Th1 or Th2 cells depends on the type of pathogen and the optimal protective response;
- produce long-lasting immunological memory (T and B cells): this is mediated by the retention of antigen on follicular dendritic cells in lymph nodes, leading to a long-term depot, and also explains why antibody levels often persist years after the primary course of immunizations have been completed, rather than decaying to zero.
- to produce 'herd immunity': the generation of a sufficiently large pool of immune individuals reduces the opportunity for wild-type disease to spread, increasing the effectiveness of the immunization programme; over 75 per cent immunization rates are required to achieve this.

Active immunization can use either purified component, e.g. toxin (inactivated = toxoid), or subcomponent or live attenuated pathogen (e.g. BCG, polio). This can be combined with passive immunization (although this may reduce the development of long-term immunological memory). This approach is used for tetanus and rabies as a strategy for treatment, post-exposure.

Toxoid/subcomponent vaccines

- Immune response frequently requires augmentation with adjuvants
- May be side-effects from adjuvants
- No risk that disease will be produced
- Inactivation may damage key epitopes and reduce protection
- Safe to use in the immunocompromised but responses (and protection) unpredictable

Attenuated vaccines

- Usually more immunogenic and do not require adjuvants
- Risk of reversion to wild type (e.g. polio)
- Side-effects from culture contaminants (demyelination from duck embryo rabies)
- May produce mild form of disease (measles, mumps)
- Contraindicated in immunosuppressed (paralytic polio in antibody deficiency)
- Unexpected viral contaminants (SV40 and polio; hepatitis B and yellow fever)

General problems of active immunization

Active immunization has a number of problems, including:
- allergy to any component (e.g. residual egg protein, often in viral vaccines from the growth media);
- reduced/absent responses in immunocompromised (including splenectomy);
- delay in achieving protection (primary and secondary immune responses require multiple injection schedules);
- preferred route of administration (site of IM; SC, ID): route of administration may determine the type of immune response and this needs to be relevant for the route of infection of the pathogen (e.g. need for mucosal immunity to enteric organisms);
- storage: most live vaccines require refrigerated storage to maintain potency; this may be a problem, especially in tropical countries;
- the age at which a vaccine is administered may alter the response. Children under the age of 24 months respond poorly to polysaccharide antigens, as do the elderly; maternal antibody and concomitant medical illness and associated drug therapy may reduce the response. Ideally responses should be checked serologically in patients where there may be a poor response. However, serological unresponsiveness does not preclude good T-cell immunity.

Additional stimulation of the immune system

Poorly immunogenic antigens may be used if combined with agents that non-specifically increase immune responses ('adjuvants').

Adjuvants
- 'Depot' of antigen (alum precipitated; oil)
- Non-specific stimulation (Freund's; MDP); Freund's adjuvant is too potent to be used in humans! It has however been safely used in microlitre quantities
- Polymerization (liposomes; ISCOMS—Quil A)
- Expression in vectors (e.g. use of vaccinia; chimeric viruses; BCG, *Salmonella*)

411

Modern approaches to vaccine development

Development of more potent but safer vaccines is always the goal. Molecular techniques have been used to modify pathogens through site-specific mutation, reducing pathogenicity, or by inserting the gene into a carrier (Vaccinia, *Salmonella*). The problem with this approach is that the development of the host response to the carrier organisms means that it can only be used once. Recombinant organisms may also be used to target antigens to particular cells: for example, *Salmonella* are rapidly taken up by macrophages, so that any additional inserted gene products will also be directed straight to antigen-presenting cells. Molecular techniques may allow the safe synthesis of bulk quantities of antigen (e.g. Hepatitis B surface antigen), although the source of antigen needs to be selected carefully to ensure that the antigen's post-translational modification (glycosylation) matches that which would be found in natural infection. Other tricks to improve the immune response include conjugation of poorly immunogenic antigens (such as polysaccharides) to immunogenic proteins, such that the humoral immune response to the polysaccharide switches from IgG2 to IgG1 and IgG3. The use of specific peptides is being used experimentally to try to stimulate specific T-cell responses; epitope mapping of antigens to determine the T- and B-cell epitopes is required.

Direct injection into muscle of nucleic acid coding for specific genes, coupled to gold microsphere carriers, has also been shown to generate an immune response. Rather than being degraded, the nucleic acid is taken up into myocytes and specific protein production can be detected for several months thereafter, leading to an excellent depot preparation. The concern is that there may be a bystander attack by the immune system upon the myocytes containing the injected DNA.

To generate an effective immune response, both host and pathogen factors need to be taken into account. Factors encouraging the development of an effective vaccine include:
- the infectious agent:
  - one or a small number of serotypes; little or no antigenic drift
  - pathogen is only moderately or poorly infectious
  - antigens for B- and T-cell epitopes are readily available
  - the immune response can be induced readily at the site of natural infection
  - wild-type infection is known to produce protective immunity
  - availability of animal models to test vaccine strategies;
- host factors:
  - humoral and cellular immunity is readily induced
  - MHC background of population is favourable to a high response
  - proposed antigens induce appropriate Th1 or Th2 response.

Factors that mitigate against an appropriate immunization response and therefore prevent the development of good vaccines include:
- infectious agent:
    - marked antigenic variation/drift; many serotypes causing disease. This limits the ability to generate an effective vaccine (e.g. pneumococcal disease)
    - potential for change in host range of the pathogen (e.g. change in cell tropism of viruses such as HIV)
    - infection may be transmitted by infected cells which are not recognized by the immune system even after immunization
    - integration of viral DNA into the host genome (latency)
    - natural infection does not induce protective immunity
    - pathogen uses 'escape' mechanisms:
        - (i) resistant external coats, e.g. mycobacteria
        - (ii) poorly immunogenic capsular polysaccharides
        - (iii) antigenic variation in response to host immune recognition, e.g. influenza virus, malaria
        - (iv) camouflage with host proteins, e.g. CMV and β2-microglobulin
        - (v) production of proteins similar to host proteins, e.g. enterobacteria; may give rise to autoimmunity
        - (vi) extracellular enzyme production to interfere with host defence (Protein A)
        - (vii) production of molecules that disrupt immune responses, e.g. superantigens
    - pathogen-induced immunosuppression; failure to form appropriate response (e.g. complement-fixing antibodies)
    - no suitable animal model;
- host factors:
    - immune response is inappropriate, e.g. antibody when cellular response is required (e.g. leishmaniasis)
    - immune response enhances infection, e.g. antibody formation may enhance infection through increased uptake into macrophages (yellow fever; ?HIV)
    - cells of immune system are target of infection
    - 'wrong' MHC background predisposes to a low response or autoimmunity.

The ultimate goal of any immunization programme is the eradication of the disease. This requires that the infection is limited only to humans, with no animal or environmental reservoir, and the absence of any subclinical or carrier state in humans. Achieving elimination requires a high level of herd immunity to prevent person-to-person spread. This requires considerable infrastructural support to ensure that all at-risk populations are targeted for immunization. This has only been achieved for smallpox, although we are close to the elimination of polio.

413

'Replacement' therapy

This is used for treatment of primary and some secondary immune deficiencies:

Type of deficiency	Replacement therapy
Humoral immune deficiency	Immunoglobulin
	(Plasma)
	α1-antitrypsin
Cellular immune deficiency	Bone marrow transplantation
	Fetal thymus transplantation
	(?thymic hormones: thymosin)
Combined immune deficiency	Immunoglobulin
	Bone marrow transplantation
	Stem-cell transplantation
	Red-cell transfusions/PEG-ADA
	IL-2 and γ-IFN
	Gene therapy (ADA deficiency)
Phagocytic cell defects	Bone marrow transplantation
	Granulocytic transfusions
	Interferons/G-CSF/GM-CSF/IL-3
	(antibiotics/antifungals)
Complement deficiency	C1-esterase inhibitor

Intravenous immunoglobulin (IVIg) for replacement therapy

IVIg is a blood product which is prepared by cold ethanol precipitation of pooled plasma, usually from a donor pool of more than 1000 donors. Subsequent purification steps vary between different manufacturers but all are based on the original Cohn fractionation process. The IgA content is variable, as is the IgG subclass content. Levels of IgA may be important when treating IgA-deficient patients, who may recognize the infused IgA as foreign and respond to it, leading to anaphylactoid responses on subsequent exposure. It is uncertain how much of a problem this, and there is no standardized method for detecting clinically significant anti-IgA antibodies. The product should have low levels of pre-kallikrein activator, fragments, and aggregates as these three contribute substantially to the generation of adverse events on infusion.

Variations of IgG subclasses do not seem to make significant differences to the effectiveness as replacement therapy. Comparing the presence of functional antibodies in individual products is difficult as there are no internationally standardized assays, but IVIg must have intact opsonic and complement-fixing function (some second-generation IVIg lacked adequate opsonic function and were relatively ineffective).

Uses

IVIg is mandatory for replacement in the major antibody deficiencies (XLA, CVID), and in combined immunodeficiencies (pre- and immediately post-BMT). Patients with secondary hypogammaglobulinaemia, such as CLL and myeloma, should also receive IVIg, although patients must be clear as to the objectives of therapy. The role of IVIg in IgG subclass and specific antibody deficiency is less secure, and regular prophylactic antibiotics might be tried first, with IVIg reserved for continuing infection despite therapy. Where there is doubt, giving a 1-year trial is reasonable, with monitoring of clinical effectiveness through the use of symptom diaries. To ensure a realistic trial, adequate dosing and frequency of infusions must be undertaken to ensure that benefit is obvious.

Dose regimes should aim to provide 0.2–0.6 g/kg/month given every 2–3 weeks; for older patients with CLL, an initial monthly schedule might be tried. However, most patients on monthly schedules find that after 2–3 weeks they start feeling non-specifically unwell or develop breakthrough infections. Under these circumstances the interval should be shortened. Rare hypercatabolic patients, or those with urinary or gastrointestinal loss, may require weekly infusions.

The dose should be adjusted according to the trough IgG level, aiming to achieve a trough IgG level within the normal range, as this has been shown to reduce lung damage; whether higher levels within the normal range are better is unknown, although most clinical immunologists will run patients with known lung disease at higher trough levels than those with no lung damage.

Adverse reactions

Most adverse reactions are determined by the speed of infusion and the presence of underlying infection. Untreated patients receiving their first infusions are most at risk. Reactions are typical immune complex reactions, with headache, myalgia, arthralgia, and fever, progressing to respiratory involvement, hypotension, collapse, and chest pain. Pretreatment of the patient with antibiotics before the first infusion reduces antigenic load, and hydrocortisone (100–200 mg IV) and an oral antihistamine before the infusion are also of benefit. The first infusion should be given at no more than two-thirds of the manufacturer's recommended rate, and it is worth starting slowly and gradually increasing. Similar precautions may be required before the second infusion.

Infection represents a major concern: hepatitis B is no longer an issue, but there have been a significant number of outbreaks of hepatitis C; the possible role of other hepatitis viruses, such as HGV, are currently being evaluated. There appears to be no risk of HIV transmission, as the process rapidly destroys the virus. The safety in respect of prion disease is not known. Newer products have specific antiviral steps such as pasteurization, solvent–detergent treatment, and nanofiltration. It should not be assumed that these products are 'safe' as a result of these measures, although they may reduce the risk.

All patients must receive counselling concerning the potential infective risks and this must be recorded in the notes (dated and signed).

Severe anaphylactoid reactions have been reported after changing brands: IVIg products are not interchangeable and once a patient is established on a product, it must not be changed except for overriding clinical reasons. Batch exposure should also be kept to a minimum, and there must be a robust system for recording batch numbers.

417

Monitoring

All patients on IVIg should have regular trough IgG levels measured, together with liver function testing, as an early warning for transmissible hepatitis. A reasonable schedule is to check every second infusion. In the event of unexpected reactions, immediate blood sampling for evidence of elevated mast-cell tryptase, complement activation (C3, C4, C3d), and checking for anti-IgA antibodies (if IgA deficient) and for infection (CRP) should be undertaken. Rare antibody-deficient patients seem to react persistently to IVIgs: changing to a different product may sometimes assist; occasionally continued prophylactic antihistamines, paracetamol, or even steroids may be required before each infusion to ensure compliance with therapy.

Intravenous immunoglobulin (IVIg) for replacement therapy *(cont.)*

Home therapy

For patients with primary immunodeficiencies, home treatment is a well-established alternative to hospital therapy. To be eligible, patients must meet the criteria in the table. Specific centres in the UK are recognized as being able to provide appropriate training: patients should not be sent home on IVIg without having been formally trained and certified by an approved centre, which will also arrange for long-term support. The Primary Immunodeficiency Association* can provide details of approved centres.

*Primary Immunodeficiency Association
Alliance House
12 Caxton Street
London SW1H 0QS
Tel: 0171 976 7640; Fax: 0171 976 7641
e-mail pimmune@dial.pipex.com

Intravenous immunoglobulin (IVIg) for replacement therapy

Criteria for home therapy	Comments
4–6 months' hospital therapy	Must be reaction free
Patient motivated	
Patient has trainable partner	Infusions must never be done alone
Patient has good venous access	Portacaths are not recommended for long-term use in immunodeficient patients
GP must be supportive	GP will be first on-call if there are difficulties
Patient must have a phone	To call for assistance
Patient must accept regular follow up by the training centre	
Patient must complete infusion logs	For batch monitoring

Intramuscular immunoglobulin (IMIg)

There is no role for IMIg in replacement therapy. Administered doses are too low to be effective in preventing infection. However, occasional older patients prefer the convenience of a weekly injection at their GP's surgery to hospital-based infusions. IMIg has been associated with an adverse reaction rate of 20%.

Subcutaneous immunoglobulin (SCIg)

For those with poor venous access, high-dose subcutaneous immunoglobulin replacement is at least equivalent to IVIg in terms of maintaining adequate trough IgG levels and preventing infection. A 16 per cent solution of immunoglobulin is used (usually preparations for IM use), and is administered in a weekly dose of 100 mg/kg via a syringe driver, in multiple sites. Tolerability is reasonable, with local irritation being the only significant side-effect. At present no products are licensed for subcutaneous use.

10 Immunotherapy

Intramuscular immunoglobulin (IMIg)
Subcutaneous immunoglobulin (SCIg)

C1-Esterase inhibitor

Deficiency of C1-esterase inhibitor causes episodic angioedema which may be fatal if involving the upper airway (see Chapter 2).

Purified C1 inhibitor is available. This is a blood-derived product that is available in the UK on a named-patient basis (Baxter-Immuno). It is steam treated as an antiviral precaution but the same precautions apply as to IVIg and patients should be counselled as for IVIg, and the fact recorded in the clinical notes. Liver function tests and hepatitis serology (HBV and HCV) should be checked prior to treatment and batch numbers recorded. The product is expensive and should be reserved for major attacks (all attacks above the shoulders); it is relatively ineffective against attacks involving the bowel, for which conservative management with fluids, analgesics, and non-steroidal anti-inflammatories is more successful. It can be used prophylactically prior to surgery.

The dose is 1000–1500 Units administered as a slow bolus IV; this should raise the C1-esterase inhibitor level in the serum to above 50 per cent for several days and will prevent attacks when used prophylactically. When used as treatment, it will prevent attacks progressing, but does *not* lead to a dramatic resolution of symptoms; accordingly laryngeal oedema may require other measures, such as tracheostomy, as urgent procedures.

Plasma can be used if the purified concentrate is unavailable, but is less effective and may even increase the oedema by providing fresh substrate for the complement and kinin cascades. Pooled virally inactivated FFP is now available, and may carry a reduced risk of infection, although this is debated.

422

α1-Antitrypsin (α1AT)

α1AT deficiency leads to progressive emphysema and to liver disease. Purified α1AT is now available on a named-patient basis. Trials have not been that encouraging, but this is because late-stage patients with established disease have been involved. No good prophylactic trials have been undertaken in asymptomatic patients so it is not yet known how effective the drug is in preventing complications. Supplementation may also be useful during acute infections when high local levels of trypsin are released by activated neutrophils. Infusions need to be given at least weekly to maintain enzyme activity.

10 Immunotherapy

C1-Esterase inhibitor
α1-Antitrypsin (α1AT)

Immune stimulation

Specific immune stimulation = immunization (see above).

Non-specific immune stimulation has been the holy grail of some clinical researchers but the results have been uniformly disappointing! A large number of agents have been tried but few have found favour in routine clinical practice. Certain nutritional supplements may have a limited role, although this is controversial. α-Interferon is probably the most successful, being a useful adjunctive therapy in the treatment of viral hepatitis. Benefit has also been claimed for levamisole in malignant disease (colonic cancer). IL-2 may have some slight benefit in renal tumours and melanoma, but is too toxic for routine use. Colony-stimulating factors have a significant effect indirectly by increasing the availability of host components (macrophages and neutrophils).

Biological immunostimulants	Synthetic immunostimulants
Thymic factors	Levamisole (unlicensed)
Tuftsin	Isoprinosine (licensed)
Transfer Factors	Azimexon (experimental)
BCG	Cimetidine (licensed, but not as an
Bestatin	immunomodulator)
Lentinan	
Muramyl dipeptide	
C parvum	
Cytokines	
(i) Interleukin-2	
(ii) Interferons (α and γ)	
(iii) Growth factors	

Immune suppression/immunomodulation

- Drugs:
  - corticosteroids
  - cytotoxics/anti-metabolites: azathioprine, cyclophosphamide, methotrexate, chlorambucil, 2-CDA, fludarabine
  - cyclosporin/tacrolimus/sirolimus/mycophenolate
  - cromoglycate
  - cimetidine
  - anti-TNF drugs (thalidomide, oxypentifylline)
  - antimalarials (hydroxychloroquine, mepacrine)
  - sulphasalazine
- Biologicals:
  - intravenous high-dose immunoglobulin
  - polyclonal xeno-antisera (rabbit ATG)
  - monoclonal antibodies (OKT3, anti-CD25); chimeric antibodies
  - blood transfusion (NB Factor VIII)
  - cytokines (γ-IFN)
  - anti-cytokines; cytokine receptor antagonists
- Physical
  - plasmapheresis
  - specific immunoadsorption (protein G columns)
  - total lymphoid irradiation
  - thoracic duct drainage

427

Corticosteroids

These drugs are based on endogenous products of the adrenal cortex and form the mainstay of immunosuppressive therapy; synthetic compounds are more potent. Natural steroids are highly plasma bound (corticosteroid binding globulin; albumin). Actions of corticosteroids are manifold.

Actions

- Transiently increased neutrophils (decreased margination and release of mature neutrophils from marrow)
- Decreased phagocytosis and release of enzymes (lysosomal stabilization)
- Marked monocytopenia and reduced monokine (IL-1) production
- Alteration of cellular gene expression (high-affinity cytoplasmic receptor translocated to nucleus) via nF-κB inhibition through increased cytoplasmic concentrations of IκBα
- Release of lipomodulin (inhibits phospholipase A2 with reduction of arachidonic acid metabolites)
- Lymphopenia due to sequestration in lymphoid tissue and interference with recirculation (CD4+ T cells > CD8+ T cells > B cells) and lymphocytotoxic effects (high doses)
- Decreased T-cell proliferative responses (inhibit entry into G1 phase)
- Reduced serum IgG and IgA
- No effect on NK or antibody-dependent cell-mediated cytotoxicity (ADCC) activity

Side-effects

- Carbohydrate metabolism: poor cellular glucose uptake; increased hepatic gluconeogenesis and glycogen deposition
- Increased lipolysis and free fatty acid (FFA); increased selective fat deposition
- Inhibit protein synthesis and enhance protein catabolism
- Increase glomerular filtration rate (GFR) and sodium retention; decrease calcium absorption, inhibit osteoblasts

Clinical side-effects are multitudinous: diabetes, hyperlipidaemia, obesity, poor wound healing, growth arrest (children), myopathy, hypertension, purpura, cataracts, glaucoma, peptic ulcer, allergy (synthetic steroids), aseptic necrosis, and psychiatric complications. Patients on medium- to long-term treatment should therefore have regular checks of blood sugar and bone mineral density. Prophylactic therapy against bone loss is highly desirable, especially in females and all older patients. Optimal therapy is yet to be determined but includes hormone replacement therapy (HRT) (if not contraindicated by underlying disease), vitamin D, and calcium, or cyclical Didronel® and calcium.

Doses of over 20 mg/day for long periods may also increase the risk of opportunist infection with *Pneumocystis carinii*; consideration should therefore be given to the use of low-dose co-trimoxazole.

Uses

- Autoimmune diseases, e.g. SLE, vasculitis, rheumatoid arthritis
- Polymyalgia rheumatica, giant-cell arthritis
- Allergic diseases (asthma, hay fever)
- Inflammatory diseases (Crohn's disease)
- Malignant disease (lymphoma)
- Allograft rejection
- Other immunological diseases (ITP, glomerulonephritis)

Dosage regimes

These are variable according to the disease being treated and up-to-date literature should always be consulted. Prednisolone is the stock drug, other steroids have little advantage but the BNF has equivalency tables. Enteric-coated tablets are kinder to patients, but may lead to erratic absorption; if plain steroids are used, gastro-protection with either an H2-antagonist or proton-pump inhibitor is most effective in preventing ulceration. The trend is now to use low-dose steroids for RhA (prednisolone 7.5 mg/day); for SLE higher doses (up to 30 mg/day) are required (larger doses for cerebral lupus). Life-threatening immunological disease requires much higher doses, 1–2 mg/kg, orally or IV. Various pulsed regimes using IV methylprednisolone have been advocated, especially in acute vasculitis. The evidence is split over their effectiveness: 10 mg/kg is advocated, pulsed at varying intervals, often in combination with IV cytotoxics. Topical steroids with limited absorption are invaluable in controlling local allergic symptoms (asthma, hay fever).

429

Where patients who have been on long-term steroids are being tailed off, they will remain adrenally suppressed for up to 6 months after cessation of therapy and should therefore have steroid cover for illnesses, operations, etc. Patients should carry warning cards.

CYTOTOXIC DRUGS

Azathioprine

Azathioprine is converted *in vivo* to 6-mercaptopurine and acts to inhibit the synthesis of inosinic acid (precursor of purines) thus inhibiting DNA synthesis and reducing cell replication.

Actions

- Preferentially inhibits T-cell activation rather than B-cell activation
- Reduces the circulation of large 'activated' lymphocytes, but has little effect on small resting lymphocytes
- In long-term use causes significant lymphopenia (T and B cells)
- Hypogammaglobulinaemia, due to inhibition of B-cell proliferation (less or no effect on T-cell proliferation)
- Suppression of monokine production

Side-effects

- Causes profound bone marrow suppression: this is related to deficiency alleles of the enzyme thiopurine methyltransferase (TPMT) involved in its metabolism. Genetic screening is now available through the Purine Research Laboratory at Guy's Hospital, London
- Toxic hepatitis (? related to TPMT deficiency)
- Opportunist infections (including HSV, papillomaviruses)
- Gastric upset (probably also related to TPMT deficiency)
- Teratogenicity
- ? Malignancy (lymphoma)

Uses

- Autoimmune diseases (SLE, rheumatoid arthritis, vasculitis, liver disease, myasthenia, inflammatory bowel disease)
- As a 'steroid-sparing' agent

Dosage

In view of the potential for severe/fatal side-effects, azathioprine must be introduced carefully. The initial dose should not exceed 1 mg/kg and the patient should receive weekly full blood counts with a differential white count for the first month of therapy. If there is any drop in platelets or white cells, it is unsafe to continue with therapy. Deficiency alleles for TPMT are present in 1 in 300 of the population: pretreatment screening is helpful, although it is unlikely to be available urgently. If it is tolerated, then the dose can be increased to 2.5 mg/kg (or in special circumstances to 4 mg/kg). The need for continuing therapy needs to be reviewed regularly. Hypogammaglobulinaemia may be severe and require replacement therapy, although recovery may eventually occur over several years.

Liver function tests must also be monitored. Allopurinol is contra-indicated with azathioprine as it interferes with elimination and raises blood levels.

Cyclophosphamide and chlorambucil (alkylating agents)

These drugs bind to and cross-link DNA and possibly also RNA, thus interfering with DNA replication and transcription. Effects are dependent on the phase of the cell cycle during exposure and the competence of the DNA repair mechanisms.

Actions

- Dose-dependent lymphopenia (T (CD8 > CD4) and B cells)
- Reduced B-cell proliferation and antibody synthesis (reduced IgG and IgM)
- Lesser effect on T cells (CD8 >> CD4, which may actually enhance T-cell responsiveness under certain circumstances)

Side-effects

- Bone marrow depression
- Alopecia
- Haemorrhagic cystitis (acrolein)—ensure good hydration and use mesna for doses above 200 mg/kg; may be less risk with pulsed IV therapy
- Sterility (males and females—offer males sperm banking and warn all patients of reproductive age and record in notes)
- Secondary lymphoid neoplasms (especially NHL (11-fold increase), bladder tumours (10 per cent long-term), skin tumours (fivefold increase), and acute myeloblastic leukaemia)
- Opportunist infections (use co-trimoxazole and antifungal prophylaxis)
- Nausea and vomiting (high dose)

Major uses

- Vasculitis, especially Wegener's granulomatosis, PAN, M-PAN, CSS
- SLE and RhA
- Glomerulonephritis (including Goodpasture's)

Dosage

There is considerable debate over the optimal regimes for use of cyclophosphamide: there are exponents of both continuous low-dose oral cyclophosphamide (2–4 mg/kg/day) versus the use of intravenous pulse therapy (10 mg/kg/pulse or 0.75–1 g/m^2 body surface area, intervals determined by protocol and blood counts). Long-term side-effects may be higher with continuous oral therapy, but this may reflect the higher total dose, and lower doses may be effective. In life-threatening conditions, high-dose IV pulses, with IV steroids, will have a faster effect (remember mesna cover and IV fluids). Chlorambucil is used orally in doses of 0.03–0.06 mg/kg/day and is less toxic to the bladder than cyclophosphamide, but probably equally toxic to the marrow in therapeutic doses. Dosages of both drugs will require adjustment in renal impairment. Regular weekly blood counts are required.

433

Methotrexate

Methotrexate is a competitive inhibitor of the enzyme dihydrofolate reductase and impairs synthesis of tetrahydrofolate from folic acid (required as co-factor for thymidine synthesis). It therefore interferes with DNA synthesis. It is also thought to interfere with other intracellular enzymes. As an immunosuppressive agent it is used in low weekly doses (much lower than the doses used as an anti-neoplastic agent).

Actions

- Variable effects on lymphocyte numbers in peripheral blood
- Possible inhibition of monokine production
- Inhibition of lipo-oxygenase pathway
- Reduction in antibody synthesis

Side-effects

- Mucositis, nausea, and vomiting
- Bone marrow suppression (megaloblastic—may be reversed by folinic acid rescue): may be worse if other anti-folate drugs are co-administered, e.g. sulphasalazine, co-trimoxazole
- Hepatic fibrosis (dose-related)
- Pneumonitis (5 per cent of patients)
- Sterility

Uses

- RhA; psoriatic arthropathy
- Polymyositis/dermatomyositis
- GvHD in BMT

Dosage

The drug is given weekly either orally or IM; initial dose is 7.5 mg (adult), increased stepwise depending upon side-effects and clinical benefit to a maximum of 20–30 mg/week. Dose may need reducing in renal impairment. Care needs to be taken with co-administration of other drugs. Folinic acid rescue may relieve severe side-effects (given 24–36 hours later).

Monitoring should include baseline Fbc, LFTs, chest radiograph, and lung function; thereafter weekly pre-dose full blood counts and regular liver function tests are required; if abnormal LFTs are noted, the drug dose should be reduced or the drug stopped. It is thought that the risks of monitoring for liver disease by biopsy outweigh any benefit. Development of pneumonitis is an absolute indication for withdrawing the drug: high-dose steroids may be required.

2-Chloro-deoxyadenosine (2CDA) and fludarabine

These two drugs act by inhibition of adenosine deaminase, i.e. effectively producing 'SCID'. Their primary use is in the treatment of haematological malignancy, but they have the potential, with careful use, to be potent immunosuppressive agents. Both produce a profound and long-lasting CD4$^+$ T-cell lymphopenia.

OTHER DRUGS

Cyclosporin/tacrolimus (FK506)/sirolimus (rapamycin)

These three agents are macrolide antibiotics derived from fungi. They act specifically on T-helper cells, but leave other cell types unaffected. Target cells are inhibited but not killed (therefore effects are fully reversible on cessation of treatment).

Modes of action

- Cyclosporin A (CyA) interacts with cyclophilin, a 17 kDa protein (peptidyl-prolyl *cis-trans* isomerase) and tacrolimus interacts with FK-BP, a 12 kDa protein, similar to cyclophilin
- The complex prevents calcineurin, a calcium- and calmodulin-dependent protein, from dephosphorylating the nuclear factor of activated T cells (NF-AT), reducing transcription of the IL-2 gene
- Immunosuppressive activity is not directly related to this activity
- CyA and tacrolimus inhibit IL-2 and IL-2Ra gene expression and prevent T-cell activation (cells arrested at G0/G1)
- Sirolimus has no effect on IL-2 production; it binds FK-BP, but the complex does not inhibit calcineurin; it appears to block calcium-independent signalling (via CD28)
- May interfere with macrophage function (lymphokine release and receptor synthesis)
- CyA interferes with B-cell proliferation and antibody production

Side-effects

- Hypertension
- Hirsutism
- Nephrotoxicity
- Hepatotoxicity
- Lymphomas (NHL—85 per cent EBV+)
- Opportunist infections (CMV, papillomaviruses, HHV-8)
- Neurotoxicity
- Multiple drug interactions (CyA and tacrolimus induce cytochrome P450(IIEI))
- Diabetes (inhibition of insulin release)

Uses

- Combination therapy for allografts
- RhA, SLE
- Autoimmune diseases (uveitis, Behçet's, inflammatory bowel disease)

Dosage

CyA and tacrolimus are available orally and intravenously, although oral bioavailability of CyA is poor (improved with Neoral® formulation). Dosage for CyA depends on the circumstances, but 10–15 mg/kg/day may be required for allograft rejection, while 5 mg/kg may suffice for autoimmune disease. Tacrolimus dosage is 0.1–0.3 mg/kg/day for allograft rejection; experience of this drug is less in autoimmune disease. Monitoring of drug levels is desirable for both drugs. Sirolimus is still experimental, but because it operates on different activation pathways it may make a useful combination treatment.

Mycophenolate mofetil

This drug is a prodrug of mycophenolic acid. In its actions it is similar to azathioprine.

Actions

- Blocks inosine monophosphate dehydrogenase and blocks synthesis of guanine
- It acts predominantly on lymphocytes, to prevent proliferation

Side-effects

- Lymphopenia
- Opportunist infections (CMV, HSV)
- Lymphoma
- Hepatotoxicity

Uses

- Prophylaxis of allograft rejection

Dosage

Dosage is 1 g twice a day. Fbc and LFTs should be monitored regularly.

Brequinar

Brequinar is an experimental drug that inhibits pyrimidine synthesis. It has the greatest effects on B cells and antibody production, especially IgE. It is effective in animal models of allograft rejection.

439

D-Penicillamine

This enigmatic drug comes and goes in terms of its utility as an immunomodulator. Its precise immunological actions are not known precisely, but it decreases antibody production and inhibits T-cell proliferation, possibly through enhanced hydrogen peroxide production or through sulphydrylation of the surface receptors of the lymphocytes. Neutrophil chemotaxis and oxidative function are impaired, and macrophage antigen-presenting function and monokine production are reduced. It is also believed to inhibit collagen synthesis, hence its use in scleroderma. It is very slow in its onset of action and actually causes a range of autoimmune diseases, including myasthenia gravis, renal disease (nephrotic), SLE, polymyositis, and Goodpasture's syndrome. It is mainly used in RhA and scleroderma. Dosage is 250 mg daily increased to 1 g daily, but with regular monitoring (every 1–2 weeks initially) of renal function, urinalysis and Fbc. Penicillin-allergic patients may be at increased risk of reacting to penicillamine.

Gold

Gold may be given either as IM injections or orally, although the evidence suggests that parenteral therapy is more effective. It is concentrated selectively in macrophages, and reduces monokine production (IL-1), hence also reducing T- and B-cell responses. It impairs endothelial expression of adhesion molecules and hence reduces cellular traffic to sites of inflammation The profile of side-effects is similar to that of penicillamine, and the onset of action is also slow. It is used only in RhA. Dosage is dependent on the route and expert advice on current regimes should be sought from a clinician experienced in its use.

10 Immunotherapy

D-Penicillamine
Gold

Hydroxychloroquine/mepacrine

Antimalarials have a particular role to play in the management of joint and skin complaints in connective tissue diseases. They are also effective in relieving the fatigue experienced in association with connective tissue diseases such as SLE and Sjögren's syndrome. The mode of action is uncertain, but there is evidence that they interfere with the production of cytokines and reduction of production of granulocyte lysosomal enzymes. Their onset of action is slow. However, they are well tolerated with few side-effects: haemolysis may occur in G6PD-deficient patients and retinal toxicity is possibly a problem, although this is mainly true for chloroquine. The evidence that there is a significant risk of ocular toxicity from hydroxychloroquine is minimal, and some authorities have indicated that ocular screening is a waste of time in patients on hydroxychloroquine. If long-term therapy is considered, then baseline screening and retinal photographs should be recorded. Mepacrine stains the skin yellow.

The preferred antimalarial is hydroxychloroquine. Starting dose for hydroxychloroquine is 400 mg/day (adult), reducing to maintenance of 200 mg/day; alternatively the maximum daily dose is calculated as 6.5 mg/kg lean body mass. Mepacrine is an unlicensed drug in the context of autoimmune disease.

Thalidomide/oxypentifylline

Thalidomide is an interesting drug which has been known to reduce the severity of conversion reactions due to treatment of lepromatous leprosy. It is a potent inhibitor of TNF-α production by monocytes, due to interference with gene transcription, and also decreases the expression of adhesion molecules. Circulating CD4$^+$ T cells are reduced. It also inhibits γ-interferon production by T cells, due to preferential stimulation of Th2 cells. Side-effects include its well-documented teratogenicity, neuropathy, and drowsiness (which may limit dose). It is used especially in the management of ulceration in Behçet's syndrome and in reducing the severity of GvHD. Dosage is 100 mg/day, reducing to 50 mg on alternate days. Nerve conduction studies should be carried out as a baseline pretreatment. Women of child-bearing age must be formally counselled over the risks and agree to take appropriate contraceptive measures. This must be recorded in the notes. Thalidomide is not a licensed drug in the UK.

Oxypentifylline is a drug originally introduced for peripheral vascular disease. It has similar but weaker actions to thalidomide in inhibiting TNF production.

443

Sulphasalazine

Sulphasalazine has been around for many years, having originally been introduced as an antibiotic. It comprises sulphapyridine coupled to 5-aminosalicylic acid via a diazo bond that can be split by enteric bacteria. The precise mode of action as an immuno-modulatory agent is uncertain. It has minor immunosuppressive activities, mainly localized to the gut, but little effect on periph-eral blood lymphocyte numbers or function. It is used predominantly in rheumatoid arthritis and seronegative arthritides, in doses of 500–2000 mg/day in divided doses. It has a significant array of side-effects including male infertility, macrocytic anaemia, rash, Stevens–Johnson syndrome, and secondary hypogamma-globulinaemia.

Colchicine

Colchicine is a useful anti-inflammatory. Its precise immunological role is uncertain, but it inhibits microtubule assembly and therefore inhibits mitosis. It is concentrated in neutrophils and inhibits chemotactic activity, thus reducing the accumulation of non-specific inflammatory cells. It is valuable in Behçet's syndrome and familial Mediterranean fever. Unfortunately its value is limited by side-effects at therapeutic doses (diarrhoea and gastrointestinal discomfort); the usual dose is up to 0.5 mg four times daily, if tolerated.

445

BIOLOGICALS

High-dose IVIg

High-dose IVIg is widely used as an immunomodulatory agent in autoimmune diseases. Unfortunately many of the uses have not been well supported by proper double-blind placebo controlled trials, and in view of the potential risks of infection (increased to volume exposure in these groups, see above), this cannot be condoned. The precise mechanisms of action clinically are uncertain, although many mechanisms have been postulated.

Actions

- Fc-receptor blockade on phagocytic cells
- Inhibition of cytokine production
- Inactivation of pathogenic autoantibodies (anti-idiotypes)
- Inhibition of autoantibody production by B cells
- Decreased T-cell proliferation
- Actions of soluble cytokines, cytokine receptors, and antagonists present in IVIg
- Inhibitory actions of stabilizing sugars

Side-effects

- Aseptic meningitis (elevated lymphocytes and protein in CSF) ?secondary to sugars
- Renal failure (secondary to osmotic load from sugars)
- Massive intravascular haemolysis (secondary to IgG isoagglutinins)
- Hyperviscosity (CVAs, MI)
- Immune complex reactions in patients with high-titre rheumatoid factors, or other immune complex disease, e.g. SLE
- Anaphylactoid reactions (IgA deficiency; infected)

Main uses

- Replacement therapy for primary and secondary immuno-deficiencies (see above)
- Autoimmune cytopenias (ITP, AIHA)
- Vasculitis: Kawasaki syndrome, Wegener's granulomatosis
- Neurological diseases (acute Guillain–Barré, CIDP, pure motor neuropathy, myasthenia gravis, LEMS, MS)
- Factor VIII and Factor IX inhibitors
- Anti-phospholipid antibodies in pregnancy
- Autoimmune skin disease (pemphigus, pemphigoid, epidermolysis bullosa acquisita)
- Polymyositis, dermatomyositis

Dosage

The dosage regimes range from 0.4 g/kg/day for 5 days, through 1 g/day for 2 days to 2 g/kg/day as a single dose. Minimal evidence is available to distinguish between the schedules. Fewer doses may be required for ITP. My own practice is to start all high-dose regimes on the 5-day schedule to assess tolerability and then increase to 1 g/kg/day for 2 days subsequently. In adults and children, risks of renal impairment and aseptic meningitis are highest with the ultra-rapid infusion schedule of 2 g/kg/day, and I tend to avoid this if possible. Rapid infusions should be avoided in all elderly patients because of the risks of hyperviscosity.

Pretreatment, IgA deficiency and high-titre rheumatoid factors should be excluded, and renal function assessed. Pretreatment Fbc, LFTs, and hepatitis serology (HBV, HCV) should also be measured. IgA-deficient patients require special care, and should be on products low in IgA (Octagam®, Alphaglobin®, Gammagard-SD®, Vigam-S®). If there is renal impairment to start with, daily creatinines should be measured, and if there is a rise of 10 per cent or more, then therapy should be discontinued. Fbc should be repeated during the course to ensure that haemolysis does not take place (haptoglobin is a sensitive indicator of intravascular haemolysis). Infusion rates should follow manufacturers' guidelines and there must be no switching of products. Batch numbers MUST be recorded.

447

Polyclonal antibodies

Xenogeneic antisera raised by the immunization of animals with purified human T cells or thymocytes (rabbit anti-thymocyte globulin (ATG) and rabbit anti-lymphocyte globulin (ALG)) are potent immunosuppressive agents and cause a profound lymphopenia. They are difficult to standardize and have significant batch-to-batch variation. They also contain cross-reactive antibodies that react with other cells types, including platelets. Their utility is limited by the development of a host-anti-rabbit response which both neutralizes the xeno-antiserum and also gives rise to a serum sickness reaction.

Actions

- Complement-mediated lymphocyte destruction
- Cause marked but variable lymphopenia
- Reduced T-cell function

Uses

- Acute graft rejection or GvHD
- Diamond–Blackfan syndrome

Dosage

Dosage depends on batch but is usually within the range of 5–30 mg/kg/day. Their effect can be monitored by absolute lymphocyte counts or flow cytometric analysis of peripheral blood lymphocytes.

Monoclonal antibodies

Monoclonal antibodies, raised in mice, can be more specific (e.g. anti-CD3, anti-CD25, anti-CD52 (Campath®), anti-CD4, anti-LFA-1, anti-ICAM-1, anti-Tcrαβ) and can be targeted at specific cells (e.g. activated T cells, anti-CD25); they can be 'humanized', so that only the antigen-binding site is mouse, the rest of the antibody being human IgG. The most widely used is anti-CD3 (OKT3, anti-CD3 ε-chain).

Uses

• Acute graft rejection (second line after ATG) or GvHD

Side-effects

• Severe lymphopenia
• Excess cytokine release (TNF)
• Opportunist infections
• Lymphoproliferative disease
• Anti-mouse response (if not humanized) and serum sickness

Recombinant proteins (chimeric proteins)   449

Genetically engineered proteins, such as CD4-Ig heavy chain, have been produced but their therapeutic roles remain to be defined.

PHYSICAL METHODS

Total lymphoid irradiation (TLI)

TLI is experimental as an immunosuppressive therapy, having been used previously for the treatment of lymphoid malignancies. It produces profound impairment of T-cell numbers and function although there is a small population of radioresistant small lymphocytes. A more modern variant is to use UV sensitizing agents and then irradiate leucocytes in an extracorporeal circulation (photopheresis). TLI may be of benefit in intractable rheumatoid arthritis, multiple sclerosis, and severe SLE.

Side-effects

- Leucopenia
- Thrombocytopenia
- Opportunist infections
- Lymphoma (NHL)

Thoracic duct drainage

This has been used in the past for treatment of severe RhA. It causes a severe and long-lasting immunosuppression. Similar effects are seen from accidental thoracic duct damage in oesophageal and cardiac surgery, where a chylous effusion is allowed to drain unchecked. A profound and persistent lymphopenia of both T and B cells is caused. Recovery of immune function may occur over a long period. Prophylaxis against Pneumocystis carinii pneumonia and fungal infections will be required if the drainage is accidental.

10 Immunotherapy

Total lymphoid irradiation
Thoracic duct drainage

Plasmapheresis

Plasmapheresis is the removal of plasma constituents using automated cell separators; the plasma components are removed by either centrifugation of membrane filtration. The erythrocytes and other cellular components are reinfused and the removed plasma replaced with either FFP or FFP + IVIg to maintain circulating volume. About 50 per cent of the plasma is removed each time and a therapeutic course is usually 3–5 daily treatments. The amount of antibody removed depends on volume of distribution and so 90 per cent of IgM but only 20 per cent of IgG is removed each time as only 40 per cent of the IgG is within the vascular space. Plasmapheresis also has the advantage of the removal of immune complexes and small mediators (toxins, anaphylotoxins, cytokines, etc.), in addition to the antibodies. Plasmapheresis is only suitable for urgent therapy, as antibody levels return rapidly and frequently overshoot to higher levels after plasmapheresis is discontinued. It is important to commence conventional immunosuppression at the same time.

Side-effects

- Leakage/air embolism
- Anticoagulation (citrate toxicity)/thrombocytopenia
- Reactions to replacement fluids

Uses

- Hyperviscosity (Waldenström's macroglobulinaemia, IgA myeloma)
- Goodpasture's syndrome/Wegener's granulomatosis
- Cryoglobulinaemia
- Myasthenia gravis
- Guillain–Barré syndrome (but IVIg is as good)

It has been tried in other autoimmune diseases (RhA, FVIII antibodies, MS, lupus nephritis) with variable anecdotal success. A limiting factor in its use is access to appropriate equipment.

Immunoadsorption

Selective removal of autoantibodies has been attempted using an extracorporeal circuit including a column of inert beads coated with Protein A or Protein G for specific adsorption of IgG. This treatment is experimental and experience is limited.

10 Immunotherapy

Plasmapheresis
Immunoadsorption

Allergy interventions

Treatment for allergic disease is divided into three major target areas, mast cells, released mediators, and the specific immune response. Treatment can be topical or systemic: topical is preferred if this is effective. The underlying chronic inflammatory component, especially of asthma, needs always to be addressed rather than just using symptomatic agents. Corticosteroids and antihistamines are more effective as prophylactic agents, taken before allergen exposure.

Mast-cell active

- Corticosteroids (interfere with synthesis of leukotrienes)
- Mast-cell stabilization: cromoglycate/nedocromil/ketotifen (prevent allergen-triggered calcium flux and hence prevent degranulation)

Released mediators

- β-Agonists (smooth muscle relaxation, some anti-inflammatory effect? (salmeterol))
- Antihistamines: use long-acting high-potency non-sedating drugs without cardiotoxicity (loratidine, cetirizine, fexofenadine)
- Corticosteroids
- Anti-PAF drugs (clinical results disappointing)
- Leukotriene antagonists (useful adjunctive treatment in asthma)

Specific IgE

- Desensitization
- Peptide therapy (experimental)
- Anti-FcRε therapy (experimental)

The mechanism of desensitization is uncertain: specific IgE may rise in early stages of treatment then fall; the role of 'blocking antibodies' (IgG4) is unknown. One hypothesis suggests that sequential exposure gradually switches the CD4+ T-cell response from Th2 to Th1, reducing IgE production and the levels of the pro-allergic cytokines IL-4 and IL-5. Traditional desensitization is done weekly until maintenance doses are reached, when the intervals between injections are spaced out. The precise protocol and total duration of therapy varies depending on the allergen, but all require long-term commitment from patients. Current UK guidelines suggest that desensitization is inappropriate for those with multiple allergies, with severe asthma, heart disease, or hypertension requiring β-blockade (difficult to resuscitate in emergencies!), or during pregnancy. Desensitization should only be carried out with purified standard allergens. Rush and ultra-rush schedules have been devised, but are rarely required in practice and significantly increase the risks of reactions. Desensitization must be carried out in hospital and staff must be conversant with emergency management of anaphylaxis and cardiac arrest procedures.

USES OF INTERFERONS AND CYTOKINES

The use of cytokines has disappointed clinical researchers: there are a number of reasons for the lack of clinical efficacy, including:

- Redundancy: multiple cytokines with the same or overlapping actions.
- Pleiotropism: cytokines may have a range of effects on different cells. Effects may be dependent on other signals.
- Range: cytokines are short-range molecules (known exceptions are IL-1, IL-6, and TNF-α). This is of clinical importance for therapy.
- Milieu: cytokines rarely work in isolation. The balance of different cytokines is critical in determining the response. Difficult to model *in vitro*.
- Biological significance: cytokine responses have evolved; apparently harmful responses serve to the advantage of species and are therefore conserved (TNF response in sepsis).
- Clinical utility: usage of single cytokines in pharmacological doses for therapy has been, in the main, disappointing (based on misconceptions over physiological roles of cytokines).

Further thought needs to be given to the use of cytokines in combination, or administration at the local level where the clinical effect is required.

CLINICAL UTILITIES OF CYTOKINES

Primary immunodeficiencies

- *CGD*: γ–IFN. Acute treatment for abscesses; low-dose prophylactic treatment. ? Acts to increase bactericidal activity of neutrophils via unknown bypass pathway.
- *Hyper-IgE*: γ–IFN. Theoretical benefit from inhibition of IgE production. Clinical trial planned (CyA is probably more effective).
- *CMC*: γ–IFN. Anecdotal reports, limited benefit.
- *CVID*: PEG–IL-2. Small clinical trial in USA; some benefit apparent.
- *Cytokine deficiency*: IL-2 and γ-IFN tried. Cases very rare.

Malignant disease

- *Melanoma*: IL-2. Trials disappointing. Significant side-effects.
- *Renal cell carcinoma*:   IL-2. Small, uncontrolled trials show some benefit in some patients, including those with metastatic disease.
- *Hairy-cell leukaemia*: α-IFN. Now established as treatment of choice; self-administered by patient at home.
- *Chronic myeloid leukaemia*: α-IFN may be beneficial (?toxic to Philadelphia chromosome positive cells).

Infectious disease

- *Hepatitis B*: α-IFN ± γ-IFN for conversion of HBeAg+ to HBeAb+; reduction in infection. γ-IFN with booster doses of vaccine when no humoral response after three doses?
- *Hepatitis C*: α-IFN may cure infection or at least lead to remission while on treatment (ribavirin may be useful in combination).
- *Papillomavirus*: α-IFN beneficial for genital and ? common warts.
- *Kaposi's sarcoma*: α-IFN tried, results disappointing and no better than chemotherapy ± radiotherapy.
- *HIV*: IL-2 and IFNs tried—no significant benefit, but further trials planned.
- *Leprosy*: γ-IFN beneficial in lepromatous leprosy.
- *Leishmaniasis*: γ-IFN beneficial in visceral leishmaniasis.
- Toxoplasma: γ-IFN used as experimental therapy.

Other diseases

- *Scleroderma*: γ-IFN tried to decrease collagen synthesis: effect dubious.
- *Multiple sclerosis*: β-IFN is effective in relapsing and remitting disease.

CLINICAL USES OF GROWTH FACTORS

Non-malignant disease

- *Renal failure*: erythropoeitin established as treatment of choice for treating anaemia of chronic renal failure (CRF), especially for patients on dialysis. Increased risk of thrombosis. Quality of life versus cost!
- *Cyclic neutropenia*: G-CSF shortens cycle from 21 to 14 days, reduces nadir for neutrophils from 3–4 days to 1 day. Not curative. Effects of long-term therapy unknown.
- *SCID*: GM-CSF/G-CSF/IL-3 shorten time to myeloid engraftment. There may be a risk of worsening GvHD.
- *HIV*: Erythropoeitin for AZT-induced and HIV-induced anaemia. Trials not encouraging.

Malignant disease

- *Post-chemotherapy*: G-CSF/GM-CSF shorten neutropenic period following myelotoxic chemotherapy. Not known whether GM-CSF has any advantages over G-CSF. NB Bone pain may be a significant side-effect during infusions. May be a risk of secondary myeloid leukaemias if high doses used.
- *Post-BMT (leukaemia and lymphoma)*: G-CSF/GM-CSF/IL-3 hasten engraftment in autologous transplants. Experimental use of IL-6 for increasing platelets. Direct effect on some leukaemias.
- *Myelodysplasia*: GM-CSF, IL-3, EPO to encourage recovery.

461

ADOPTIVE IMMUNOTHERAPY

Bone marrow transplantation

See Chapter 9.

Interleukin-2 and LAK therapy

LAK therapy (lymphokine activated killer cells) has been proposed as a treatment for malignant disease. Peripheral blood lymphocytes are harvested and then stimulated *in vitro* with high-dose IL-2 and reinfused into the patient with additional IL-2. Side-effects are severe and tumoricidal activity limited. A better approach may be to expand tumour-invading lymphocytes. The therapy is moderately toxic in therapeutic doses (fluid retention; capillary leak syndrome). There is some evidence of benefit in melanoma and renal cell carcinoma (salvage therapy).

Part 2

11 Immunochemistry

Introduction

Electrophoresis, immunoelectrophoresis, immunofixation, isoelectric focusing, and immunoblotting

The most basic technique for the detection of serum proteins is that of serum electrophoresis, in which serum is applied to a electrolyte containing agarose gel and a current applied across the gel. Proteins are separated largely on the basis of their surface charge. The separated proteins are then visualized by incubating the gel with a protein-binding dye. As the amount of dye bound is proportional to the protein present, the amount of protein present in each band can be calculated from the absorbance of the dye if the total protein concentration is known. This is the method used for paraprotein quantitation.

In the electrophoretic strip, individual proteins may be identified either by immunoelectrophoresis, in which troughs cut parallel to the electrophoretic strip are filled with antisera which is allowed to diffuse towards the separated proteins. Reaction at the point of equivalence gives an arc of precipitation. A faster technique is immunofixation, in which the antisera are laid over the electrophoretic separation and unreacted proteins washed out before staining with a protein-binding dye. Both these techniques are used principally to identify monoclonal immunoglobulins. Serum is preferred as the mobility of fibrinogen is such that it runs in the same region as some immunoglobulins.

More sensitive techniques are required for CSF, as the concentration of immunoglobulins are lower. Here the electrophoretic separation is carried out by isoelectric focusing. The gel contains ampholytes which move under the current to set up a pH gradient across the gel. Proteins applied subsequently then move to the part of the gel where the pH ensures that they become electrically neutral. They then cease to move in the current. The gel is then blotted onto nitrocellulose filters which are reacted with antisera against immunoglobulins (immunoblotting).

Radial immunodiffusion (RID)

This is a simple, although slow, method for the measurement of any protein for which an antiserum exists. The antiserum is incorporated into an agar gel, which is poured onto a plate and allowed to set. Regular holes are then cut into the gel and the serum containing the protein of interest placed in the holes. The serum diffuses into the gel and forms an immunoprecipitate which can be seen as a white halo around the well. The log(concentration) is proportional to the diameter of the ring. The ring diameter can be measured using an eyepiece graticule.

There are a number of pitfalls to this technique, particularly if it is used to measure concentrations of immunoglobulins, as variations in molecular weight (for example if serum contains monomeric rather than polymeric IgM, as may happen in Waldenström's macroglobulinaemia) or the presence of immune complexes may cause falsely low or falsely high values. IgA-deficient individuals often have antibodies to ruminant proteins, including immunoglobulins, and as the antisera that are incorporated in the gel are often raised in ruminants, this may cause reverse precipitation in the gel and lead to entirely spurious results.

Nephelometry and turbidimetry

These techniques are the mainstay of specific protein measurement. As with other techniques, they rely upon immune complex formation when antibodies and antigens react. This alters the optical properties of the solution and the light absorbance or scatter can be measured. The reactions can be enhanced by using reaction diluents containing polyethylene glycol (PEG) which stabilizes the immune complex. Accuracy may be enhanced by using kinetic assays (rate nephelometry). This technique is suitable for automation, but is dependent on high-grade monospecific antisera of high potency. Monoclonal antibodies are rarely suitable for this type of system. Anything that causes the serum to be turbid before the reaction begins, or interferes with the optical properties of the solution, will cause difficulties. This includes lipaemic sera or haemolysed samples with excess free haemoglobin (with haemoglobin–haptoglobin complexes).

α_1-Acid glycoprotein

This protein is also known as orosomucoid. Its significance is as an acute-phase protein. It used to be used extensively in the diagnosis and monitoring of inflammatory bowel disease, and it was felt that it was more specific for this category of disease. There is no strong evidence to support this assertion and CRP probably provides all the information required. It is induced by IL-1, IL-6, and TNF-α. However, its dynamic range is only twofold, compared to >100-fold for CRP. There is a sex difference, with levels in females being lower. Levels are also reduced in pregnancy and in patients receiving oestrogens. It is known to bind certain drugs such as propranolol. There are probably few indications for its regular measurement at present.

α_1-Antichymotrypsin

• Normal adult range: 0.3–0.6 g/l.
This protein is one of the SERPIN family (serine protease inhibitors) whose major role is the protection of tissues from proteolysis by neutrophil and macrophage enzymes. It is particularly active against cathepsin G. It rises rapidly during an acute-phase response (within 8 hours) and has a dynamic range of fivefold (much less than CRP). It remains elevated for longer. It, too, has been suggested as a useful marker for inflammatory bowel disease, but there is little evidence to support this and it is not widely used.

α_1-Antitrypsin (α1AT)

- Normal adult range: 1.0–1.9 g/l.

This is a proteolytic inhibitor with a wide range of inhibitory activities. It is a member of the SERPIN family. It comprises the major part of the α-1 fraction on serum electrophoresis and deficiency may be detected readily on an electrophoretic strip. Occasionally split α-1 bands may be noted due to allelic variants of α1AT with different mobilities. In conditions where there are high levels of circulating proteases, protease–α1AT complexes may form, with loss of the α-1 band; the complex moves in the α-2–β region of the electrophoretic strip. Low levels are associated with cirrhosis, emphysema, and neonatal jaundice, and also adult liver disease. Deficiency may also be associated with vasculitis (particularly of the skin) and with membranoproliferative glomerulonephritis. There are a number of deficiency alleles, and when a low value is detected, the phenotype should be determined. Other members of the family should be screened and phenotyped. This represents the only clinical utility of α1AT measurements. High levels are seen as part of the acute-phase response, and particularly in chronic infections (bronchiectasis). Levels are also increased in pregnancy, in patients on oestrogens, and in certain malignant diseases, including some germ-cell tumours. However, it is not useful clinically in any of these situations. It has been suggested that measurement of α1AT in faeces may give information on gut protein loss, as it is resistant to degradation, although there appears to be a high false negative rate. It may be a useful alternative to radioisotopic methods for proving the presence of a protein-losing enteropathy. Measurements are usually made by nephelometry.

α_1-Antitrypsin phenotypes

The gene for α1AT is located on chromosome 14, close to the immunoglobulin heavy chain locus (*PI* gene system, for protease inhibitor). A large number of variant alleles have been described. The identification is usually undertaken by isoelectric focusing , but for some rare alleles functional studies may also be required. In the UK, deficiency alleles occur with an incidence of about 1 in 2000. Many variants are seen in other racial groups and, as a consequence, are found only exceedingly rarely in the UK. The important deficiency alleles include *S*, *P*, *W*, *Z*, *Mmalton* and *null* (no expressed α1AT). Homozygosity for one or heterozygosity for any two of these alleles leads to severe deficiency. Heterozygosity with any non-deficiency alleles leads to a reduction but not absence of α1AT. The allele *Mduarte* gives rise to a functional deficiency with normal antigenic concentrations. Studies should always be undertaken on family members and referring clinicians should always be asked for a family tree. Antenatal diagnosis is also possible, by *PI* typing a fetal blood sample.

In the UK, *PI* typing is undertaken by the Protein Reference Units in Birmingham and Sheffield, and their excellent handbook gives more detail on the genetic system.

α_2-Macroglobulin

This has anti-protease activity. It is an acute-phase protein and also acts as the carrier for IL-6. It is a major component of the α-2 band on electrophoresis and contributes significantly to the elevation of α-2 seen in chronic inflammatory conditions. As it is a very high molecular weight protein (725 kDa), it is preferentially retained in the nephrotic syndrome, giving a relative increase in relation to other areas of the electrophoretic strip. Levels are also reported to be elevated in ataxia telangiectasia, diabetes mellitus, oestrogen therapy, and pregnancy. Reduced levels have been found in pre-eclampsia and acute pancreatitis. Deficiency has been reported but is exceptionally rare. There is no value in routine measurement at present.

Avian precipitins

IgG-precipitating antibodies to avian antigens are found in cases of bird-fancier's lung. These react particularly with avian serum and faecal proteins. It is important to recognize that the presence of precipitins is a marker of exposure and does not automatically mean that disease will be present. However, the presence of multiple precipitin lines tends to be a feature of disease. Any bird is capable of inducing precipitins, but the most common causes of problems are pigeons (in pigeon-breeders), psittacine cage birds, and domestic poultry (as an occupational disease). The antibodies are usually detected by double diffusion assays in agar, although ELISA and fluorescent assays are also used.

Bacterial antibodies

- Normal adult ranges:
  - Tetanus: >0.1 IU/ml
  - Diphtheria: >0.1 IU/ml
  - Pneumovax®: >20 U/ml
  - Hib: >0.15 µg/ml (>1 µg/ml is protective)

Antibodies to tetanus, diphtheria, pneumococcal polysaccharide, *Haemophilus influenzae* type b (Hib) capsular polysaccharide, and meningococcal polysaccharide are available as a screen of specific immune function. These tests are also useful for investigating the level of protection following immunization, in particular for patients who have had previous adverse reactions and are due for re-immunization. They are a valuable *in vivo* test of humoral immune function following test immunization in patients with suspected immunodeficiency. Under these circumstances, a baseline, pre-immunization, and a 3–4 week post-immunization sample are required. There is no good agreement as to what constitutes an acceptable response, but a minimum requirement would be a post-immunization response above the minimum protective level and at least a twofold rise in titre. However, greater than a fourfold rise is achieved by most adults. When investigating suspected immuno-deficiency it is worth bearing in mind that a small minority of patients make a good initial response but that the antibodies decline rapidly, so that within 3–6 months they have become undetectable. These patients may also be at risk of infections. If there is doubt, then late samples should also be looked at.

These antibodies are usually detected by ELISA. International standards are available for Hib, tetanus, and diphtheria antibodies, and it is anticipated that agreement will soon be reached for an international standard for pneumococcal polysaccharide antibodies. There are no standards for meningococcal polysaccharide antibodies.

When Pneumovax® is used as the immunogen and antigen for the detection of specific antibodies, it should be remembered that this product also contains a variable amount of cell wall polysaccharide, antibodies to which are not protective. However, if the question being asked is 'is this patient capable of recognizing polysaccharide antigens?' then this is irrelevant. It does matter, however, if the question being asked is 'is this patient protected against pneumo-coccal disease?'; the assay can be modified to adsorb out the cell wall polysaccharide and measure only antibodies to the capsular polysaccharide. As Pneumovax® is a mixture of 23 differ-ent serotypes of varying immunogenicity, it is also possible for there to be a poor response to one serotype which is masked by adequate responses to other serotypes. Measurement of antibodies to specific serotypes is available as a research tool, but it may be that it will also become necessary as a routine tool. Likewise, measurement of IgG-subclasses of specific antibodies may, in future, prove to be of clinical value, although this has not yet been proved.

Specific deficiency of antibodies to outer membrane proteins of *Moraxella catarrhalis* in association with recurrent respira-tory infections has been reported. At present, routine assays for antibodies to these proteins are not available. Antibodies to *Pseudomonas* have been used in the monitoring of patients with cystic fibrosis and there is interest in antibodies to *Salmonella* poly-saccharides as a marker of humoral immune responsiveness.

Bence Jones proteins

See Urinary free light chains and Urinary electrophoresis, below.

β2-Microglobulin (β2MG)

- Normal adult range: 1–3 mg/l.

β2-Microglobulin serves as the light chain of the MHC class I molecule and is a member of the immunoglobulin superfamily as it comprises a single domain. It appears in soluble form in the serum and is usually rapidly cleared through the glomeruli, as it is of low molecular weight (11–12 kDa); it is also readsorbed in the proximal tubules. Measurement is by RID, RIA, enzyme-linked immuno-assay (EIA), or nephelometry, but there is no preferred method. It is useful for monitoring lymphocyte activation and turnover in myeloma, lymphoma, and HIV-related disease. Elevated levels identify patients with common variable immunodeficiency (CVID) who have granulomatous disease. Serum levels rise when there is renal impairment and very high levels are seen in patients on chronic dialysis: this may be associated with amyloid formation. Very high urinary levels can be found when there is renal tubular dysfunction, such as damage from aminoglycoside drugs. Measurement of urinary β2MG is not valuable as the protein is degraded in acid urine. High levels are found in allograft recipients undergoing rejection, although viral infections may also increase the levels. Levels fall with successful treatment.

In myeloma, serial measurement of β2MG is a useful adjunct in terms of monitoring tumour burden and cell turnover. However, interpretation of levels is complicated by the need to consider renal function, particularly as free light chains are nephrotoxic and may damage tubules, thus inhibiting readsorption, and there may also be glomerular damage preventing filtration: the effects on β2MG serum levels in myeloma are therefore complex. However, levels below 4 mg/l are associated with a good prognosis, while levels above 20 mg/l are associated with a poor prognosis, although this may well represent the effects of renal damage. Treatment with α-interferon elevates serum levels, which needs to be considered in monitoring levels.

Elevated levels of β2MG are seen in connective tissue diseases such as Sjögren's syndrome and rheumatoid arthritis, and in granulomatous diseases such as sarcoidosis and granulomatous CVID. Levels fall when patients are treated with corticosteroids or other lymphocytotoxic chemotherapy.

In HIV disease, β2MG is said to be a useful surrogate predictor of disease progression, and gives similar information to the absolute CD4+ T-cell count. However, the dynamic range in HIV is small compared to that in lymphoproliferative diseases. The CD4+ T-cell count and viral load are preferred in the UK.

Caeruloplasmin

• Normal adult range: 0.19–0.71 g/l.

Caeruloplasmin is a copper-binding protein, of molecular weight 150 kDa, with an α-2 mobility on electrophoresis. Levels are reduced in most cases of Wilson's disease (hepatolenticular degeneration), although a few patients will have normal values, usually when there is an intercurrent stimulus to the acute-phase response. As it is synthesized in the liver, levels will be reduced in severe liver disease (hepatitis and primary biliary cirrhosis); levels are also reduced in severe malabsorptive syndromes where there is copper deficiency. Levels will be elevated in acute-phase responses, in particular in rheumatoid arthritis and vasculitis (giving a green colour to serum), and in pregnancy, oral contraceptive use, and thyrotoxicosis. Measurement is usually by nephelometry. Clinically, the most important indication for measurement is in suspected Wilson's disease. It has been proposed as a useful marker in the monitoring of vasculitis, although it is doubtful whether it gives any additional information over measurement of CRP.

C3, C4, and Factor B

- Normal adult range:
  - C3: 0.68–1.80 g/l
  - C4: 0.18–0.60 g/l.

These are the complement components most regularly measured. As they are present in significant concentrations, measurement by rate nephelometry is the usual method. Care needs to be taken over taking and transportation of the samples for complement assays, as traumatic venepuncture or delay in transport may lead to falsely low levels, due to *in vitro* activation, particularly of C4 and C3. This may be prevented by taking samples into EDTA, as the breakdown is calcium dependent. Measurement of all three components allows one to look for activation of the complement system by either the classical pathway (C4) or alternate pathway (Factor B): see table for typical changes. In practice few laboratories bother with measurement of Factor B. Measurement of C3 is valuable in monitoring SLE. C4 null alleles are common and affect the baseline level of C4: it is not possible to use C4 levels as a marker of activity in SLE without knowing how many null alleles there are. It is useful in the diagnosis of SBE (reduced C3), post-streptococcal glomerulonephritis (low C3), and other conditions of complement activation. A persistently low C3 may indicate the presence of a C3-nephritic factor (see Chapter 12). In patients with angioedema, a low C4 may indicate C1-esterase inhibitor deficiency. Both C3 and C4 are acute-phase proteins, and may therefore be normal even at times of rapid consumption: assessment of C3 breakdown products is advised. C4 is often reduced in pre-eclampsia.

Low C4, normal C3	Normal C4, low C3	Low C4, low C3
Genetic deficiency	Post-streptococcal GN	Sepsis
SLE (active—check C3d)	C3-nephritic factor	SLE (active)
Hereditary angioedema	Gram-negative sepsis (alternate pathway activation)	Rheumatoid arthritis (rare)
Type II cryoglobulinaemia	SBE	
Eclampsia		

Complement allotypes

The locations for the complement genes are known. C2, Factor B, C4A, and C4B form part of the MHC genes (class III) encoded on chromosome 6, linked to HLA-DR. C3 is encoded by an autosomal co-dominant system on chromosome 19. Null alleles are common, particularly for C2 and C4. Determination of the complement allotypes is sometime undertaken as part of extended MHC phenotyping/genotyping when looking at disease association and specifically at complement deficiency states. C4 null alleles confer an increased risk of developing SLE and also drug-induced lupus. C4 null alleles have also been associated with systemic sclerosis, rheumatoid arthritis, common variable immunodeficiency, and selective IgA deficiency.

CH100 and APCH100

These test the integrity of the classical (CH100) and alternate (APCH100) pathways of complement activation. Their use is therefore limited to the investigation of suspected complement deficiency. Any patient with recurrent meningococcal disease should be screened, as there is a strong possibility of a complement deficiency. Rarely, patients with atypical lupus may also be deficient in either C1 or C2. Serial monitoring of the CH100 in SLE provides no information that cannot be obtained from C3, C4, and C3d measurement and is therefore not recommended. If the CH100 or APCH100 are absent, the laboratory will automatically perform additional tests to identify the missing components. Two methods are in use: gel assays, based on a modified RID, dependent on 100 per cent haemolysis, or the tube haemolytic assay dependent on 50% haemolysis (giving a CH50/APCH50). In both types of assay the classical pathway activity is detected by using antibody-coated sheep red cells, while for the alternate pathway, guinea-pig red cells are used, as these are susceptible to direct lysis via the alternate pathway. Both assays are dependent on the terminal lytic sequence. Activity can be reported in terms of units/ml or compared to a standard serum and reported as a percentage. However, it is probably adequate to report as 'normal', 'low', or 'absent'. Abnormal results will often be found if patients are screened too soon after acute infection: leave at least 3–4 weeks.

485

C1-esterase inhibitor (immunochemical)

- Normal adult range: 0.18–0.54 g/l.

C1-esterase inhibitor is one of the control proteins of the classical pathway of complement activation. It is also an important control protein for the coagulation, fibrinolytic, and kinin pathways. It is likely that the angioedema seen in hereditary deficiency is due to unregulated kinin production rather than the activation of the C1. C1-esterase inhibitor is reduced in hereditary angioedema. If during an attack of angioedema, the C4 is reduced, the C1-esterase inhibitor should be measured. Eighty per cent of patients with hereditary angioedema (HANE) lack the inhibitor (type I deficiency); the remaining 20 per cent (type II deficiency) have normal or high levels of a functionally inactive inhibitor, due to point mutations at the active site of the enzyme. It is reported that levels of C1q are reduced in acquired angioedema, while they are normal in HANE. However, this test is not always reliable. Measurement is usually by RID or nephelometry.

C1-esterase inhibitor (functional)

- Normal adult range: 80–120 per cent (expressed as a percentage of control serum).

This should be measured in cases of angioedema with low C4, when the total immunochemical C1-esterase inhibitor is normal or high. The purpose of the assay is to detect type II hereditary angioedema. There are a number of specific assays, including commercial colorimetric assays: some require citrated plasma while others require serum, and it is important to check which samples are required by the local laboratory. The inhibitor is labile and samples should be separated as soon as possible to avoid artefactually reduced levels.

Acquired C1-inhibitor deficiency may occur in older patients. This is due to the production of a paraprotein that interferes with the function of C1-esterase inhibitor, and is associated with both myeloma and lymphoma. The development of new angioedema in an older patient should lead to a search for such a paraprotein (immunoglobulins, electrophoresis, paraprotein, and β2-microglobulin) and for its source, as well for evidence of complement consumption. As noted above, C1q may be reduced in acquired but not in hereditary angioedema. Autoantibodies may also occur, albeit very rarely, in patients with SLE.

487

C3d (C3 breakdown products)

• Normal range: 1.8–12.0 mg/l.

Measurement of C3d is a better measure of the activation of the complement system than measurement of immune complexes. C3d levels correlate with disease activity in SLE, and are also elevated in patients with severe diffuse cutaneous disease associated with systemic sclerosis. They are valuable because, as noted above, C3 is an acute-phase protein and levels may remain within the normal range despite significant consumption if there is an acute-phase response. Measurement is by RID. Because some activation of C3 occurs with blood clotting, it is essential that samples are taken into EDTA which chelates the calcium required for C3 degradation.

Other assays have been studied to see whether they have a better predictive value. The best seems to be a multistage sandwich ELISA to detect the terminal lytic complex C5b–C9. This also correlates well with disease activity, but is a more expensive and complicated assay.

C1 and C2, alternate pathway components and terminal components

• Normal adult range: reported as a percentage of control serum.

Measurement of individual complement components requires the availability of specific antisera. They are usually detected by either double diffusion or RID. It may be necessary to carry out functional assays, with complementation by other sera with known complement deficiencies. Measurement of individual components should follow, not precede, a functional evaluation by CH100/APCH100, to determine the location of the missing component. They are of value in the investigation of recurrent meningococcal disease and atypical lupus.

C2 levels will be reduced in activation of the classical pathway. However, C2 deficiency is the most common deficiency of the complement pathway, with C2 null alleles occurring at a frequency of between 1 in 100 to 1 in 500. C2 deficiency often leads to an atypical form of lupus in which skin manifestations are common. As active lupus will lower C2 levels through consumption, it is often difficult to be sure whether complete C2 deficiency is present. However, in complete deficiency the CH100 will be absent. Genetic studies may be necessary to confirm the diagnosis.

11 Immunochemistry
C3d (C3 breakdown products)
C1 and C2, alternate pathway components and terminal components
C3a, C4a, and C5a (anaphylotoxins)

C3a, C4a, and C5a (anaphylotoxins)

The anaphylotoxins are released as part of the activation process of
the complement cascade, being cleaved off their parent molecules.
All share a terminal arginine, which is essential for biological
activity and which is removed by carboxypeptidase-N, the enzyme
responsible for their inactivation. All are potent triggers for histamine release and smooth muscle constrictors, and they increase
vascular permeability. They also act as chemotactic factors and
aggregate neutrophils. Measurement is usually by radioimmunoassay, but as they are labile, special collection tubes are required
containing a protease inhibitor, nafamostat (Futhan®) as well as
EDTA. The commercial source of these tubes has now ceased
production. Immediate separation and freezing of the plasma is
required for accurate measurement. The clinical utility of measurements of the anaphylotoxins is limited, although they may be valuable in monitoring shocked patients, patients with respiratory
distress syndrome, and in patients undergoing extracorporeal circulation. Although they change in other conditions with complement
activation, such as SLE, there are other, more convenient assays that
will give the same information.

C-reactive protein (CRP)

- Normal adult range: <4 mg/l.

CRP is named from its reactivity with the C-substance poly-saccharide of streptococci. It is a member of the pentraxin family and functions as a non-specific opsonin for bacteria. It also binds to free DNA. Mononuclear phagocytes have specific CRP receptors. No cases of CRP deficiency have been reported, suggesting that its absence is incompatible with survival. CRP is the most useful marker of the acute-phase response. It rises within hours of the onset of an inflammatory stimulus and has a circulating half-life of about 8 hours. It is therefore useful in both diagnosis and monitoring. Normal levels are seen in most viral infections and in degenerative arthropathy. Levels of up to 100 mg/l are seen in inflammatory arthritides; some viral infections, such as EBV, CMV, and adenovirus; in polymyalgia rheumatica; and sometimes in malignant disease (lymphoma, hypernephroma). Moderate elevations of CRP (100–300 mg/l) are seen in active vasculitis, including temporal arteritis, in moderate bacterial infections, and occasionally as a result of lymphoma. Levels of CRP above 300 mg/l usually only occur in response to serious bacterial sepsis, very severe vasculitis, and certain atypical infections, such as *Legionella*. It does not give the same information as the ESR, as other factors such as red cell number, size, shape, charge, and other high molecular weight serum proteins such as IgM may affect the latter. In general terms, the ESR, as an acute-phase marker, is dependent on fibrinogen, which rises only slowly and falls equally slowly. The half-life of fibrinogen is approximately a week. The CRP tells you what has happened to the patient within the past 6–8 hours, while the ESR tells you what happened to them last week.

The stimuli to the production of CRP are IL-1, IL-6, and TNF-α. As raised IL-6 levels may also be involved in the pathogenesis of myeloma, through an autocrine mechanism of self-stimulation, CRP levels may be elevated in myeloma and relate to the plasma cell burden.

It has been suggested that the normal range usually quoted (<4–6 mg/l) may be misleading. There are some patients who, when tested with ultrasensitive assays for CRP, have exceptionally low basal CRP which rises by the normal increment (up 100-fold), while still remaining within the normal quoted range. This may explain the rare patients with severe inflammatory disease such as giant-cell arteritis who never have an 'abnormal' CRP, even with active disease. The normal range in the neonatal period may also need revision, as levels are found above the 'normal' range without evidence of disease.

Cryofibrinogens

Cryofibrinogen is an abnormally cold-insoluble fibrin–fibrinogen complex, with fibrin being the key component. It can lead to typical vasculitic lesions on cold extremities and is also associated with thrombophlebitis migrans. Its most common underlying association is with occult malignancy (myeloma, leukaemia, prostatic carcinoma). It is also associated with connective tissue disease, pregnancy, oral contraceptives, diabetes mellitus, and cold-induced urticaria. Cryofibrinogenaemia is said to be common in IgA nephropathy. A separate form may also be seen in heparin-treated patients, when the heparin acts as a co-factor for the precipitation. To detect a cryofibrinogen, paired EDTA and clotted samples (*not* heparin) must be taken at 37 °C and transported at that temperature to the laboratory, where the serum and plasma will be separated warm and then cooled to 4 °C. The cryoprecipitate will form only in the EDTA plasma. This will be washed, redissolved, and its identity confirmed either by direct measurement or by immunofixation on electrophoresis.

Cryoglobulins

Cryoglobulins are cold-insoluble immunoglobulins. All immunoglobulins are cold-insoluble to a significant degree and it is the temperature at which precipitation occurs that determines whether disease will result. Usually proteins that precipitate above 21 °C cause problems, as this is the lowest skin temperature that is compatible with survival. The higher the temperature at which precipitation takes place, the more problems will occur. Most cryoglobulins are IgG or IgM; IgA and light chains only are much rarer. The reasons for abnormal cryoprecipitability are not known, but include abnormal amino acid structure (paraproteins) and abnormal glycosylation, as well as abnormal physicochemical interactions with solvents.

Three types of cryoglobulins are recognized: type I, composed of monoclonal immunoglobulins and associated with lymphoproliferative diseases, Waldenström's macroglobulinaemia, and myeloma. Type II cryoglobulins are comprised of a monoclonal component which has rheumatoid factor activity and hence binds to polyclonal immunoglobulins. This type is often associated with B lymphoproliferative diseases, but also occurs with chronic infections (e.g. SBE) and connective tissue diseases. Type III cryoglobulins consist exclusively of polyclonal immunoglobulins with rheumatoid factor activity and are associated with connective tissue diseases and chronic infections. The precipitates may also include other serum components, including complement and fibronectin; C4 levels may be reduced. In certain parts of the world, such as northern Italy, many cases of mixed essential cryoglobulinaemia have been found to be associated with hepatitis C infection. In infection-related cases the immunoglobulin in the cryoprecipitate may have specificity against the infection. Investigation for cryoglobulins should take place in any patient with cutaneous vasculitis and in patients with glomerulonephritis accompanied by low C4 but normal C3. Only 7 per cent of patients with Raynaud's syndrome have cryoglobulins.

It is necessary to take the blood sample at 37 °C and to transport it to the laboratory at this temperature, where the serum is separated by allowing clot retraction to take place, also at 37 °C. The serum is then cooled to 4 °C for 48–72 hours. Normally the precipitate forms within 24 hours but occasionally it may form slowly. A cryocrit may be determined by centrifuging the precipitate and serum in a graduated tube: this is reported as a percentage of the serum volume. The components of the cryoglobulin should be determined by washing the precipitate in ice-cold buffer and then redissolving it in warm buffer, prior to electrophoresis and immunofixation (the electrophoresis may have to be carried out on a constant-temperature plate). Nephelometry may give misleading results unless it can be carried out at 37 °C, so warm RID is preferred. The precipitate should be tested for rheumatoid factor activity.

Cryoglobulins and cold agglutinins are often confused: see Chapter 12 for further information on cold agglutinins.

CSF IgG and albumin (oligoclonal banding)

- Normal adult range:
    - IgG: 0.01–0.05 g/l
    - Albumin: 0.06–0.26 g/l
    - IgG : albumin ratio: <22 per cent.

Measurement of CSF IgG, albumin, and detection of oligoclonal bands are useful as adjunctive tests in the diagnosis of multiple sclerosis. When the blood–brain barrier is intact, mainly low molecular weight proteins are found in the CSF. Any inflammatory disease increases the passage of proteins into the CSF, including those of higher molecular weight. Certain conditions are associated with the presence of plasma cells within the brain, leading to local immunoglobulin production, which is oligoclonal. Contamination of the CSF with blood, through poor lumbar puncture (LP) technique renders the test uninterpretable. Elevation of the CSF IgG or a ratio of CSF IgG/CSF albumin >22 per cent is strongly suggestive of intrathecal synthesis. Detection of oligoclonal immunoglobulins is now usually carried out by isoelectric focusing of paired serum and CSF, followed by immunoblotting. Intrathecal synthesis is present if IEF bands are detected in CSF but not serum. Oligoclonal IgG bands in the CSF are not specific for MS but may also occur in encephalitis, neurosarcoid, neurosyphilis, meningitis, polyneuritis, subacute sclerosing panencephalitis, SLE, and tumours. If a paraprotein is present in serum, then this may also be found in the CSF.

Complex calculations of other indices, based on CSF and serum IgG, IgM and albumin concentrations, and on the IgG synthetic rate have been proposed. However, they add little information to that obtained from the CSF IgG : albumin ratio, which costs half as much. Where unusual infections are suspected it may be valuable to compare the ratio of specific antiviral titres in the CSF and serum with the equivalent ratio for IgG: if the ratio is higher for the specific antibody, then it suggests that there is a CNS infection.

497

Fungal precipitins

Precipitating IgG antibodies to fungal antigens are usually detected by immunodiffusion, although ELISA techniques may also be used. They are associated with hypersensitivity pneumonitis. Farmer's lung is typically associated with antibodies to *Aspergillus fumigatus*, *Thermoactinomyces vulgaris*, and *Micropolyspora faeni*. Other occupational lung diseases (malt-workers lung, etc.) may be associated with other fungi, including *Aspergillus clavatus*. The antigens are predominantly low molecular weight. The antibodies are not, however, diagnostic, but are markers of exposure and should always be interpreted in the light of clinical findings. Usually few precipitin lines are present. Concentration of the sera may be required to reveal weak lines. The antibody response is reduced in smokers. However, when an aspergilloma (fungus ball) is present, often in an old tuberculous cavity, antibodies to high molecular weight antigens may be detected. Here there are multiple precipitin lines and the antibodies are frequently readily detectable, even in unconcentrated sera.

Allergic bronchopulmonary aspergillosis (ABPA) is an eosinophilic pneumonia which is also associated with precipitating antibodies to *Aspergillus fumigatus*. However, total IgE and *Aspergillus*-specific IgE are elevated. Other fungi that are associated with an IgE-mediated response include *Cladosporium*, *Alternaria*, and *Penicillium* species. These are associated mainly with asthmatic symptoms (e.g. in inhabitants of damp, mouldy accommodation). Some hypersensitivity pneumonitides (cheese-worker's lung, humidifier fever (*Penicillium*); wood-worker's lung (*Alternaria*)) may be associated with precipitins to these fungi, but the tests are not reliable for diagnoses, as the fungi are ubiquitous and many healthy individuals have antibodies.

IgG antibodies to *Candida* species may be found in otherwise healthy individuals, indicating the ubiquitous nature of the yeast. These include antibodies against the mannan component (polysaccharide), as well as protein antigens. Indeed, absence of antibodies to *Candida albicans* mannan may suggest the possibility of a humoral immune deficiency. Patients with chronic mucocutaneous candidiasis (Chapter 2) often have very high levels of IgG precipitins to *Candida*, with multiple precipitin lines, and this is helpful in diagnosis. Testing for antibodies to *Candida* in other immunodeficiencies, such as HIV infection, when yeast infection is suspected, is unreliable. Similar constraints apply to detection of antibodies to *Nocardia*.

Haptoglobin

• Normal adult range: 1.0–3.0 g/l.

Haptoglobin is an α-2 globulin that is involved in the recycling of haem iron, by binding liberated haemoglobin. Levels are markedly reduced in the presence of haemolysis. Other diseases leading to increased red cell fragility, such as sickle-cell disease, thalassaemia, and G6PD deficiency, are also associated with reduced haptoglobin levels. Genetic lack of haptoglobin has been reported. Elevated levels are seen in biliary obstruction, aplastic anaemia, and as part of an acute-phase response. Haptoglobin exists in polymeric forms, which gives rise to difficulties in measurement by RID.

ICAM-1, soluble

Serum sICAM-1 levels reflect endothelial activation, and may therefore be valuable in monitoring liver and cardiac allograft recipients for rejection, in conjunction with CRP, β2-microglobulin and sIL-2 receptors. Assay is by EIA. The problem with this approach is the need for rapid turnaround, which with most EIA systems, as used for ICAM-1 and s-IL2 receptors, makes the test very expensive. Measurement of β2-microglobulin and CRP, which can be run on a nephelometer, may be of more practical use.

501

IgA antibodies

Anti-IgA antibodies have been reported as a cause of adverse reactions to blood products, including intravenous immunoglobulins. These will only occur in those who are completely deficient in IgA and will therefore see infused IgA as 'foreign'. These reactions may occur in otherwise healthy individuals with selective IgA deficiency, and also in some patients with common variable immunodeficiency or IgG subclass deficiency who are also completely deficient in IgA. All three groups have an increased tendency to form autoantibodies. It is less likely that anti-IgA antibodies will form in patient with XLA, who will have no capacity to synthesize IgG. IgE-anti-IgA antibodies have been described, although their significance is uncertain. The antibodies are usually detected by agglutination of tanned red cells coated with IgA.

Similar problems of transfusion reactions have been found in patients with deficiencies of either C4A or C4B (Chido and Rodgers blood groups), as they may also see infused C4 as foreign and make an antibody response.

IgA subclasses

IgA exists as two subclasses, IgA1, the predominant serum IgA, and IgA2, which occurs in secretions with IgA1 in roughly equal amounts. Specific deficiencies of IgA1 and IgA2, either alone or in combination with other immunoglobulin abnormalities, have been described. It has been suggested that measurement of IgA subclasses may be valuable in the investigation of recurrent *Haemophilus* infection of the respiratory tract. It may also be valuable in the investigation of transfusion reactions where some IgA is detected, as the patient may be deficient in only one subclass and hence see the other subclass as 'foreign'.

502

IgG subclasses

- Normal adult ranges:
  - IgG1: 2.0–10.0 g/l
  - IgG2: 0.5–7.5 g/l
  - IgG3: 0.05–0.9 g/l
  - IgG4: 0.0–2.2 g/l.

The only indication for the measurement of IgG subclasses is in the investigation of suspected primary immunodeficiency and as an adjunct to the diagnosis of Sjögren's syndrome, where the polyclonal increase in IgG is restricted to IgG1. IgG1, IgG3, and IgG4 antibodies are predominantly directed against proteins, while IgG2 antibodies are directed against polysaccharides. Antiviral antibodies are of IgG1 or IgG3 subclass, depending on the virus. As IgG1 is the major contributor to total IgG, IgG1 deficiency is clinically severe (effectively as CVID). IgG2 deficiency is complex: complete genetic deficiency is compatible with normal health and low IgG2 does not always lead to infections. IgG2 levels may be slow to develop in children. Levels are related to Gm allotypes, which in turn are racially distributed. Total IgG2 levels correlate poorly with responses to test immunization to polysaccharide antigens (such as pneumococcal polysaccharide). IgG2 deficiency and IgG4 deficiency are often associated. IgG3 deficiency has been proposed to be associated with asthma, possibly due to increased susceptibility to viral infections, intractable epilepsy, and chronic sinusitis. IgG4 deficiency has been difficult to define, because levels are anyway very low; however, using newer, more sensitive assays, it is possible to differentiate low IgG4, which appears to be of little significance, from complete deficiency, which is associated with chronic suppurative lung disease. It must be understood that normal total immunoglobulins and IgG subclasses does not exclude significant humoral immune deficiency (specific antibody deficiency; see Chapter 2).

Other than the unusual pattern of elevation of IgG1 and relative suppression of other subclasses in Sjögren's syndrome, there are no other indications for the investigation of IgG subclasses in states when the total IgG is high, although it must be remembered that a high total IgG, in a patient with recurrent infections, may be masking a subclass or specific antibody deficiency.

Immune complexes

The formation of immune complexes is a key part of the normal immune response and complexes are being formed and cleared all the time. Pathological immune complexes tend to be formed when there is low-affinity antibody or when there are abnormalities or deficiencies of the complement system. Many assays of immune complex formation have been described. However, they are difficult to standardize, have poor reproducibility, and the different assays give different results in the same clinical circumstances. Such assays are not recommended for routine clinical use and the use of more specific markers of complement activation, such as C3d or C5b–C9 complexes, are recommended.

Immunoglobulins (IgG, IgA, IgM)

- Normal adult range:
  - IgG: 5.8–15.4 g/l
  - IgA: 0.64–2.97 g/l
  - IgM: 0.24–1.90 g/l (male)
    IgM: 0.71–2.30 g/l (female)

Measurement of serum immunoglobulins is indicated in the investigation of suspected myeloma, Waldenström's macroglobulinaemia, lymphoma, connective tissue diseases, and primary or secondary immunodeficiency. Elevation of IgA may occur in cirrhotic liver disease, chronic infections, and in the elderly. IgM may be significantly elevated in primary biliary cirrhosis and in acute infections, especially EBV and CMV, as well as chronic infections such as TB. Very marked polyclonal elevations of all classes of immunoglobulin are seen in HIV infection, in Sjögren's syndrome (where it is predominantly IgG1, with a suppression of other IgG subclasses), and sarcoidosis. Less marked increases are seen in other inflammatory or chronic infective conditions. Transient severe reductions in all isotypes may be seen in acute severe bacterial infections: this may lead to spurious diagnoses of humoral immunodeficiency. IgA deficiency is the most common primary immunodeficiency disease and may be asymptomatic. Significant immunodeficiency may be present with normal immunoglobulins, and measurement of IgG subclasses and specific antibodies may be helpful. It is important to note that there is a sex difference in the normal range of IgM: this is frequently ignored where immunoglobulins are not measured in immunology laboratories, leading to misleading reports.

It is essential that measurement of immunoglobulins is accompanied by electrophoresis of the serum, as this will give essential additional information that will assist in the interpretation of low or high immunoglobulins. For example, where low IgG and IgA are noted, the electrophoresis may show other signs of nephrotic syndrome (reduction of albumin, increase in α-2 band). Equally, where high immunoglobulin levels are found, it is essential to determine whether there is any monoclonal component present, and whether this is on the background of humoral immune suppression (suggesting myeloma) or a generalized polyclonal increase (suggesting chronic infection/inflammation).

Where low IgA is found, it is important to carry out further tests to determine whether IgA is completely absent, or merely reduced. Those found to be completely deficient should be screened for anti-IgA antibodies and should be issued with a transfusion warning card to carry.

507

Immunofixation

Immunofixation has now replaced immunoelectrophoresis as the technique of choice for the identification of proteins on electrophoresis, as it is far quicker and easier to perform. It is mainly used to identify monoclonal bands detected on electrophoresis. These will mainly be immunoglobulin bands, but the technique can be applied to any protein for which a suitable polyclonal antiserum is available. Because the mobility of fibrinogen and CRP on electrophoresis falls in the β–γ region, these proteins, if elevated, may cause confusion and their specific identification may be necessary. Usually, provided well-clotted serum is used, fibrinogen does not cause problems. In acute bacterial infections, the CRP may be sufficiently high to appear as a discrete band. A proportion of patients will have more than one discrete paraprotein band, which may be of different heavy and light chains.

It is essential to fix for both heavy and light chains. Usually IgG, IgA, and IgM, as well as the light chains, are screened first. If light-chain bands with no corresponding heavy chains are detected, then the process should be repeated with IgD and IgE. Where monoclonal immunoglobulin bands are detected, it is also essential to look at the urine. When the paraprotein levels are very high, it may be necessary to dilute the serum to get good immunofixation (prozone effect). Heavy chains in the absence of light chains are extremely rare and this is more often due to abnormal light chains failing to react with one particular antiserum than to a true heavy-chain disease. Before diagnosing heavy-chain disease, it is therefore worth trying several different anti-light-chain antisera.

Interleukin-2 receptors, soluble (sCD25)

Serum levels of soluble IL-2 receptors are useful in monitoring solid organ allograft recipients, as levels rise early in rejection episodes. Levels also rise in acute graft-versus-host disease. Elevated levels are seen in other conditions associated with lymphocyte activation, but are not, on the whole, clinically useful. Measurement is usually by EIA, but this approach is expensive and not easily given to the very rapid turnaround required for monitoring of graft rejection at reasonable cost.

Isohaemagglutinins

Isohaemagglutinins are mainly of the IgM class, although IgG antibodies may also be detected. It is useful to measure them in the context of the investigation of someone with suspected humoral immune deficiency, as low or absent agglutinins is an indicator of poor IgM synthesis. This test is, of course, unusable in individuals of blood group AB. Titres are very low in small infants aged under 1 year.

The presence of high titres of IgG isohaemagglutinins in intravenous immunoglobulin has been associated with significant haemolysis in isolated case reports. Where very high doses are used, it may be appropriate to 'cross-match' the IVIg against the patient's red cells first.

Mannan-binding protein (mannan-binding lectin, MBP)

MBP is one of the collectin family of carbohydrate-binding proteins. Structurally it strongly resembles C1q and is capable of activating complement directly (collectin pathway). It functions as a soluble non-specific opsonin, binding to oligosaccharides. Deficiency has been described, but its association with clinical disease is uncertain, as deficiency alleles are relatively common and most carriers are asymptomatic. It has been suggested that the deficiency is only significant if other aspects of the innate or specific immune system are impaired, when chronic infections, in particular otitis media and chronic diarrhoea, may occur. The role of MBP measurements in the investigation of recurrent infections is thus not wholly established at present. Measurement is usually by RID.

Neopterin

Neopterin is a pteridine which is synthesized predominantly in macrophages, and levels are increased in diseases when macrophages are active. It can be measured in CSF and urine in addition to serum. It has been proposed to be a useful surrogate marker in HIV disease. However, levels correlate closely with those of β2-microglobulin and only one or other need be measured. Levels have also been reported to be elevated in other viral, proto-zoal, and bacterial infections, especially TB, inflammatory bowel disease, tumours, and chronic fatigue syndromes. It is thus not a specific marker of HIV infection or progress. Commercial ELISA assays are available.

Orosomucoid

See α_1-Acid glycoprotein, above.

11 Immunochemistry

Mannan-binding protein (mannan-binding lectin, MBP)
Neopterin
Orosomucoid

513

Paraprotein by densitometry

This measures the amount of monoclonal immunoglobulin by scanning a stained electrophoretic strip. The measurement of the total protein is also required. The results from paraprotein measurement may not correlate well with the immunochemical measurements, particularly for IgM and IgA paraproteins, where polymerization may occur in the serum and give erroneous results by nephelometry. Healthy adults do not have detectable levels of paraproteins, but up to 20 per cent of elderly patients over the age of 75 will have low levels of paraproteins (<10 g/l). Chronic infections and chronic inflammatory conditions may also cause low levels of paraproteins; transient monoclonal bands may appear after bone marrow transplantation.

Pneumococcal polysaccharide antibodies

See Bacterial antibodies, above.

Salivary IgA and secretory piece

This is a qualitative test for the presence of mucosal antibody and may be helpful in the work-up of suspected immunodeficiency. True secretory piece deficiency is exceptionally rare. The usual technique for detection is by double diffusion.

Serum amyloid A and serum amyloid P (SAA and SAP)

SAA, which is the circulating precursor of the secondary (AA) type of amyloid and whose physiological function is currently unknown, is an acute-phase protein with a very wide dynamic range. The normal level is approximately 2 mg/l and this may increase by 1000-fold during the acute-phase response (compared to a tenfold increase of CRP). Monitoring is said to be valuable in disease known to predispose to the development of AA amyloid, such as chronic infections and inflammation. However, the CRP test is more widely available and probably gives the same information, although in allograft rejection the two markers may move independently. SAP is related to CRP structurally and is a member of the pentraxin family. Despite this similarity, its function is not fully understood and it does not function as a major acute-phase protein. Routine measurement is not justified at present, although labelled SAP has been used as a tracer for amyloid deposits.

Serum electrophoresis

Serum electrophoresis is primarily used to detect the presence of monoclonal bands due to the presence of paraproteins, although it will provide a host of other information about the patient provided that it is read by a skilled individual. Where myeloma is suspected, both urine and serum should be sent. Serum electrophoresis will also provide evidence of an acute phase response, hypogamma-globulinaemia and alpha-1-antitrypsin deficiency.

Transferrin

• Normal adult range: 2.0–4.0 g/l.

Serum transferrin is increased in iron deficiency and pregnancy, and reduced in anaemia of chronic disease, chronic infections, burns, and rare genetic absence. It is a 'negative' acute-phase protein. Measurement of transferrin is also used in calculating the urine selectivity (see below).

11 Immunochemistry

Serum amyloid A and serum anymloid P (SAA and SAP)
Serum electrophoresis
Transferrin

Urinary free light chain quantitation

Quantitation of urinary free light chains is essential in myeloma when an excess of monoclonal free light chains have been detected by immunoelectrophoresis, particularly when the tumour cells only produce light chains (Bence Jones myeloma). Unfortunately this is difficult and there is no generally accepted technique in use. Nephelometric assays use antisera that are calibrated for use mainly against bound, not free, light chains, and in serum, not urine; so it is necessary to undertake an arithmetic correction. However, the latter is based on some assumptions, including that one-sixth of the mass of intact immunoglobulin is light chain and that all the light chain is either free or bound, but not both, and that if there is whole Ig, it contains only one type of light chain. The correction is to multiply the nephelometric result by 0.17. In urines where both free κ and free λ are detected the $\kappa:\lambda$ ratio should be in the range 1.0–4.0; values outside this range are highly suggestive of the presence of excess free light chains. Alternatives to nephelometry for light-chain quantitation include scanning densitometry, but this is less accurate in urine than in serum, unless there is significant proteinuria. However, the most important aspect is serial monitoring in an individual patient, so the absolute value is less important than the change in value against time. β2MG is a more useful marker of tumour burden.

Urine electrophoresis and immunofixation

This is the screening test to detect free light chains in the urine. Random urine is usually satisfactory, but a 24-hour urine is more sensitive. It used to be necessary to concentrate urine prior to electrophoresis, but modern electrophoretic systems have increased sensitivity and have rendered this step unnecessary. Monoclonal free light chains are associated with myeloma, Waldenström's macroglobulinaemia, and, rarely, with lymphoma. Polyclonal free light chains may be found in the urine when there is renal tubular damage, and as a consequence of old age and chronic inflammatory conditions (e.g. rheumatoid arthritis). Interpretation of urine electrophoresis is difficult as other discrete proteins may be present that give an appearance similar to monoclonal light chains. In particular, prostatic proteins may appear in the urine in older men. Immunofixation is essential to confirm the nature of any discrete bands found in the urine.

11 Immunochemistry
Urinary free light chain quantitation
Urine electrophoresis and immunofixation
Urine selectivity (IgG and transferrin)

Urine selectivity (IgG and transferrin)

This test may be useful in determining whether the predominant
protein in the urine is low molecular weight (as may occur in minimal change disease) or includes higher molecular weight proteins.
IgG and transferrin are measured and the urine-to-serum ratio of
IgG is divided by the urine-to-serum ratio of transferrin to give the
selectivity. A value of >0.15 indicates 'non-selective' proteinuria
and is against a diagnosis of minimal change disease. This test is
only reliable if proteinuria >1 g/l is present. It is no longer widely
requested by renal physicians.

Viral antibodies

Antibodies against exposure and immunization viral antigens should form part of the work-up of patients suspected of having a humoral immune deficiency. Absence of detectable antibodies in patients who have a clear exposure or immunization history is highly suspicious. The panel should include measles, mumps, rubella, chickenpox, herpes simplex, EBV, CMV, polio, and hepatitis A and B. However, it is important only to select those where exposure/immunization is documented.

Remember that test immunization with live vaccines in suspected immunodeficiency is **contraindicated**!

Viscosity

• Normal adult range: 1.4–1.9 (ratio to water).

Measurement of serum viscosity is helpful in monitoring Waldenström's macroglobulinaemia and other myelomas, where hyperviscosity occurs. Hyperviscosity may lead to serious end-organ damage if undetected: cardiac failure, cerebral infarction, retinal vein occlusion, and renal failure being the major complications. IgA myelomas are prone to develop hyperviscosity because the IgA paraprotein frequently polymerizes *in vivo*. This is detected on electrophoresis as a stepladder of multiple bands. If a cryoglobulin is present, the viscosity must be measured under warm conditions. Serial monitoring is helpful, particularly when plasmapheresis is being undertaken. In many laboratories measurement of viscosity has replaced measurement of the ESR as a general acute-phase test, as automated viscometers are available.

12 Autoantibodies

523

Introduction

There are many hundreds of reported autoantibodies, not all of clinical value. The repertoire of the typical regional immunology laboratory will cover most of the ones described below. Some will only be available through specialist referral laboratories, or through research laboratories. When requesting tests, it is essential to decide in advance what clinically useful information will be obtained by carrying out the test: just because a test is available does not mean that it is of value under a given circumstance. If a test result is not going to affect clinical management in any way, then it is a waste of time and money doing it, even though it may satisfy the intellectual curiosity of the requester.

Autoantibodies are divided broadly into two categories: organ-specific, where the target antigen has a restricted distribution, usually limited to one organ such as the thyroid gland; and organ-non-specific, where the target antigen has a wide distribution. Organ-non-specific antibodies may none the less be associated with a disease of restricted organ involvement, for example primary biliary cirrhosis, where the target antigen is in the mitochondria which are widely distributed, but the disease is limited to the liver. It is not clear why autoantibodies to a widely distributed antigen should be associated with an organ-specific disease. Neither is it clear why autoantibodies arise that are directed against intracellular components, as intact cells should exclude antibodies from reacting with the component. However, it is now known that autoantibodies may in some circumstances cross intact cell membranes.

Autoantibodies may also be divided into:

- primary pathogenic antibodies, where the antibody mediates a functional effect either by interfering with a cellular or molecular function (for example, the blocking of neuromuscular transmission by antibodies to the acetylcholine receptor on muscle endplates) or by direct damage to tissues (for example, anti-glomerular basement membrane antibodies); or
- secondary antibodies, which are not directly involved in the disease process, but are markers for the existence of the process, for example anti-thyroglobulin antibodies.

The latter may still be useful diagnostic tools. However, not all autoantibodies are diagnostically useful, as they may have low sensitivity and specificity. Recent evidence has indicated that a number of autoantibodies may penetrate viable cells (previously this was not thought to occur), and this may change our views about the pathogenicity of some antibodies.

A number of techniques are used for the detection of autoantibodies. The nature of the antigen will largely dictate the type of assay, although it is frequently possible to use more than one method to measure a given antibody. This always gives rise to difficulties in the comparison of results from different methods. Too little work has been done on proper comparisons, not only at the technical level, but also to evaluate the tests in terms of their clinical performance. For each type of antibody there needs to be a 'gold standard assay' to which all other assays are compared, and if differences are detected, then the differences must be fully evaluated in the clinical context. This is frequently ignored, particularly where commercially produced assays are concerned, and this leads to confusing or misleading results being produced when small, non-specialist laboratories take on autoantibody testing.

Autoantibodies can be of any class, although in most circumstances the diagnostic process focuses on IgG antibodies. IgM autoantibodies seem to be of little relevance under most circumstances, although there are occasional exceptions, such as IgM anti-cardiolipin antibodies. IgA autoantibodies are rare but may be diagnostically useful, for example in coeliac disease where IgA endomysial antibodies have the highest sensitivity and specificity. Attempts have been made to link IgA autoantibodies of other specificities to particular variants of disease, for example IgA rheumatoid factors in rheumatoid arthritis and IgA ANCA in vasculitis. It is worth bearing in mind that autoantibodies may appear transiently after certain infections, particularly EBV and adenovirus infections. Any specificity may appear but the most common are rheumatoid factors and anti-nuclear antibodies. Such autoantibodies are not usually associated with disease and usually disappear over about 6 months.

TECHNIQUES

Particle agglutination assays

Although the technique is old, it is reliable and still widely used. It is relatively cheap. The antigen (either pure or as an extract) is coated onto an inert carrier particle, usually gelatin or latex but originally tanned red cells. When mixed with serum containing the appropriate antibody, the particles are agglutinated. The principle is simple but reading the end-point of a particle agglutination titration requires some skill. IgM antibodies tend to be picked up preferentially because of their pentameric shape, which allows better cross-linking. The assay is still widely used for antibodies to thyroid antigens and rheumatoid factors, and provides the basis of the direct Coombs test (DCT) for anti-red cell antibodies in the investigation of haemolytic anaemia.

Immunoprecipitation assays

These depend upon the formation of insoluble immune complexes where an antibody encounters the optimum concentration of antigen. The prototype assay is the Ouchterlony double diffusion assay, where the antigen and antibody are added to wells cut in agar gels and allowed to diffuse towards one another. Line(s) of precipitation form at the point of equivalence, indicating the presence of an antibody against the antigen. The process is slow and may take up to 72 hours to form lines. The technique may be improved by using electrolyte containing agarose and applying a current across the gel, forcing the antibody and antigen together (counter-current immunoelectrophoresis). This modification is used extensively for the detection of antibodies to extractable nuclear antigens. If the immune complex formation takes place in the liquid phase, then the light absorbing/scattering properties of the solution will be altered and can be measured. Thus nephelometry can be used for antibody detection, although in practice it is only used for rheumatoid factor detection. As for specific protein measurement, the stability of the immune complex may be poor and agents such as polyethylene glycol (PEG) may be added to ensure a stable reaction. PEG may also be used in gels to enhance and stabilize the immune complex.

527

Indirect immunofluorescence

This is the standard technique for the detection of many serum autoantibodies. An appropriate tissue block is snap-frozen and is cut on a cryostat to provide sections (usually 4 μm thick) that are mounted on a slide and air-dried. Other fixation techniques may be used under special circumstances (e.g. acetone or ethanol). Similar methods can be used on cell suspensions prepared on slides using a cytocentrifuge (for example neutrophils for ANCA or HEp-2 cells). The slides can then be incubated with appropriate dilutions of test and control sera, washed, and then incubated with anti-human immunoglobulin (isotype-specific) antiserum which is conjugated with fluorescein isothiocyanate (FITC). This technique allows the tissue and intracellular distribution of autoantibody binding to be visualized. Alternatives may be used for FITC in the second stage, such as enzymes (immunoperoxidase) which will give a colour reaction when the slides are incubated with an appropriate substrate. These methods have the advantage that the slides can be fixed and counter-stained to reveal the tissue structure and that an ordinary transmission light microscope is all that is required. However, the processing has an extra incubation step.

Key features that are essential to obtaining reliable results are:
- Good tissue selection and processing.
- Appropriate starting dilution (to avoid non-specific serum binding).
- Use of serum not plasma, as fibrinogen causes non-specific fluorescence.
- Appropriate FITC-conjugated antiserum selection. This is mostly from commercial sources but there is usually considerable batch to batch variation. The fluorescein molecule to protein ratio needs to be between 1 and 4.5 to give reasonable results. Too low and the intensity is inadequate, too high and the non-specific fluorescence swamps the specific staining. Optimal dilution needs to be determined by a chequerboard titration (see Chapter 16).
- Appropriate internal/external controls (quantitative as well as qualitative).
- A good-quality fluorescence microscope, properly maintained, with a properly adjusted light source.
- Finally, and most importantly, an experienced microscopist who is familiar with the relevant patterns.

For laboratory convenience, it is standard practice to test for the basic autoantibodies using a tissue multiblock, containing liver, stomach, and kidney (some laboratories also include thyroid), usually of rodent origin. This allows the detection of most anti-nuclear antibodies, smooth muscle, mitochondrial, reticulin, gastric parietal cell, ribosomal, and LKM antibodies. Screening will often be carried out at a single dilution with a conjugated antiserum that recognizes IgG, IgA, and IgM. Positive samples will then be titrated using a monospecific anti-IgG antiserum. The disadvantage of this multiblock screen is that it encourages clinicians to request 'auto-antibody screens' without thinking about what they are specifically looking for. It is important to get into the habit of thinking through the differential diagnosis and requesting specific autoantibodies (even though the laboratory may still give you the others anyway).

The technique is the same whatever other tissues are used: for other autoantibodies human, monkey, or other animal tissue may be required. Provided that the blocks for frozen section are prepared carefully and stored in sealed vials, they will last for long periods if stored at -80 °C.

Attempts have been made to use flow cytometry for autoantibody detection, where the antibodies are bound to cellular components of the blood. This is not widely used at present.

Direct immunofluorescence

The technique here is very similar to that used for indirect immuno-fluorescence, except that in this case the tissue is obtained directly from the patient, snap-frozen, and sectioned prior to incubation with the FITC-conjugated anti-serum. This allows the detection of tissue-bound antibody in the patient. This is important, because tissue-bound antibody may be present even when there is insufficient antibody to be detected free in the serum. In addition, other tissue reactants such as complement and fibrinogen may be detected. Patterns of reaction may be absolutely diagnostic, for instance in the diagnosis of bullous skin diseases. Direct immuno-fluorescence is used extensively in the diagnosis of skin diseases (because of the accessibility of the tissue for biopsy) and renal disease.

529

Radioimmunoassay (RIA)

These assays have been used for many years for the detection of
antibodies and are highly sensitive. However, they do require pure
antigen. Many variants have been described. Because of the desire
to cut down on the use of radioisotopes, many RIA-based assays
have been switched to fluorescent or enzyme-linked immunoassays.
However, RIA remains the gold-standard assay for acetylcholine
receptor and intrinsic factor antibodies, and is still widely used for
antibodies to dsDNA.

Enzyme-linked and fluorescent
immunoassays

These have taken over from RIA, and to some extent from indirect
immunofluorescence, and use antigen bound on to a solid phase
(bead or plate) which is reacted with serum, then washed and
reacted with the antiserum against human immunoglobulin, which
is coupled either to an enzyme or to a fluorescent dye. In the former,
the next stage is reaction with the substrate, either directly or via an
amplification step to give a colour that can be measured spectro-
photometrically; and in the latter, the plate can be read directly
using an appropriate exciting light source (which will be of a
different wavelength to the emitted light). These assays tend to be
more sensitive than immunofluorescence, but often lose specificity
as a result. They are unlikely to replace multiblock screening, as this
is cheap and gives a huge range of information that cannot be
obtained from a single EIA, particularly related to patterns of
nuclear and cytoplasmic reactivity. To be effective, pure (recombinant) antigens should be used, but this adds to the cost. Very different results may be obtained, for example, when ENAs are detected
by EIA compared to counter-current immunoelectrophoresis. The
clinical relevance of these difference in long-term management has
not been evaluated.

531

Western blotting

In this technique, crude antigen preparations are electrophoresed and then blotted onto nitrocellulose paper , which can then be reacted with sera: unbound antibody is washed off, while bound antibody is detected with an enzyme-conjugated antiserum, which will give an appropriate colour reaction at the site of bound antibody. This is a useful technique when antibodies to multiple specificities are being sought and the antigens are only available as a crude homogenate. It has been applied in the research setting to ENA antibody detection, but is expensive and labour intensive, so not suited to high-volume diagnostic screening.

ANTIBODIES

Acetylcholine-receptor antibodies (AChRAb)

AChRAbs are the marker for myasthenia gravis. Two types of antibodies have been described, those that bind to the receptor at sites distinct from the binding site for acetylcholine, and those that block the binding of the neurotransmitter or α-bungarotoxin. Some of the antibodies are capable of modulating the removal of the receptors from the surface of the muscle through cross-linking followed by internalization. They are detected by a quantitative competitive radioimmunoassay. Levels above 5×10^{-10} mol/l are regarded as positive; levels of $2–5 \times 10^{-10}$ mol/l are regarded as equivocal, and may be seen in ocular myasthenia. Some laboratories report the levels only semi-quantitatively (high, low, etc.). The highest levels are seen in young patients (<40 years with generalized disease), while lower levels are seen in older patients, those with thymoma, and in penicillamine-induced myasthenia. Approximately 15 per cent of typical myasthenic patients are negative for AChRAb; it is thought that some may have IgM antibodies. In ocular myasthenia, about 20 per cent of patients will be seronegative. Antibodies persist in 60 per cent of patients even if the disease is in remission.

AChRAbs have also been detected in the myasthenic syndrome associated with penicillamine usage (about 1 per cent of treated patients); these antibodies disappear when the drug is stopped. Very rarely, they may appear transiently during the immunological reconstitution phase of bone marrow transplantation.

Adrenal antibodies

Autoantibodies to adrenal cortex (any or all of the three layers) are found in approximately 50 per cent of patients with Addisonian adrenal insufficiency where there are other autoimmune diseases, although the prevalence drops when the autoimmune adrenalitis occurs alone. They are virtually never found in patients with tuberculous adrenal destruction. The target antigen is usually the adrenal microsomes, although antibodies to the ACTH receptor have also been described in a few patients with Cushing's syndrome (paralleling thyroid-stimulating antibodies). 21-Hydroxylase is the major target antigen in Addison's disease and type I APGS. There is frequent cross-reactivity of the antibodies with the steroid-producing cells of the theca interna of the ovary and the Leydig cells of the testis: in the former case there may be ovarian failure. Other antigenic enzymes in steroid-producing cells include the P450 side-chain cleavage enzyme (P450 scc) and 17α-hydroxylase. Autoimmune adrenal disease is closely associated with other organ-specific autoimmune disease, including thyrogastric (Schmidt's syndrome) and parathyroid autoimmune disease, and it is therefore important to screen for thyroid antibodies and gastric parietal cell antibodies. Multiple endocrine autoantibodies may be found in chronic mucocutaneous candidiasis with endocrinopathy. Screening such patients is important, as the autoantibodies may appear before overt manifestations of endocrine insufficiency. Detection is by immunofluorescence.

Anti-nuclear antibodies (ANA)

See Nuclear antibodies, below.

ANCA

See Neutrophil cytoplasmic antibodies, below.

12 Autoantibodies

Auerbach's plexus

Antibodies against the myenteric plexus of the oesophagus have been reported to be detected by immunofluorescence in patients with achalasia of the cardia, a motility disorder of the oesophagus. However, the diagnostic role of these antibodies remains to be confirmed.

β2-GPI antibodies

These antibodies have been reported as part of the anti-phospholipid antibody spectrum (see Cardiolipin antibodies, below). Few laboratories are offering this test on a routine basis at present.

C1q antibodies

Antibodies to C1q have been described in hypocomplementaemic urticarial vasculitis, rheumatoid vasculitis, and SLE. Antibodies to the neoantigen formed by activation of C1q have also been associated with types of glomerulonephritis.

Cardiac antibodies

These antibodies are positive in a proportion of patients with Dressler's syndrome after myocardial infarction, after cardiac surgery, in some cardiomyopathies, and after acute rheumatic fever. Multiple antigens have been identified. Their diagnostic value is low. They are detected by immunofluorescence.

538

12 Autoantibodies

Cardiolipin (anti-phospholipid) antibodies

Cardiolipin is a phospholipid and antibodies to it form part of the spectrum of anti-phospholipid antibodies, along with false positive VDRL, lupus anticoagulants, and antibodies to derived phospholipids. Anti-cardiolipin antibodies are usually detected by EIA. However, standardization and reproducibility of the assays has always been a major problem, as demonstrated by the wide scatter of results in QA schemes. This probably relates to the requirement for β2-GPI (apolipoprotein H) from serum as a co-factor for the binding of cardiolipin antibodies, although autoantibodies have also been detected to the co-factor itself. This co-factor binds anionic phospholipids *in vivo* and its normal function is to inhibit coagulation and platelet aggregation. Anti-phospholipid antibodies are strongly associated with livedo reticularis, SLE, Sneddon's syndrome (cerebral events and livedo), Budd–Chiari syndrome, recurrent fetal loss, and the anti-phospholipid syndrome (major venous and arterial thrombosis, stroke, TIA, and multi-infarct dementia, in the absence of other features of lupus). There is no strong correlation with premature myocardial infarction or with cerebral lupus (despite the fact that the brain is full of phospholipid!). Symptoms are mainly associated with IgG-class antibodies; however, rare patients with typical symptoms will be encountered who have only IgM-class antibodies, and never make IgG antibodies. The amount of the antibody in units does not seem to relate to the severity of the disease, nor does immunosuppression usually have a significant effect on the level. Transient positive antibodies may be found after viral infections (especially EBV). Anti-phospholipid antibodies associated with syphilis and other infections do not usually react with β2-GPI and are rarely associated with a clotting disorder.

Lupus anticoagulants are antibodies that interfere with the clotting process *in vitro* and are usually detected by prolongation of the APTT, but the test of choice is the dilute Russell viper venom test (dRVVT). Because cardiolipin antibodies and lupus anticoagulants recognize different phospholipid specificities, it is important to test for both, as either may be present independently of the other and present with similar clinical problems. Although it has been suggested that lupus anticoagulants are more specific for recurrent fetal loss than cardiolipin antibodies, both may be associated with the syndrome. Women with lupus who are planning pregnancy should be screened for both anti-cardiolipin antibodies and lupus anticoagulants, in addition to testing for anti-Ro antibodies.

Cartilage antibodies

Antibodies to collagens types I, II, and III have been found in a range of inflammatory conditions where there is cartilage damage, including rheumatoid arthritis, relapsing polychondritis, and a whole range of other connective tissue diseases. They therefore have a low specificity and are of little diagnostic value.

Centriole antibodies

These antibodies will only be detected reliably if HEp-2 cells are used as the substrate for ANA detection. There are two brightly staining polar dots. They are found very rarely in patients with scleroderma and related overlap syndromes, but are said to occur commonly in mycoplasmal pneumonia.

12 Autoantibodies

Cartilage antibodies
Centriole antibodfies

543

Centromere antibodies

These antibodies can only be detected on HEp-2 cells; they are sometimes referred to as kinetochore antibodies, as they react with antigens located at the inner and outer kinetochore plates. The antigens are 17, 80, and 140 kDa proteins involved in the attachment of the spindle fibres. This gives the diagnostic condensation of fluorescence along the metaphase plate in dividing cells, which distinguishes the staining from other speckled-pattern ANAs. These are usually found in the CREST syndrome and limited cutaneous scleroderma (sometimes referred to as limited scleroderma). About 70–80 per cent of patients with features of CREST will have anti-centromere antibodies, while 1 per cent of patients with progressive systemic sclerosis (PSS) will be positive. Patients with severe Raynaud's phenomenon and features of scleroderma should also be screened for the ENA Scl-70, associated with PSS, as well as centromere antibodies. Detection of anti-centromere antibodies is of prognostic significance. Scl-70 and anti-centromere antibodies seem to be mutually exclusive.

It has been reported that up to 12 per cent of patients with primary biliary cirrhosis may be positive for anti-centromere antibodies, of whom about half will have clinical signs of scleroderma. However, it is possible that this is a misinterpretation of the immunofluorescence pattern, as M2-antibody-negative PBC is often positive for a pattern of multiple nuclear dots which is sometimes referred to as pseudo-centromere, because of its resemblance to the centromere staining. However, the metaphase plate is not stained. It is important that dividing cells are present in each cytospin used when HEp-2 immunofluorescence is undertaken.

Cold agglutinins

These are often confused with cryoglobulins. They are autoanti-bodies that reversibly agglutinate erythrocytes in the cold, causing small-vessel obstruction in the skin of the extremities, Raynaud's phenomenon, and haemolytic anaemia. The most common speci-ficity is anti-i but other specificities such as anti-I or anti-Pr occur. They are often triggered by infections, especially *Mycoplasma pneumoniae*, rickettsia, *Listeria*, and EBV. These are usually poly-clonal IgMκ, although EBV may be associated with a polyclonal IgMλ anti-i response. They may also occur in association with lym-phoproliferative diseases where the agglutinin is usually mono-clonal (invariably IgMκ); this is typically a disease of the elderly. The cold agglutinins may precede the overt development of lymphoma by many years. Paroxysmal cold haemoglobinuria is associated with anti-P antibody which binds to the red cell and fixes complement in the cold. Red cell lysis takes place when the cell is rewarmed. It is rare and was originally described in association with syphilis (Donath–Landsteiner antibody). It is now more commonly associated with viral infections such as mumps, measles, and chickenpox. As for cryoglobulins, samples must be taken and trans-ported to the laboratory at 37 °C.

dsDNA antibodies

- Normal adult range:
  - Negative: <30 IU/ml
  - Borderline: 30–50 IU/ml
  - Positive: 50–300 IU/ml
  - Strongly positive: >300 IU/ml.

This test is confirmatory for SLE. Only antibodies to double-stranded DNA are measured. Elevated levels occur predominantly in SLE, but also in 'lupoid' chronic active hepatitis. These antibodies are not found in other connective tissue diseases, nor in all patients with SLE. Because the antibodies have a circulating half-life of 3 weeks, serial measurements are not useful in monitoring the activity of SLE. However, it has now been shown that a rising titre may predict clinical relapse and that treatment on a rising titre before symptoms reappear may reduce the total amount of immuno suppression required. When assaying for dsDNA antibodies, it is essential that the substrate is free of single-stranded DNA. The Farr technique (a radioimmunoassay using DNA precipitated by ammonium sulphate) is the gold standard, but ELISA methods are available, although some are significantly contaminated with ssDNA and give misleading results. Misleading results may be obtained in some assays related to the presence of low-affinity antibody. The kinetoplast of the organism *Crithidia lucilla* contains pure dsDNA: this test allows the rapid fluorescent detection of dsDNA antibodies, although it is less sensitive than the Farr assay.

ssDNA antibodies

Antibodies to single-stranded DNA and other forms (Z-DNA) have been reported in a wide range of connective tissue diseases, but they have a low sensitivity and specificity. Antibodies to ssDNA may occur in drug-induced lupus, but they also occur in idiopathic lupus. Other diseases in which there is a high prevalence of anti-ssDNA antibodies are rheumatoid arthritis, scleroderma, and polymyositis. They are more important as a factor reducing the sensitivity and specificity of assays for dsDNA, because the substrate in assays for the latter may be contaminated with ssDNA, produced during the purification process. A number of commercial assays have been shown to be contaminated in this way, leading to erroneous diagnoses of lupus on the basis of false positive reports of antibodies to dsDNA. While assays to ssDNA are available, they do not have routine use except in assessing samples for quality control of assays for dsDNA assays.

549

ENA antibodies

These antibodies recognize saline extracted cellular antigens and cause speckled-pattern anti-nuclear antibody staining. Six major specificities are tested for routinely: anti-Ro (associated with Sjögren's, SLE, cutaneous lupus, neonatal lupus, and congenital complete heart block), anti-La (associated with Sjögren's, SLE, and neonatal lupus), anti-Sm (specific for SLE, but common only in West Indians), anti-RNP (associated with SLE and, when occurring alone, said to identify mixed connective tissue disease), anti-Scl-70 (associated with progressive systemic sclerosis), and anti-Jo-1 (associated with polymyositis and dermatomyositis). The individual antibodies are discussed separately. Many other specificities have been identified. Antibodies to ENA are detected by a variety of methods, including double diffusion, counter-current immuno-electrophoresis, EIA, and immunoblotting. There is currently considerable debate about the optimal method: newer methods, in particular EIA, seem to be more sensitive, although the significance of the increased number of positives in terms of clinical utility remains to be determined. QA performance tends to be poor.

Endomysial antibodies (EMA)

This test is valuable in the diagnosis of coeliac disease; IgA-class antibodies are looked for routinely, unless IgA deficiency is present, in which case IgG-EMA should be sought. IgA-EMA will be positive in 60–70 per cent of patients with dermatitis herpetiformis and 100 per cent of untreated coeliac patients. Monitoring of IgA-EMA is valuable in confirming adherence to a gluten-free diet (GFD), as the antibody disappears, along with anti-gliadin antibodies, on a GFD and returns if there is a gluten challenge, even in the absence of overt symptoms. The antibodies are usually detected by immunofluorescence on monkey oesophagus sections, although umbilical cord has also been used. The antigen is now known to be tissue transglutaminase and solid-phase assays have been tested, although they do not perform appreciably better. The very high sensitivity and specificity of IgA-EMA in coeliac disease (100 per cent for both) has led to suggestions that jejunal biopsy may no longer be required. This is particularly attractive to paediatricians who wish to avoid invasive and unpleasant investigations in children. The Newcastle experience over some 5 years, where we have monitored biopsy findings against EMA results, has shown no false positive diagnoses on the basis of IgA-EMA. However, recent evidence has suggested that IgA-EMA may be negative in children under the age of 1 year, who may subsequently go on to develop biopsy-proven coeliac disease; these children may have IgG antibodies to gliadin. Such a finding needs confirmation, as it would have implications for the substitution of EMA testing for biopsy in very young children.

In cases of proven coeliac disease, treatment with a strict gluten-free diet leads to the gradual disappearance of the anti-gliadin and anti-EMA antibodies, usually in the order of IgA antibodies first and IgG antibodies later. Thus monitoring at intervals is useful in assessing dietary compliance. This is important as persistent exposure to gluten is thought to be a factor predisposing to the development of small bowel lymphoma in coeliac disease.

Patients with coeliac disease may have autoantibodies to the crypt basement membrane of human fetal jejunum. These antibodies appear to be of identical specificity to those detected as endomysial antibodies.

Endothelial antibodies

Antibodies against a variety of endothelial antigens have been described in a variety of vasculitic syndromes, especially SLE, haemolytic uraemic syndrome, Kawasaki syndrome, Wegener's granulomatosis, microscopic polyarteritis, and during solid organ graft rejection. The diagnostic significance is therefore low. The few laboratories offering this test have now withdrawn the service.

553

Epidermal antibodies (including direct immunofluorescence of skin)

These are useful in the diagnosis of blistering skin diseases. In bullous pemphigoid, herpes gestationis, and epidermolysis bullosa, there is an autoantibody directed against the basement membrane zone. In bullous pemphigoid, the autoantibodies recognize two keratinocyte hemidesmosomal proteins, BP230 and BP180. On direct immunofluorescence (DIF) up to 90 per cent of cases have typical linear IgG deposition; when serum is tested only 70 per cent will be positive (using monkey oesophagus as a substrate). In herpes gestationis, the antigen is the BP180 protein, but IgG deposition is seen on DIF in only 25 per cent of cases, although 100 per cent will have C3 deposition; serum is rarely positive. Epidermolysis bullosa acquisita will also give linear IgG and C3 on DIF that has no distinguishing features unless the biopsy is split between the dermis and epidermis by using a high-salt incubation, in which cases the immunofluorescence appears on the dermal side. The antigen is type VII procollagen.

Antibodies that recognize the intercellular substance of the epidermis give a typical chickenwire staining, both by direct and indirect immunofluorescence. These antibodies are typically found in pemphigus vulgaris and pemphigus foliaceus. In pemphigus vulgaris the antigen is desmoglein-1, an intercellular adhesion molecule of the cadherin family. The antigen in pemphigus foliaceus appears to be different by immunoblotting, but the two conditions are not readily distinguishable by routine immunofluorescence. A paraneoplastic form of pemphigus has been described with autoantibodies to desmoplakin I, a desmosomal protein.

Dermatitis herpetiformis causes the deposition of granular IgA, and sometimes C3 along the dermal papillae on DIF. Endomysial and gliadin antibodies may be present in serum. DH must be distinguished from linear IgA disease (a bullous disease) where there is linear IgA deposition, often with IgG and C3, at the dermo-epidermal junction.

DIF of the skin from patients with SLE usually shows coarse irregular granular deposition of IgG, IgM, C3, and C4 along the dermo-epidermal junction. However, similar features may be found in chronically sun-exposed skin from individuals without lupus. DIF of skin from patients with lichen planus shows characteristic flame-shaped deposits of fibrin and IgM in the epidermis.

Epidermal antibodies (including direct immunofluorescence of skin)

555

Erythrocyte antibodies

Anti-red cell antibodies are investigated to test for the temperature of maximal activity, specificity for red cell antigens, whether they are complement binding, and whether the activity is agglutinating or haemolytic. This involves looking at the patient's red cells, serum, and the eluate of the cells. Cells may also be treated with enzymes to enhance reactivity with certain antigenic systems (e.g. Ii or Pr). In warm haemolytic anaemia the major target antigens are of the rhesus system, although many other antigens have been reported as involved. Warm haemolytic anaemia may be associated with idiopathic haemolysis or secondary to SLE, CLL, lymphomas, and viral infections. In drug-induced haemolysis, there are often antibodies to drug–cell neoantigens (e.g. quinine, penicillins, and cephalosporins). See also cold agglutinins, above.

Ganglioside antibodies

Antibodies to gangliosides (sialylated glycolipids which form part of the myelin sheath) have been associated with a number of neurological diseases. Antibodies to GM1 (and asialo-GM1) and other gangliosides have been associated with Guillain–Barré syndrome, chronic demyelinating polyneuropathy, and multifocal motor neuropathy (see Chapter 5). In paraproteinaemic neuropathies anti-GM1 antibodies may appear as the paraprotein specificity; usually the antibody is IgM. It has been suggested that the presence of anti-GM1 antibodies may be a predictor of response to intravenous immunoglobulin, although this is not compelling at present. Antibodies to GQ1b have been associated with the Miller Fisher variant of Guillain–Barré syndrome (external ophthalmoplegia, ataxia, and arreflexia).

12 Autoantibodies

Erythrocyte antibodies
Ganglioside antibodies

557

Gastric parietal cell (GPC) antibodies

Antibodies to gastric parietal cells are found in almost all patients with pernicious anaemia (PA) in the early stages, although the frequency diminishes with disease progression. The target auto-antigens are the α- and β-subunits of the H^+,K^+-ATPase (proton pump). The antibodies are associated with atrophic gastritis (type A), but not with antral gastritis (type B), although the latter may be associated with antibodies to the gastrin-producing cells. The antibodies may be found in asymptomatic individuals; however, about 3 per cent per annum will go on to develop PA. There is a strong association of PA with thyroid disease, and 50 per cent of patients with PA will also have anti-thyroid antibodies, while 30 per cent of patients with thyroiditis with have GPC antibodies. The antibodies are best detected by fluorescence on a tissue multiblock containing a section of stomach. There is no correlation of the titre of antibody with disease.

Antibodies to gastrin-producing cells and gastrin receptors (blocking gastrin binding) have also been described in patients with pernicious anaemia (8–30 per cent), but these are of no routine clinical value at present.

559

Gliadin antibodies (IgG and IgA)

Gliadin antibodies are found in coeliac disease and dermatitis herpetiformis, but are not specific, being found also in other bowel diseases where there is breakdown of mucosal integrity. In children IgA-AGA may be seen in cow's milk intolerance and post-infective malabsorption. IgA anti-gliadin antibodies are more specific than IgG antibodies, except when IgA deficiency is present. IgG anti-gliadin antibodies occurring alone are of no particular diagnostic significance, and may be present in a wide range of inflammatory and infective bowel conditions. The sensitivity and specificity of IgA anti-gliadin antibodies are approximately 100 per cent and 95 per cent, respectively; while the figures for IgG antibodies are 50 per cent and 60 per cent, respectively. However, it has been noted that IgA antibodies to endomysium (EMA) are even more accurate. Because there is a higher false-positive rate for gliadin antibodies, it is likely that EMA testing will replace them. Gliadin antibodies are most usefully detected by ELISA, which is also helpful in screening large numbers of samples rapidly. Positive samples can then be run for EMA by immunofluorescence.

Because IgA deficiency increases the risk of developing coeliac disease by about 15-fold, it is essential that cases where there is a positive IgG anti-gliadin antibody but negative IgA anti-gliadin antibody are screened for IgA deficiency (by double immuno-diffusion). In complete IgA deficiency, IgG anti-gliadin antibodies (and IgG anti-endomysial antibodies) assume the same diagnostic significance as their IgA counterparts.

IgA anti-gliadin antibodies are also found in IgA mesangial glomerulonephritis, and may be useful as a diagnostic test. The disease itself is not affected by adherence to a gluten-free diet. Positive results are seen in children and adults with diabetes mellitus (type I), in first-degree relatives of patients with coeliac disease, and in patients with Down's syndrome, all of whom have an increased risk of developing coeliac disease.

Glomerular basement membrane antibodies

Anti-GBM antibodies are the marker for GBM disease or Goodpasture's syndrome. The usual presentation is with a rapidly progressive glomerulonephritis. The antibodies are directed against the non-collagenous domains of type IV collagen, although it is possible that there are other target antigens (entactin /nidogen?). These antibodies are examples of primary pathogenic antibodies which are directly involved in the disease process. Complement fixation takes place at sites of antibody localization. The same antigen is present in both glomerular and alveolar basement membranes, although alveolar haemorrhage is usually limited to patients who smoke or are exposed to other irritants (solvent fumes). Antibodies can be detected in serum by indirect immunofluorescence, usually using human kidney: there is a typical linear glomerular staining. Direct immunofluorescence on both kidney and lung biopsies will usually be positive for IgG and C3, and occasionally IgA, with the same staining pattern. It is much more difficult to get adequate lung biopsies and the deposition of antibody may be patchy in lung. Indirect immunofluorescence is, however, less sensitive than other types of immunoassay (ELISA or RIA), being positive in only about 75 per cent of biopsy-proven cases of GBM disease. However, immunofluorescence is much more amenable to being done as a one-off emergency test: this is important, as early aggressive plasmapheresis is essential to preserving renal function, and knowing that the patient is positive for anti-GBM antibodies influences therapy. It has been noted that 10–35 per cent of patients with anti-GBM antibodies may also have anti-neutrophil cytoplasmic antibodies (ANCAs), with a P-ANCA pattern, usually due to myeloperoxidase antibodies. The significance is uncertain. It is worth remembering that Wegener's granulomatosis may present with pulmonary haemorrhage and glomerulonephritis. The screen for all such patients should include both ANCA and GBM antibodies. These patients require urgent immunological investigations—one of the few occasions that this is necessary.

563

Glutamic acid decarboxylase antibodies

Anti-GAD antibodies have been found in more than 60 per cent of patients with the stiff-man syndrome. It is known that the enzyme is concentrated in the GABAergic neurones involved in the control of muscle tone. The enzyme is also found in pancreatic islet cells and is the target antigen in type I diabetes mellitus. Clearly, the enzyme must be distinct in the two sites as not all diabetics develop the stiff-man syndrome.

Gut antibodies

Antibodies to gut epithelium have been described in inflammatory bowel disease and may appear transiently post-bone marrow transplantation. In both cases the significance is uncertain. Antibodies to brush border have been described in ulcerative colitis and in some patients with *Yersinia enterocolitis*. There are reports of high levels of antibodies to colonic epithelial cells in ulcerative colitis, with between 70 and 80 per cent of patients positive, depending on the assay system. This is not used routinely for diagnosis at present and its value is uncertain.

Heterophile antibodies

These are not true 'autoantibodies' but represent a source of confusion with real autoantibodies. They are antibodies that may normally be present in serum and bind to tissue sections, particularly rodent tissues. They are particularly common in patients who have been transfused or alloimmunized in other ways (multiple pregnancies, organ grafts).

12 Autoantibodies

Glutamic acid decarboxylase antibodies
Gut antibodies
Heterophile antibodies

565

Histone antibodies

Antibodies to histones are the marker for drug-induced lupus. These cause a homogeneous anti-nuclear staining pattern on immunofluorescence. The target antigens are invariably the histones H2A-H2B in procainamide-induced lupus, while in hydrallazine-induced lupus H3 and H4 have been proposed as the targets. Virtually all procainamide-treated patients with lupus will have histone antibodies, while about 20 per cent of asymptomatic treated patients and untreated patient with lupus will be positive. Most cases of drug-induced lupus are negative for antibodies to dsDNA, although antibodies to ssDNA may be present. Commercial ELISA assays are available. However, it is essential to ensure that the histone is entirely free of contaminating DNA: this is difficult to do, as the DNA has to be digested in the presence of protease inhibitors to prevent damage to the histones.

Hsp-90 antibodies

Antibodies to the 90 kDa mammalian heat-shock protein have been described in up to 50 per cent of lupus patients and a few patients with polymyositis. The antigen is located in the cytoplasm and on the surface membrane. They are not sought routinely.

Hu antibodies

A variety of anti-neuronal antibodies have been described under various circumstances. Anti-Yo (Purkinje cell) antibodies and anti-neuronal antibodies are discussed elsewhere. Antibodies specific for neuronal cell nuclei (anti-Hu ANNA) have been described in some patients with small cell carcinoma of the lung accompanied by paraneoplastic syndromes of sensory neuropathies or encephalomyelitis. These antibodies recognize a 36–42 kDa protein of neuronal nuclei, especially of Purkinje cells. They must be distinguished from non-neurone-specific antinuclear antibodies. The immunofluorescence staining pattern is homogeneous. Another rare anti-neuronal nuclear specificity, anti-Ri, has been documented in a few women with breast cancer, together with ataxia, myoclonus and opsoclonus.

12 Autoantibodies

567

Inner-ear antibodies

It has been suggested that certain rare cases of progressive deafness may be due to an autoimmune process directed against antigens of the inner ear. These can be detected by immunofluorescence on sections of the inner ear (either bovine or guinea-pig), although obtaining suitable material is exceptionally difficult. Originally it was thought that antibodies to type II collagen formed the basis of this autoimmune process, but more recently it has been shown that the antigen is a heat-shock protein (Hsp-2). A commercial immunoblot system is now available for this antigen.

Insulin antibodies

Autoantibodies to insulin have been described as a cause of insulin resistance and are highly specific. Antibodies to the insulin receptor have also been described in insulin resistance, usually associated with acanthosis nigricans.

Intrinsic factor antibodies

Antibodies to intrinsic factor are highly specific for pernicious anaemia and are found in up to 75 per cent of patients (see Chapter 5). Two types of antibodies can be detected, those that block the binding of B12 to intrinsic factor and those that block the uptake of the IF–B12 complex. Assay of IF antibodies has usually been carried out by RIA. Attempts to develop reliable EIAs have not been satisfactory. The value of testing for IF antibodies is uncertain as the diagnosis of pernicious anaemia depends on demonstrating abnormal uptake of B_{12} in a Schilling test.

12 Autoantibodies

Inner-ear antibodies
Insulin antibodies
Intrinsic factor antibodies

Islet-cell antibodies

These may be found early in the course of type I diabetes mellitus, but gradually disappear with time; they are not found in type II diabetes. They are usually detectable within the first year after diagnosis. A small group of patients with multiple autoimmune endocrine disease maintain their antibody levels. They are also useful for screening first-degree relatives for risk of developing diabetes: their presence increases the relative risk 75-fold. They are usually detected by immunofluorescence on human pancreatic tissue (Group O) and there is an international standard with unitage (JDF units), although there is no good evidence that quantitation offers any particularly useful clinical information. One of the antigens is now thought to be glutamic acid decarboxylase.

Jo-1 antibodies

These antibodies are found in approximately 25 per cent of adult patients with autoimmune myositis, rising to 68 per cent in patients with myositis, Raynaud's, arthritis, and interstitial lung disease (anti-synthetase syndrome). In sera contain anti-Jo-1, the antinuclear antibody may be negative, without the speckled pattern seen with other antibodies to ENA: however, variable faint cytoplasmic staining may be seen on HEp-2 cells. Antibodies to Jo-1 should therefore be specifically requested. The target antigen is histidyl-tRNA synthetase. Autoantibodies to other tRNA synthetases (threonyl (PL-7), alanyl (PL-12), isoleucyl (OJ), glycyl (EJ), and lysyl) are also associated with variant myositis syndromes, but occur in very small numbers of patients overall. In clinical practice only antibodies to Jo-1 are readily available, and the antibodies are usually detected by immunodiffusion or ELISA. Antibodies to signal recognition particles (SRPs) may also be associated, especially in dermatomyositis and polymyositis without the additional features of the anti-synthetase syndrome. Anti-SRP antibodies give a granular cytoplasmic staining on HEp-2 cells.

Ku antibodies

Antibodies to this ENA are found in patients with SLE, MCTD, Sjögren's syndrome, and scleroderma (often with myositis). It is thus of little diagnostic value. The target antigen appears to be a 86kDa DNA-binding protein. It appears to be identical to the specificity previously called Ki. This antigen gives fine, speckled nuclear and nucleolar staining, depending on the stage of the cell cycle.

La (SS-B) antibodies

Antibodies to the ENA La recognize a 48 kDa protein complexed to small RNAs and is probably involved in processing of RNA Pol III transcripts. Most interestingly this protein has sequence homology with a retroviral protein. This antibody is found mainly in primary Sjögren's syndrome, but is very rare in Sjögren's syndrome secondary to rheumatoid arthritis, systemic sclerosis, or primary biliary cirrhosis. About 15 per cent of patients with SLE will have antibodies to La. Antibodies to this specificity have been associated with neonatal congenital complete heart block, although this is less common than with anti-Ro antibodies. For techniques, see under ENA.

Liver–kidney microsomal (LKM) antibodies

These antibodies bind to microsomes in the cytoplasm of hepatocytes and the cells of the proximal renal tubules, but do not stain distal renal tubules. They are often confused with mitochondrial antibodies, but the latter will also stain both the stomach and other tubules in the kidney. Three types of LKM antibodies have been described. LKM-1 antibodies recognize the cytochrome P450IIID6 and are associated with type 2a and 2b autoimmune chronic active hepatitis. Type 2a disease begins in childhood in 50 per cent of cases and is associated with autoimmunity to thyroid and gastric parietal cells. Type 2b is associated with antibodies to hepatitis C in addition to the LKM antibodies. LKM-2 recognize the cytochrome P450IIC9 and are associated with hepatitis induced by the diuretic ticrynafen (tienilic acid). LKM-3 have been reported in hepatitis-δ: the antigen is unknown; δ-infection is also associated with antibodies to the lamins of the nuclear envelope. Antibodies have also been recognized that react only with liver microsomes (LM antibodies), where the target antigen in cytochrome P450IA2. The fluorescence staining is most marked in perivenous hepatocytes. These antibodies have been associated with hepatitis induced by the drug dihydrallazine.

12 Autoantibodies

La (SS-B) antibodies
Liver–kidney microsomal (LKM) antibodies

Loop of Henle antibodies

This pattern is extremely rare and is probably of low diagnostic value. Reported cases have had renal tubular acidosis, pernicious anaemia, and primary biliary cirrhosis.

Lupus anticoagulant

See under Cardiolipin antibodies, above.

Lymphocytotoxic antibodies

Autoantibodies (as opposed to alloantibodies induced by pregnancy or transfusion) to lymphocytes have been detected in rheumatoid arthritis, systemic sclerosis, and SLE, although their role in the generation of lymphopenia is uncertain. There is no evidence to support their role in the lymphopenia of common variable immunodeficiency as has previously been suggested. Routine search for these antibodies is probably of little clinical value.

Mi-2 antibodies

Antibodies to this ENA are found typically in patients with a steroid-responsive dermatomyositis, and recognize a 220 kDa nuclear antigen. They are found only in a small subset of patients with inflammatory myositis. Homogeneous nuclear staining is usually seen.

12 Autoantibodies

575

Mitochondrial antibodies

• Normal adult range: titre < 1/40.

Mitochondrial antibodies are detected by their typical granular staining on the cytoplasm of all cells in the tissue multiblock, although they may be confused with LKM, ribosomal, and signal recognition particle antibodies. Nine discrete reactivities have been described, although these are not all detectable on standard tissue sections. Even for those patterns that are detectable, the distinction is dependent on recognizing quantitative differences in the level of staining of different cell populations. M1 antibodies are associated with syphilis, M2 antibodies with primary biliary cirrhosis, M3 with lupus-like disease, M5 with miscellaneous connective tissue disease, M6 with drug-induced hepatitis (iproniazid), M7 possibly with myocarditis and cardiomyopathy, and M9 with either early or variant PBC. M2 antibodies are strongly associated with primary biliary cirrhosis, and more than 95 per cent of PBC patients will be positive. Because of the difficulty in distinguishing the different antigenic specificities on their fluorescence patterns, new mitochondrial antibodies should be put up against the E2 antigen (see mitochondrial M2 antibodies) to confirm the specificity. Patients with type 3 autoimmune chronic active hepatitis (usually associated with antibodies to soluble liver antigens) will often have anti-mitochondrial antibodies and this entity may be an overlap syndrome of CAH and PBC. Mitochondrial antibodies are often detected in patients with autoimmune thyroiditis and Sjögren's syndrome, both of which diseases are associated clinically with PBC.

Mitochondrial M2 antibodies

The antigen of the M2 mitochondrial autoantibodies is now known to be the E2 component of the pyruvate dehydrogenase complex, although other components, E1-α and E1-β, as well the E2 subunit of branched-chain dehydrogenase, are target antigens. It has been suggested, but not confirmed, that the M9 autoantigen is sulphite oxidase. In view of the association of mitochondrial antibodies with diseases other than PBC it is now advisable to screen AMA-positive sera for antibodies to the M2 antigen, to confirm the specificity. This is usually done by EIA. Immunofluorescence remains the screening test of choice for primary biliary cirrhosis because of its simplicity and low cost.

12 Autoantibodies

Mitochondrial antibodies
Mitochondrial M2 antibodies

577

Multiple nuclear dot antibody

Two patterns of multiple nuclear dots are recognized. The pattern of 2–6 dots located close to the nucleolus is associated with antibodies to p80 coilin (anti-coiled body antibodies); this is the Nsp-II pattern. The pattern of 5–10 dots is associated with antibodies to a soluble nuclear protein Sp100; this is sometimes referred to as Nsp-I or pseudo-centromere, but there is no staining of the metaphase plate as in a true centromere antibody. This pattern is associated with a subgroup of patients with primary biliary cirrhosis, especially those who are anti-M2 antibody negative.

Myelin-associated glycoprotein antibodies (MAG)

IgM anti-MAG antibodies are associated with paraproteinaemic polyneuropathies, where the paraprotein is IgM (but not IgG or IgA). Levels of antibody do not correlate with severity of the nerve disease. Rarely anti-MAG antibodies are found in Guillain–Barré, MS, and myasthenia gravis.

Nephritic factors

Nephritic factors are autoantibodies of either IgG or IgM class which stabilize activated complement components and prevent their normal inactivation by the control proteins. Four types are recognized.

C3-nephritic factor

This is an autoantibody to the alternate pathway C3 convertase (C3bBb), which stabilizes the convertase and prevents its natural destruction by Factors H and I; the antibody recognizes the Bb component of the convertase. This allows continuous and unregulated activation of C3. It is usually detected by its effect on C3 mobility on electrophoresis, detected by immunofixation, and is reported as present or absent. Patients with mesangiocapillary glomerulonephritis type II and/or partial lipodystrophy who have a markedly reduced C3 should be screened for the presence of a C3-nephritic factor. Not all patients with partial lipodystrophy who have a C3-nephritic factor will have renal disease, although there is an increased risk of them developing it. Conversely not all patients with C3-nephritic factor have partial lipodystrophy.

C4-nephritic factor

This is also an autoantibody, very rarely described, that stabilizes the active form of C4 (C4bC2a) and leads to increased activation of the first part of the classical pathway, although, because the normal regulatory processes are intact at the level of C3, the reaction proceeds no further. C4 and C3 are usually reduced. It has been associated with SLE and other types of glomerulonephritis. It is detected by electrophoretic studies of activated serum using immunofixation.

Properdin-dependent nephritic factor

This is another nephritic factor of the alternate pathway, which slowly cleaves C3, C5, and C9 and is dependent on the presence of properdin. It is heat labile. It occurs in other types of mesangiocapillary glomerulonephritis.

C1q antibodies

These antibodies occur in SLE and mesangiocapillary GN; they recognize activated C1q (bound to antibody or solid phase).

Neuronal antibodies

These antibodies react with a 96 kDa surface antigen of neuronal cells and occur mainly in patients with neuropsychiatric lupus. They may be detected by immunofluorescence or by Western blotting. Although they may be detected in CSF, they are always present in the serum, and their presence in CSF is a manifestation of the leakiness of the blood–brain barrier. There is little advantage in looking at CSF rather than serum. Approximately 74 per cent of patients with neuropsychiatric lupus will have these antibodies, but about 11 per cent of patients without neuropsychiatric manifestations will also have them. It has been suggested that the titre of antibodies correlates with degree of neuropsychiatric impairment. They seem to be more specific for neuropsychiatric lupus than ribosomal P antibodies.

Neutrophil antibodies

Antibodies against neutrophil surface antigens may occur in autoimmune neutropenia. However, because of the presence of Fc receptors for IgG on neutrophils, it is very difficult to prove unequivocally that anti-neutrophil antibodies are present, and none of the current techniques are entirely satisfactory. Tests include neutrophil agglutination, antibody-mediated phagocytosis of neutrophils by macrophages, antibody-dependent lysis, and flow cytometry.

Antibodies specific for neutrophil nuclei, reacting with unknown antigens, are found in rheumatoid arthritis with vasculitis, particularly in Felty's syndrome (RhA, splenomegaly, vasculitis and leg ulceration, neutropenia). There is homogenous nuclear staining present only on neutrophils, but not liver or HEp-2 cells. Their importance is more in their potential to cause misinterpretation in tests for ANCA, where they may be confused, by the inexperienced, with the perinuclear pattern.

Neutrophil cytoplasmic antibodies (ANCA)

• Normal adult range: titre <1/10.

This is a test for Wegener's granulomatosis and microscopic polyarteritis: these patients will usually have a cytoplasmic ANCA (C-ANCA) pattern; 5–10 per cent of WG patients will be negative for ANCA. The antibodies are present in both the systemic and localized forms of Wegener's. The antigen is known to be proteinase 3 (Pr3), a granule protein that is also expressed on the neutrophil surface. As a test for Wegener's, meta-analysis of all published data has shown a sensitivity of 66 per cent and a specificity of 98 per cent. The perinuclear (P-ANCA) pattern is found less commonly in WG and M-PAN, but mainly in other forms of severe vasculitis, including Churg–Strauss syndrome, SLE, and rheumatoid vasculitis. It also occurs in inflammatory bowel disease, particularly where there is liver involvement (primary sclerosing cholangitis (PSC)). This pattern results from a redistribution of certain cytoplasmic antigens when cold ethanol is used as a fixative for the human neutrophils. Multiple antigens are involved in producing this pattern, including antibodies to myeloperoxidase, lactoferrin, elastase, and cathepsins. Anti-lactoferrin antibodies have been reported to be associated with inflammatory bowel disease and PSC. Antibodies to nuclear antigens and to GBM may co-exist with ANCA, making diagnosis difficult. The gold standard method for detection is immunofluorescence on cold-ethanol-fixed neutrophils. Other fixatives such acetone or formalin give unreliable results and do not distinguish reliably between C-ANCA and P-ANCA. Solid-phase assays for purified antigens (Pr3, myeloperoxidase, and lactoferrin) are available but are expensive. It is therefore still appropriate to screen on neutrophils, as more information can be gathered from this test, and then use a confirmatory test only on positive samples. Serial monitoring of C-ANCA is useful as a rising titre may herald a relapse of Wegener's. Whether there is any value in serial monitoring of P-ANCA is less certain.

585

Nuclear antibodies (ANA)

- Normal ranges:
  - age < 18: titre < 1/20
  - age 18–65: titre < 1/40
  - age > 65: titre < 1/80.

Nuclear antibodies are associated with the connective tissue diseases. Only IgG antibodies are significant: IgM ANA are non-specific and frequently occur after viral infections, although occasional patients with connective tissue disease produce only IgM ANA. IgM ANA are said to be the most common type of ANA in rheumatoid arthritis, although some of these are due to cross-reactive IgM rheumatoid factors. A significant titre of IgG ANA is dependent on age, and low-titre positive ANAs in the elderly must be carefully interpreted in the context of relevant clinical symptoms and signs. The pattern of ANA will give diagnostic pointers: speckled ANA are found in Sjögren's syndrome, SLE, and mixed connective tissue disease (MCTD); homogeneous ANA are associated with SLE and drug-induced LE: while nucleolar ANA are associated with scleroderma and systemic sclerosis. It is therefore important that the pattern should be reported. Homogeneous ANAs are usually associated with antibodies to dsDNA and histones, while speckled ANAs are associated with antibodies to the ENAs Ro, La, and Sm/RNP complex. The ENAs, Jo-1 and Scl-70 are not usually detectable on rodent liver and on HEp-2 cells give distinctive cytoplasmic and speckled nuclear staining, respectively. Because of the long circulating half-life of the autoantibodies, measurement does not need to be carried out more frequently than once every 3 weeks (unless the patient has been plasmapheresed).

Detection of ANA is usually carried out by immunofluorescence on rodent liver sections. HEp-2 cells are an alternative, though usually more expensive. The advantage of HEp-2 cells is that the nuclei are very large, so it is far easier to identify the patterns of nuclear reactivity; HEp-2 cells also provide a more sensitive substrate, as well as being essential for the detection of anti-centromere antibodies (although very experienced microscopists can usually pick up the pattern on liver sections). This increased sensitivity means that screening on HEp-2 cells will pick up more ANAs in healthy individuals (about 6.9 per cent in one study). One of the disadvantages of liver is that it has low amounts of the Ro antigen, which is cytoplasmic in location, very saline soluble, and hence easily washed out. This phenomenon gave rise to the concept of ANA-negative lupus, as about 20 per cent of patients with clinically unequivocal lupus were negative for ANA when screened on rodent liver. However, if HEp-2 cells are used, this figure drops to almost zero, as there are higher levels of Ro antigen and it is mainly intranuclear in its distribution, making it more resistant to leaching. A genetically modified HEp-2 cell (HEp-2000) is supposed to have higher levels of Ro antigen, but in the UK National External Quality Assurance Scheme (NEQAS) performance it was no better than standard HEp-2 cells. On HEp-2 cells, Sm/RNP complex antibodies give a very coarse granular staining, which spares the nucleoli, while Ro and La antibodies give a finer staining pattern. Other staining patterns detected on HEp-2 cells, and discussed elsewhere, include centriole, centromere, nuclear matrix, nuclear pore, proliferating cell nuclear antigen (PCNA), multiple nuclear dots (pseudocentromere), and nucleolar. On HEp-2 cells antibodies may also be detected to lysosomes and Golgi bodies: these have no major significance. A pattern of cytoplasmic radiating fibres may be associated with anti-actin or anti-vimentin antibodies. The latter have been associated with SLE.

The detection of a strong positive ANA should lead to further tests to investigate the specificity, as this will help clarify the likely clinical diagnosis. Further tests should always include a search for antibodies to dsDNA and ENA, particularly if homogeneous or speckled patterns are identified. If drug-induced LE is suspected, anti-histone antibodies are appropriate.

Perinuclear ANAs are described, particularly in rheumatoid arthritis and other connective tissue diseases, and may occur in both RhF positive and negative patients. Similar antibodies are often found as a result of EBV infection. Antibodies to lamins A, B, and C also give this type of staining pattern and are found in some SLE patients and in patients with the constellation of hepatitis, anti-phospholipid antibodies, cytopenias, and leucocytoclastic vasculitis.

Because of the multiplicity of different antigens recognized, it has proven difficult to standardize testing for ANA, although there is an agreed WHO standard for homogeneous ANA.

Nuclear matrix antibodies

These antibodies give large, coarse speckles on HEp-2 cells; the specificity appears to be against heterogeneous nuclear RNA and matrix proteins: by immunoblotting at least four proteins are recognized, of molecular weight 70, 31, 23, and 19 kDa. The 70 kDa determinant is U1-RNP. The antibodies are rarely seen but occur in lupus as well as undifferentiated connective tissue diseases.

Nuclear mitotic spindle antibodies

These antibodies, which will only be seen on HEp-2 cells, are rare and not specific, being found in SLE, rheumatoid arthritis, CREST, MCTD, and Sjögren's syndrome. Various patterns have been described. NuMA (nuclear mitotic apparatus protein) shows fluorescence concentrated at the spindle poles. Anti-tubulin antibodies stain the spindle fibres. Antibodies to mitotic spindle antigens (MSA) show two patterns of staining: MSA-2 does not stain interphase cells and is sometimes referred to as the midbody pattern, while MSA-3 shows fine, dense nuclear staining in some interphase cells and two sets of discrete granules on either side of the metaphase plate in dividing cells.

Nuclear pore antibodies

Antibodies to a 210 kDa nuclear pore antigen have been described in up to 27 per cent of cases of primary biliary cirrhosis (in addition to the multiple nuclear dot pattern). The immunofluorescence here gives a perinuclear staining pattern, best seen on HEp-2 cells.

12 Autoantibodies

Nuclear matrix antibodies
Nuclear mitotic spindle antibodies
Nuclear pore antibodies

Nucleolar antibodies

Nucleolar antibodies will be detected on routine screening on rodent liver. However, they are much easier to see on HEp-2 cells, where three discrete staining patterns may be identified:
- speckled nucleolar staining with fine, speckled nuclear staining;
- homogeneous nucleolar staining;
- clumpy nucleolar staining with nuclear dots.

The speckled pattern is associated with antibodies to RNA polymerase I and is present in 4 per cent of patients with systemic sclerosis, associated with the diffuse form of the disease. The homogeneous staining is seen with antibodies to PM-Scl (see below) and the clumpy form is associated with antibodies to fibrillarin, which is a component of the U3-RNP. The latter is found in 8 per cent of patients with systemic sclerosis, particularly disease with cardiopulmonary involvement but little joint involvement.

Other nucleolar antigens to which autoantibodies have been detected include Nor-90, a 90 kDa protein of the nucleolar organizer region; To, a 40 kDa protein complexed to 7S or 8S RNA; and an RNP particle that includes RNA polymerase III.

Ovarian antibodies

This test is useful for identifying primary autoimmune ovarian failure as a cause of infertility and may be found in 15–50 per cent of patients with premature ovarian failure. Patients may also be positive for adrenal antibodies (cross-reactive steroid cell antibodies) and for thyroid antibodies. Detection is usually by immunofluorescence. Recent data suggests that antibodies to 3β-hydroxysteroid dehydrogenase may be a more sensitive marker of premature (autoimmune) ovarian failure.

12 Autoantibodies

Nucleolar antibodies
Ovarian antibodies

591

Parathyroid antibodies

These are found in patients with idiopathic hypoparathyroidism, hypoparathyoidism associated with other endocrinopathies, and in chronic mucocutaneous candidiasis. They are usually detected on group O human parathyroid by immunofluorescence. However, they are impossible to detect if ANA or mitochondrial antibodies are present. Testing should therefore be carried out in parallel with testing on the standard tissue multiblock.

PCNA (proliferating cell nuclear antigen) antibodies

This antigen is expressed only at certain times in the cell cycle. It is readily detectable only on HEp-2 cells, where it gives variable-sized speckles in only some cells. The antigen (cyclin) is an $33\,kDa$ auxiliary protein for DNA polymerase-δ. It is seen in about 3 per cent of patients with SLE, but does not appear to identify any particular clinical subgroup.

Pituitary gland antibodies

Antibodies to pituitary components have been described in a variety of centrally mediated endocrine disorders, in the empty sella syndrome, in some pituitary tumours, and in some patients with insulin-dependent diabetes mellitus. They are usually detected by immunofluorescence on pituitary sections or on pituitary cell lines. The diagnostic value is uncertain.

12 Autoantibodies

Parathyroid antibodies
PCNA (proliferating cell nuclear antigen) antibodies
Pituitary gland antibodies

Platelet antibodies

Platelets autoantibodies (as opposed to alloantibodies) are found in patients with ITP, but are also found in other conditions associated with thrombocytopenia, such as HIV, connective tissue diseases, thrombotic thrombocytopenic purpura (TTP), and heparin-induced thrombocytopenia. Many techniques have been described to detect such antibodies, including phagocytosis by neutrophils, lymphocyte activation, RIA, EIA, and flow cytometry. Using sensitive techniques, over 90 per cent of patients with ITP will be shown to have platelet-associated IgG. However, there is no consensus on the best technique or on the value of routine testing. The target antigens are varied but include platelet GP Ib, IIb, and IIIa. Alloantibodies to platelets react with PL^{A1} antigen.

PM-Scl antibodies

PM-Scl antibodies are found in the polymyositis–scleroderma overlap syndrome, although they may also be found in patients with dermatomyositis/polymyositis or systemic sclerosis occurring alone. There may be an increased risk of renal disease in the overlap patients. The target antigen appears to be a complex of 11 proteins occurring in the nucleolus and elsewhere. The pattern of immunofluorescence on HEp-2 cells is variable, with homogeneous nucleolar staining, with some atypical nuclear speckling and cytoplasmic staining. Detection is usually by immunodiffusion or immunoblotting.

Poly-(ADP-ribose) polymerase antibodies

These antibodies to the 116 kDa protein have been reported in Sjögren's syndrome and in association with neuropathy. They are not sought routinely.

12 Autoantibodies

Platelet antibodies
PM-Scl antibodies
Poly-(ADP-ribose) polymerase antibodies

Purkinje cell antibodies

See Yo antibodies, below.

RA-33 antibodies

These antibodies have been described as specific for rheumatoid arthritis. They react with a 33 kDa non-histone nuclear antigen of HeLa cells. There are insufficient data to evaluate their utility.

Rheumatoid-associated nuclear antibodies (RANA)

If EBV-transformed cell lines are used as a target, antibodies can be detected in serum of patients with rheumatoid arthritis and other connective tissue diseases that react only with EBV-infected nuclei, but not normal nuclei. There is no routine value to this test.

12 Autoantibodies

Purkinje cell antibodies
RA-33 antibodies
Rheumatoid-associated nuclear antibodies (RANA)

Renal biopsy (snap-frozen)

Direct immunofluorescence of renal biopsies is an essential part of the evaluation of renal disease. This should always take place in parallel with examination of biopsies with standard stains and by electron microscopy. Staining should include the use of antisera to IgG, IgA, IgM, C3, C4, and fibrinogen. Linear deposition of IgG in the glomeruli is a feature of anti-GBM disease. IgA deposition is heavy in a segmental pattern in IgA nephropathy, and Henoch–Schönlein purpura is also associated with IgA deposition, often with fibrin deposition. In type II MPGN, associated with a nephritic factor, there is heavy C3 deposition in the GBM, without immunoglobulin. Patchy IgG and C3, or C3 alone is a feature of post-streptococcal GN. SLE may give any pattern of renal disease, and is usually accompanied by IgG, IgM, and complement deposition with a variable distribution. In tubulo-interstitial nephritis, there may be antibodies to the tubular basement membrane that are visible by DIF.

Reticulin antibodies

- Normal range:
    - adults: <1/40
    - adults > 65: <1/80.

These antibodies are non-specific: they are found in coeliac disease, but also in inflammatory bowel disease, particularly where there is concomitant liver disease. They may occur in the absence of clinical disease in the elderly. They will be detected as part of the 'autoimmune screen', but if coeliac disease is suspected, endomysial and gliadin antibodies should be requested. IgA reticulin antibodies are slightly more specific for coeliac disease than IgG antibodies. Up to five different patterns of anti-reticulin antibodies have been described using immunofluorescence. Only the R1 pattern is associated with coeliac disease. IgA-R1-reticulin antibodies are reported to have a specificity of 98 per cent but a sensitivity of only 25 per cent for coeliac disease. Some laboratories report the different patterns. However, there is little value in this now that anti-gliadin and anti-EMA antibodies are available, as these are the preferred diagnostic tests. Detection of high-titre anti-reticulin antibodies should automatically prompt screening for gliadin and EMA antibodies.

599

Retinal S100 antibodies

Antibodies against retinal antigens (S100) have been identified in many types of chronic inflammatory eye disease affecting the uveal tract, including the Vogt–Koyanagi–Harada syndrome, but are not disease-specific. Their diagnostic value is uncertain at present. Other anti-retinal antibodies have been described as a paraneoplastic phenomenon in patients with a cancer-associated retinopathy syndrome, seen rarely in association with small cell lung carcinoma. The antibodies may induce demyelination of the optic nerve. Lens-induced uveitis, a rare condition that may follow trauma or surgery, is associated with circulating antibodies to lens proteins.

Rheumatoid factor

• Normal adult range: titre < 1/80 (also IU).

This is a non-specific test; it detects immunoglobulins of any class reactive with the Fc region of other immunoglobulins. Rheumatoid factors (RhFs) occur in a wide variety of conditions, such as viral infections, chronic bacterial infections (SBE, TB), myelomas, lymphomas, and many connective tissue diseases. In myeloma the paraproteins with RhF activity may also be associated with cryoglobulins (type II), while in infections and connective tissue diseases the polyclonal RhFs may cause a type III cryoglobulin. Healthy elderly people may also have rheumatoid factors. Rheumatoid arthritis patients may be positive or negative for RhFs, but those with progressive disease, and with vasculitis, usually have high-titre RhFs. There is little value in serial monitoring of RhF, as the titre correlates poorly with disease activity: the CRP is more useful. Requesting RhFs in the elderly is not helpful, as positive results do not necessarily indicate disease. At present there is no conclusive evidence that detecting IgA RhFs are of particular value. RhFs may be detected by latex or particle agglutination, by EIA, or by nephelometry. The older sheep-cell agglutination test (SCAT, Rose–Waaler) is no longer used.

12 Autoantibodies

Retinal S100 antibodies
Rheumatoid factor

Ribosomal antibodies

Antibodies to ribosomes, particularly to ribosomal ribonucleo-protein (rRNP) are associated particularly with SLE (about 5–12 per cent of patients), although they may also be found in rheumatoid arthritis. It has been suggested that ribosomal antibodies in lupus may be associated with nephritis. They frequently cause diagnostic confusion as they may be misinterpreted as mitochondrial antibodies by inexperienced microscopists. However, they react particularly strongly with the chief cells of rodent stomach, and also with pancreatic tissue. The antigens are distinct from those recognized by antibodies to nuclear RNPs.

Ribosomal P protein antibodies

Antibodies to the ribosomal P protein have been associated frequently with neuropsychiatric lupus. However, there is no evidence that they are a sensitive or specific marker for this complication, as they occur frequently in patients with no evidence of cerebral involvement. They may, however, be a specific marker for lupus in general as they do not occur in other connective tissue diseases. Few laboratories have this test available routinely, so their utility is small. If neuropsychiatric lupus is suspected then anti-neuronal antibodies are probably of more value.

RNP antibodies

These antibodies are usually taken to refer to antibodies recognizing nuclear, rather than ribosomal RNPs. There are a number of such complexes (U1–U6-RNPs), which comprise a number of proteins with small nuclear RNAs. The same protein components may occur in more than one RNP complex. The most important antibodies are those against the U1-RNP, which recognize the 70 kDa A and C protein components. These give rise to a coarse, speckled pattern on immunofluorescence and occur in SLE and mixed connective tissue disease (MCTD). When they occur in the absence of antibodies to dsDNA and Sm, this is supposed to indicate MCTD, although some authorities doubt that MCTD is truly a distinct entity and prefer to think of it as a subset of SLE. There is no relation between anti-RNP antibody titres and disease activity, unlike antibodies to dsDNA.

Some sera from patients with SLE contain antibodies that react with both Sm and U1-RNP. Antibodies have been also been described that react with both U1- and U2-RNP, recognizing the U1-A and U2-B' proteins: these are seen in SLE and SLE overlap syndromes, particularly where myositis is a feature. However, distinction of the fine specificities of antibodies to nuclear RNPs is not available routinely. Normally, antibodies to RNP will be detected by immunodiffusion, countercurrent immunoelectrophoresis, ELISA, or Western blotting. The latter technique offers the possibility of distinguishing the subsets of anti-RNP antibodies.

Ro (SS-A) antibodies

Antibodies to the ENA antigen Ro recognize two proteins of 60 and 52 kDa complexed with Y1–Y5 RNAs. Antibodies have been described which recognize either protein. It is associated with Sjögren's syndrome, with the highest levels in primary disease, SLE, cutaneous LE, and C2-deficient lupus. Antibodies are of particular importance in pregnancy, as they are usually of IgG class and cross the placenta, where they can cause neonatal lupus or congenital complete heart block in the fetus. It is known that the antigen is expressed transiently in the developing cardiac conducting system. The antigen is also inducible in keratinocytes by UV light, explaining the strong association of anti-Ro with photosensitivity and with cutaneous disease. Anti-Ro is often the specificity detected in so-called ANA-negative lupus. This concept arose because the Ro antigen is present at lower levels and is mainly cytoplasmic in hepatocytes and is thus easily washed out of the tissue during processing. In HEp-2 cells there are higher nuclear levels; on this substrate there is a fine, nuclear, speckled staining. For techniques of detection see ENA antibodies (above). Immunoblotting allows distinction of antibodies against the two antigens.

605

Salivary gland antibodies

It is not possible to test for these in the presence of antinuclear or anti-mitochondrial antibodies. These are associated with Sjögren's syndrome and are more likely to occur in secondary rather than primary disease. They are detected by immunofluorescence on rodent salivary gland.

Scl-70 (PM-1) antibodies

These are found in 20–40 per cent of patients with progressive systemic sclerosis (PSS) and 20 per cent of patients with limited scleroderma, and are associated particularly with severe skin disease, musculoskeletal, and cardiopulmonary disease. It has also been suggested that the antibody is a marker for the development of carcinoma of the lung in PSS. They do not predict the development of renal disease, although their presence in patients with isolated Raynaud's predicts the subsequent development of PSS and hence is a poor prognostic marker. The antigen recognized is topoisomerase I, an enzyme involved in supercoiling DNA; the autoantibody interferes with the function of the target antigen. Scl-70 and anti-centromere antibodies appear to be mutually exclusive, as only two cases have ever been reported of co-existence of both specificities. Scl-70 antibodies give an atypical nuclear speckled pattern on HEp-2 staining; definitive proof of their presence is obtained either by immunodiffusion, ELISA, or immunoblotting.

Signal recognition particle (SRP) antibodies

These antibodies produce a cytoplasmic staining pattern on HEp-2 cells that may be mistaken for mitochondrial antibodies. The antigen is a 54 kDa protein complexed with RNA. This pattern is associated with polymyositis and dermatomyositis.

12 Autoantibodies

Salivary gland antibodies
Scl-70 (PM-1) antibodies
Signal recognition particle (SRP) antibodies

607

Skin and mucosal biopsies: direct immunofluorescence

See Epidermal antibodies, above.

Sm (Smith) antibodies

These antibodies, named after the patient in whom they were first described, are specific for SLE, and tend to be seen most frequently in West Indians with SLE; they are rare in Caucasians. The antibodies react with the B'/B and D proteins shared by U1-, U2- and U4–U6-RNPs. These specificities are often seen with antibodies to U1-RNP. Whether occurring alone or with anti-RNP, these antibodies are accepted as a diagnostic criterion for lupus. They are usually detected by the same techniques as other ENAs (Ro, La, RNP).

Smooth-muscle antibodies (SMA)

• Normal adult range: titre <1/40.
These are present in high titre in 50–70 per cent of patients with autoimmune 'lupoid' hepatitis (type 1). Twenty-five per cent of patients may also be positive for nuclear and dsDNA antibodies. They are also found sometimes in type 3 autoimmune hepatitis, although the predominant marker of this type of hepatitis is antibody to soluble liver antigens (SLA), which may be the only autoantibody in up to 25 per cent of cases. The target antigen(s) for SLA antibodies are not known, and different patterns of fluorescence have been obtained, including the liver–pancreas antigen (undefined) and the liver cytosol antibody (LC-1). High-titre SMA antibodies against F-actin are seen in type 4 hepatitis, which affects predominantly young children. Other smooth-muscle antibodies directed against tropomyosin may be found. SMAs typically stain the muscular coats of arteries and the muscular layer of the stomach section, where there is also staining of the intergastric gland fibres. On HEp-2 cells, a meshwork of fine cytoplasmic fibres may be seen. The primary substrate for detection is the tissue multiblock.

12 Autoantibodies

Skin and mucosal biopsies: direct immunofluorescence
Sm (Smith) antibodies
Smooth-muscle antibodies (SMA)

609

Sp100 antibodies

Antibodies to this antigen of nucleus give rise to the multiple nuclear dot (5–10 dots) pattern of staining on HEp-2 cells (pseudo-centromere). It is found in AMA-negative primary biliary cirrhosis. A commercial ELISA assay for antibodies to this antigen is available.

Sperm antibodies

Both agglutinating and immobilizing antibodies have been described. Multiple antigens seem to be involved and only some seem to be important in interfering with fertility. They are common after vasectomy (50 per cent of men) and may occur after trauma to the testes. They may be detected in 1–12 per cent of women and 10–20 per cent of women with infertility. Antibodies may be of IgG or IgA class and may be found in serum or seminal/cervical secretions.

Steroid cell antibodies

See Adrenal antibodies and Ovarian antibodies, above.

Striated-muscle antibodies

These are present in some patients with myasthenia gravis: almost all (80–100 per cent) patients with myasthenia with thymoma are positive. They are thus an important simple screening test in myasthenia for the presence of a thymoma and should form part of the diagnostic work-up. The antigen is thought to be a protein of the I-band of the myocyte, called titin.

12 Autoantibodies

Thyroid microsomal (peroxidase) antibodies

• Normal adult range: titre <1/800 (particle agglutination).

These are present in high titre in 95 per cent of patients with Hashimoto's thyroiditis, 18 per cent of patients with Graves' disease, and 90 per cent of patients with primary myxoedema. They are also present in low titres in patients with colloidal goitre, thyroid carcinoma, transiently in de Quervain's thyroiditis, and occasionally in normal people. They may also be found in patients with other organ-specific autoimmune diseases, such as pernicious anaemia, Addison's disease, etc. The antigen is now known to be thyroid peroxidase. The assay is usually carried out by particle agglutination or tanned red cell agglutination using crude microsomal antigens, although EIA assays using purified or recombinant TPO are now available, although whether there are any significant advantages to using these newer assays is still questionable. Some laboratories use sections of thyroid tissue in their tissue multiblock and detect thyroid antibodies by immunofluorescence. This becomes impossible in the presence of other specificities such as ANA and AMA which obscure the thyroid-specific pattern.

Thyroglobulin antibodies

• Normal adult range: titre <1/400.

Occurrence is similar to that of thyroid microsomal antibodies but thyroglobulin antibodies are less sensitive and specific. There is probably little additional information to be gained from performing this test and many laboratories have dropped it from their repertoire.

12 Autoantibodies
Thyroid microsomal (peroxidase) antibodies
Thyroglobulin antibodies
Thyroid-binding (stimulating/blocking) antibodies
Thyroid orbital antibodies

Thyroid-binding (stimulating/blocking) antibodies

Three classes of functional antibodies have also been described:
- thyroid stimulating antibodies, that increase cAMP levels in thyrocytes;
- thyroid growth-promoting antibodies, which increase tritiated thymidine uptake into DNA by isolated thyrocytes; and
- thyroid blocking antibodies that block the binding of TSH to its receptor on thyrocytes.

Several sites of antibody binding to the TSH-R have been demonstrated. All three types of antibody have been strongly associated with Graves' disease and rarely occur in other types of thyroid disease. They may be of clinical significance through correlation with response to therapy and outcome.

Their detection involves *in vitro* culture of thyrocytes, and usually some type of competitive RIA.

Thyroid orbital antibodies

These antibodies are found in Graves' disease and bind to the retro-orbital fat or fibroblasts, causing hypertrophy and resulting in exophthalmos. The antigen(s) is/are unknown. These antibodies may persist even when the thyroid disease is treated. There is no routine screen for these antibodies.

Ubiquitin antibodies

These antibodies occur in up to 80 per cent of cases of SLE and are said to be specific. At present, however, they are not measured routinely.

Voltage-gated calcium-channel antibodies

It is now accepted that IgG antibodies against the presynaptic calcium channel on the nerve terminal is the pathogenic factor in the Lambert–Eaton myasthenic syndrome (LEMS). The number of channels is reduced due to cross-linking and internalization and this impairs release of acetylcholine; complement is also involved. It is now recognized that LEMS may occur in patients who do not have small cell carcinoma of the lung, which was the association first described. Several types of calcium channels exist and the antibody is specific for the neuronal (N) type. About 90 per cent of small cell carcinoma associated LEMS will have detectable antibodies. About 40 per cent of patients with LEMS have no obvious tumour at presentation, but the tumours often become apparent over the next 4 years. Similar antibodies have also been documented in amyotrophic lateral sclerosis, although the significance is uncertain (anti-ganglioside antibodies may also occur in these patients). The assay is only available through specialist referral centres.

Voltage-gated potassium-channel antibodies

The precise value of this antibody is yet to be established, but it has been associated with acquired neuromyotonia. The potassium channels are located on the nerve terminal and control nerve excitability.

12 Autoantibodies

Ubiquitin antibodies
Voltage-gated calcium-channel antibodies
Voltage-gated potassium-channel antibodies

Yo antibodies

Yo antibodies have been associated with paraneoplastic cerebellar degeneration, seen typically with ovarian cancer, and less commonly with breast cancer or Hodgkin's lymphoma, but not in the cerebellar syndrome seen in small cell carcinoma of the lung. The antigen in question is found in the cytoplasm of Purkinje cells, and gives a coarse, granular staining by immunofluorescence. The putative target antigen (CDR34) is expressed on epithelial tumours as well as neuronal tissue, making it likely that the antibody is a cross-reactive anti-tumour antibody. The antibodies are detectable in the CSF as well as serum and disappear with successful treatment of the primary tumour.

12 Autoantibodies

Yo antibodies

617

13 Allergy

Introduction

The techniques used for allergy diagnosis *in vitro* are those already discussed in Chapters 11 and 12, and include RIA, EIA. The principles are identical.

Allergen-specific IgE (RAST, etc.)

Detection of allergen-specific IgE in the blood can be undertaken by sensitive RIA, EIA, or fluorescent assay. There are numerous acronyms for this process, depending on the method (RAST, MAST, FAST tests, etc.). The principles of all the tests are identical, with allergen bound onto a solid phase which is then incubated with a labelled anti-IgE antibody. The newer Pharmacia CAP system has a much higher sensitivity and specificity than the older systems. These tests are expensive, mainly because of the cost of preparing suitable allergens for coating onto the solid phase. Such tests should be used for confirming equivocal skin tests and for testing in patients in whom skin testing is impossible or contraindicated. Patients with very low total IgE (<20 kU/l) have a very low probability of having positive allergen-specific IgE. Conversely, patients with very high total IgE levels (>1000 kU/l) may have false-positive tests for allergen-specific IgE, due to nonspecific binding of IgE to the solid phase. This applies particularly to food allergens. However, this seems to be less of a problem with newer assays such as the CAP system. The assays can be carried out quantitatively and reported in units. However, it is more usual for the results to be graded on a scale of 0–6, where 0–1 represent no significant specific IgE and 2–6 represent increasing levels of positivity. The units are standardized against an international standard for a birch pollen allergen, but this cannot validly be applied to reactions with other allergens. Attempts are being made to standardize allergens in terms of defined proteins and protein nitrogen. With a potentially limitless list of allergens, this is a slow process. The important clinical implication is that the detection of a grade 3 response to two different allergens does not indicate that the same amount of IgE is present against both and the equivalent reactions might be expected. There is no close relationship between the grade and the severity of reactions (either past or future): indeed, the presence of allergen-specific IgE is a marker only of exposure, and positives may be detected where there is no evidence of any clinical reaction. Levels will fall with time if the offending allergen is avoided over a long period, so low or negative results may be obtained even with sensitized patients. As with skin-prick tests, if the allergic reaction is highly localized, there may be insufficient spillover of specific IgE into the circulation to be detected, leading to a false negative. Results must always be interpreted in the light of the clinical history (blood tests are not a substitute for proper history taking!).

Most manufacturers have comprehensive lists of allergens, including inhalants, foods, venoms, and occupational allergens. Tests are available for a few drugs: penicillin, amoxycillin, suxamethonium, and thiopentone. The penicillin reagent contains only the major determinants, so a negative test does not exclude significant allergy.

Allergen-specific IgG

It has been suggested that desensitization procedures work, in part, by producing blocking IgG antibodies, which prevent the allergen binding to cytophilic IgE. These have been proposed to be of the IgG4 subclass. It is further suggested that the success and duration of desensitization may be determined by measurement of such antibodies. This is controversial. It is, however, possible to measure allergen-specific IgG antibodies to allergens such as bee, or wasp venom, grass pollen, and house dust mite. Whether the results provide any clinically useful information is still unproven.

CD23, soluble (Fcε receptor)

Measurement of soluble CD23, the shed form of the Fcε receptor which has B-cell stimulatory activity, has been proposed as a useful marker of the activity of chronic allergic disease. In asthma, elevated sCD23 may denote underlying chronic inflammatory activity even when the peak flow may be near predicted. Whether long-term treatment aimed at normalizing sCD23 levels has a beneficial effect in preventing progression of the inflammatory process to irreversible lung disease remains to be determined. Measurement of this marker cannot yet be recommended without reservation. Assay is by EIA.

C3a, C4a, and C5a (anaphylotoxins)

See Chapter 11. Measurement of the anaphylotoxins may be of value in the investigation of suspected acute allergic reactions, as a marker of complement activation. This is particularly valuable in circumstances where IgE is not involved (anaphylactoid reactions). The difficulty is the need to collect the samples into Futhan–EDTA, as the tubes will not be available at the time and site of the reaction: this seriously limits the utility of the tests. Tests for C3d require EDTA samples and are therefore more useful as a marker of complement activation during a reaction.

13 Allergy

Allergen-specific IgG
CD23, soluble (Fcε receptor)
C3a, C4a, and C5a (anaphylotoxins)

Challenge tests

Challenge tests form an important part of the diagnosis of allergic disease. Clearly, identification of the site of the reaction is important. Nasal, bronchial, and oral challenge may be performed. It is wise to avoid challenging someone who has had a severe systemic reaction, or who has pre-existent severe asthma, with allergens. As for skin testing, it is essential that patients are not taking antihistamines and have been off treatment for a length of time appropriate to the half-life of their antihistamine (up to 4 weeks in some cases). Challenge tests are potentially dangerous and should be carried out by experienced staff prepared to deal with any adverse reactions that may arise. Informed consent should always be sought from the patient prior to the test.

Nasal challenge tests are usually performed by spraying a diluted solution (1:1000 of SPT solution) of the test allergen into one nostril, while spraying a similarly diluted solution of the buffer only into the other nostril. Patients' symptoms are then recorded (running nose, sneezing, itching eyes, etc.) and the nasal mucosa is inspected for signs of inflammation and oedema. Each nostril is inspected. This process is clearly limited to one allergen at a time, which restricts its use to confirming sensitivity to a single suspect allergen. More complex challenge tests involve measurement of nasal airflow (rhinomanometry) but this is rarely available outside specialist research centres.

The most common bronchial challenge is with methacholine or histamine. This is carried out by starting with very dilute solutions and gradually increasing the dose, while measuring the forced expired volume (FEV1) sequentially. A reduction of 20 per cent from the control value is viewed as a positive test and is indicative of hyperreactive airways. The dose causing this reduction is the PD20. If a dose of methacholine of 25 mg/ml is tolerated without achieving a 20 per cent reduction in FEV1, the test is unequivocally negative. Allergen solutions may be substituted for methacholine, but the principles are the same. However, it is important to remember the possibility of developing late reactions 6–8 hours after the challenge, as part of type I response. Enthusiasts may carry out endobronchial challenge through a bronchoscope, which allows them to observe the changes in the bronchial mucosa and also to carry out bronchoalveolar lavage to look at the release of mediators and the cellular response. This is important in research but not for routine diagnosis.

Food challenge is more complex. The initial step is usually withdrawal of the suspect food(s) followed by open challenge. Where multiple foods are suspected, an oligoallergenic diet may be instituted for a period to see whether symptoms remit. Foods may then be reintroduced one at a time and the patient's symptom response noted. The gold-standard for confirming food allergy is the double-blind placebo-controlled food challenge, where the patient, on an oligoallergenic diet is challenged with the suspect food concealed in opaque gelatin capsules, interspersed with identical capsules containing an innocuous substance. Both the patient and the doctor should be unaware of the contents of the capsules This is time consuming, as some food allergic symptoms may require exposure for several days before they appear and, equally, may take several days to disappear when the food is withdrawn. There needs to be a washout period between the placebo and the active capsules. A method of scoring symptoms needs to be decided in advance. Needless to say, dietary manipulation and challenges should always be carried out with the direct involvement of an experienced dietician. As for bronchial challenges, enthusiasts have directly instilled allergens into the small bowel and watched for inflammatory reactions.

Eosinophil cationic protein (ECP)

This is a granule protein of eosinophils, and its presence in serum is a marker of eosinophil activation. Levels are elevated in asthma and other allergic diseases, including urticaria, and correlate with the degree of underlying inflammation. It has been suggested that regular monitoring of ECP levels in asthma may provide evidence of the adequacy of the inhaled steroid treatment in suppressing the inflammatory process, thus allowing steroid therapy to be more accurately adjusted. ECP is the neurotoxic agent in Churg–Strauss vasculitis, and levels are elevated in acute disease. ECP levels are raised in synovial fluid from patients with rheumatoid arthritis and ankylosing spondylitis. Levels in urine are elevated by carcinoma of the bladder and in the CSF by malignant but not by benign tumours. Unfortunately, the specimen requirements require timed separation of samples, although the assay itself uses very similar methodology to that used for detecting allergen-specific IgE. This is because ECP may be released during the coagulation process. This somewhat limits its usefulness.

Eosinophil count

When investigating suspected allergic disease it is worth requesting a specific eosinophil count. This may be available routinely on the newer automated haematology counters, which are capable of providing a five-part differential; where older counters are used an additional manual differential with special stains may be required. Levels of up to $0.44 \times 10^9/l$ are normal in adults, up to $0.7 \times 10^9/l$ in children aged 1–3 years and up to $0.85 \times 10^9/l$ in the newborn. Raised eosinophil counts are not specific for allergic disease and moderate elevations are seen in parasitic infestations, as part of drug reactions, in lymphoma (especially Hodgkin's lymphoma), after radiation therapy, in certain vasculitides (Churg–Strauss vasculitis, polyarteritis nodosa), in dermatitis herpetiformis, in primary immunodeficiencies (Omenn's syndrome, materno-fetal engraftment), and in hepatic cirrhosis. Exceptionally high eosinophil counts are seen in larva migrans, hypereosinophilic syndromes, and occasionally in lymphoma, PAN, and cirrhosis. The eosinophil count is reduced by acute infection, stress, fasting for more than 24 hours, and by corticosteroids.

Examination of nasal and conjunctival secretions for the presence of eosinophils may provide confirmatory evidence for an allergic cause for local symptoms.

Histamine release assays

In vitro release of histamine by basophils in response to stimulation by cytokines or by allergens is a complex test, requiring the ability to measure free histamine. These assays are of value in the research setting, and in the clinical setting have been used for investigating the histamine releasing properties of certain drugs. Like all bioassays, they suffer from difficulties in standardization. Few routine laboratories are able to offer these tests.

Immunoglobulin E (IgE)

- Normal ranges:
  - age <1 year: <11 kU/l
  - age <2 years: <29 kU/l
  - age 2–3 years: <42 kU/l
  - age 4–5 years: <52 kU/l
  - age 6–7 years: <56 kU/l
  - age 8–10 years: <63 kU/l
  - age 11–12 years: <45 kU/l
  - age 13–14 years: <70 kU/l
  - age >14 years: <100 kU/l.

Measurement of total IgE may be helpful in diagnosing allergic disease; however, the normal range is very wide and levels correlate poorly with clinical disease. A high level of specific IgE to a single allergen may occur with a total IgE within the 'normal' range. In asthmatic patients, a level of >150 kU/l is suggestive of an allergic basis, while a level <20 kU/l is very much against it. The severity of asthmatic symptoms correlates very poorly with total IgE (but better with eosinophil count). In the investigation of dermatitis, a level of >400 kU/l is usual while a level of <20 kU/l is against atopic dermatitis. Very high levels of IgE are seen in atopic eczema, allergic bronchopulmonary aspergillosis (ABPA), parasitic infections (larva migrans, hookworm, schistosomiasis, and filariasis), lymphoma (especially Hodgkin's disease), and liver disease. In ABPA a rise in the level of IgE precedes relapse, and the level falls with appropriate therapy. Regularly monitoring of IgE is justified in this condition (the only condition in which IgE monitoring is justified!). Levels may be elevated in EBV infection, the Churg–Strauss syndrome, systemic sclerosis, and bullous pemphigoid, although this is a poor marker of disease activity. Some primary immunodeficiencies are associated with raised IgE, such as Wiskott–Aldrich syndrome and Omenn's syndrome. However, the highest levels are seen in the hyper-IgE syndrome (Job syndrome, Buckley's syndrome): here levels frequently exceed 50 000 kU/l, a level rarely, if ever, seen in atopic disease. IgE myeloma is exceedingly rare. Levels are often higher in Asians, although this it is not clear whether this is just due to a higher risk of parasitic diseases. Specific IgE testing becomes inaccurate with very high levels of IgE (>1000 kU/l], due to non-specific binding. Conversely, where the total IgE is very low, it is not useful to perform tests for specific IgE. Total IgE is usually measured by EIA or RIA.

IgE antibodies/ IgE receptor antibodies

These have been reported in patients with allergic problems. In particular, antibodies to the IgE receptor have been reported as a possible cause of chronic urticaria. Routine assays are not available at present and the clinical utility needs to be confirmed in further studies.

Mast cell tryptase

Tryptase is a specific marker for the granules of mast cells and therefore its measurement in serum provides evidence of mast cell degranulation. It is relatively stable in serum, being catabolized in the liver with a half-life of approximately 3 hours. Levels may therefore be significantly raised for 24 hours after an acute reaction involving mast cell degranulation. There is a good correlation between plasma histamine and mast cell tryptase, making mast cell tryptase the preferred marker for mast cell activation. Elevated levels may also be detected in nasal and bronchial lavage fluids after allergen challenge. Measurement is usually by ELISA or other solid-phase immunoassay. In order to assess the significance of a result taken during an acute reaction in a given patient, it is important to have a sample taken when the patient has fully recovered.

Patch testing

The purpose of patch testing is to identify type IV hypersensitivity, usually in the context of contact hypersensitivity to environmental agents. As for skin-prick testing, an area of normal skin is required: the upper and mid zone of the back is usually appropriate. The allergens are made up in petrolatum jelly and applied under occlusion in a small metal chamber (Finn chamber), which is secured firmly to the back with hypoallergenic tape. They are left in place for 48 hours and the patients are told not to wash the area. When the chambers are removed, the application areas are inspected for erythema, vesiculation, and evidence of cellular infiltrate. However, there may be false positives at this stage due to reactions of types I and III. It is therefore advisable to reread the sites at 72–96 hours. False-positive reactions at 48 hours will have disappeared on the later reading.

It is usual for a standard panel to be used in the initial screen, unless there are clear indications of the most likely allergens (e.g. through the occupation and exposure history, site of eczema, etc.). This panel will include metals (nickel, chromium), preservatives, fragrances, rubber mix, lanolin, formaldehyde, balsam of Peru, and colophony. Where there are positive reactions to one of the mixed reagents (rubber mix, fragrances) there are usually supplementary panels of the individual ingredients. If the patient is exposed to an unusual substance, then it or its contents may be made into extemporaneous patch tests, provided that appropriate safety data can be obtained from the manufacturers.

Some allergens only cause reactions when there is concomitant exposure to sunlight. This can be reproduced in the clinic using a photopatch test. Here duplicates of each allergen are applied and, after 24–48 hours, one of the pair is taken off and the back exposed to UV-A light (10 joules). The other one of the pair is then taken off and the sites read as for an ordinary patch test. The unexposed member of the pair serves as the control.

Results can be roughly graded as 0 = no response, 1+ = erythema and oedema, 2+ = erythema, papules, and small vesicles, and 3+ = marked erythema, induration, and large blisters. Grades 2+ and 3+ are positive. Antihistamines have no effect on the responses, but topical steroids applied to the sites of application or systemic steroids will significantly reduce or abolish the responses.

Skin-prick testing

This remains the most cost-effective method for determining whether someone is sensitized to an allergen. It also has the major advantage that the patient sees the results as they develop, and it takes only 15 minutes to read. Testing can either be carried out by prick testing or by intradermal testing. The latter is more sensitive, but involves the injection of a larger amount of allergen, and adverse reactions are more common. Both tests are dependent on the release of histamine from sensitized mast cells and the tests will give spurious results in patients taking antihistamines; it is important to stop the antihistamines at least 48 hours before testing, or 7 days for the long-acting antihistamines. Astemizole and terfenadine produce such prolonged blockade that four drug-free weeks are required to give meaningful SPT results. If patients cannot stop their antihistamines, then blood tests may be the only way of diagnosis. As sensitization is dependent on circulating IgE reaching the mast cells at the test site, it is possible, where the allergic reaction is highly localized, to get negative results, as insufficient IgE is present in the circulation. The degree of reactivity of the skin is variable, decreasing up the arm and differing between the dorsal and volar aspects, due to numbers of mast cells present. Mostly the volar aspect of the forearm is used, although the back is an alternative, when many tests are required. Whealing decreases with age. Patients with extensive skin disease or dermographism are unsuitable for testing. Topical or systemic steroids do not have a major effect on the immediate hypersensitivity, although they will reduce late reactions and DTH reactions.

For prick testing, the chosen site is marked out into numbered squares with a biro (this has the advantage of demonstrating dermographism if present) and the allergens are applied as a single, small drop. This is pricked through with a slight lifting motion to a uniform depth with a sharp lancet, of which several specially designed ones are available. A separate lancet should be used for each allergen and disposed of immediately. It is poor practice to use a single lancet and wipe it between allergens, as this may give misleading results due to cross-contamination. A histamine control (1 or 10 mg/ml for SPT and 0.01 mg/ml for intradermal testing) and negative control (glycerinated carrier) should always be applied. If the negative control comes up positive, or if the histamine control produces no reaction, the tests are impossible to interpret, although some would suggest that test results greater than the 'positive' negative control might be considered positive. This is risky, and confirmatory blood tests would be advisable. Tests are read after 15 minutes, with the size of the wheal (not the surrounding flare) being measured. The control should give a response of at least 4 mm and positive test results require at least 2 mm greater than the negative control. It is helpful to place a strip of wide micropore tape over the test sites and draw round the wheals. This gives a permanent record that can be transferred to the notes, and allows calculation when the wheal is an eccentric shape. For irregular wheals, the diameter across the widest part can be measured and then the diameter at right angles.

Intradermal tests (IDT) expose patients to doses 100–1000-fold higher than SPT. They may be valuable where SPT has given equivocal results. A dose (0.02 ml) of diluted allergen (a 100-fold dilution of the SPT reagent) is injected intradermally, with the test read at 15–30 minutes. If multiple IDTs are carried out at the same time with positive results, the cumulative effect may lead to systemic symptoms. IDT tends to be used more for testing for drug reactions, usually with an incremental scale of dilutions.

It is advisable to avoid any form of skin testing in patients known to have had a severe systemic reaction to any of the proposed test agents, as even the small amount of allergen introduced during SPT may be enough to trigger a reaction in a susceptible individual. Equally, skin testing should only be carried out by staff familiar with resuscitation and with appropriate facilities close at hand.

False-positive tests may often be found to food allergens, although the rate is lower with SPT than ID testing. Where commercial food allergens give an unexpected false negative, use of the fresh food may be possible (e.g. by pricking the food with the lancet, then pricking the patient).

Allergen solutions to a wide range of allergens are available commercially from several manufacturers. They should be checked regularly to see that they are still within date. At present there is no agreed standardization of the reagents, in terms of reactivity and allergen content, although steps are being taken to improve this aspect. Allergen solutions may express the allergen concentration in protein nitrogen units (PNU) or as weight/volume. Standardization is best carried out by immunochemical methods such as RAST inhibition which will give a biological potency (BU/ml). Consistent results will be obtained if trained staff carry out all tests.

Thromboxanes/prostaglandins

Assays of these short-lived mediators are available in the research setting but do not have much applicability to the routine management of allergic problems at the present time. Assays are usually by RIA.

Unvalidated tests

A large number of other tests are used for the purported diagnosis of allergic disease, often outwith conventional medical services. These are frequently promoted directly to the public. Many of these techniques have not been validated scientifically or use techniques that will not provide information on the presence or absence of key allergic mediators. Members of the public may be offered 'allergy treatments' based on the results of these tests. The Royal College of Physicians has reviewed the evidence for these tests in a recent publication (*Allergy—conventional and alternative concepts*) and this College, together with the Royal College of Pathologists and the British Society for Allergy and Clinical Immunology, have produced a booklet of guidance called *Good allergy practice*. Tests where there is limited or no current evidence of value in the diagnosis of IgE-mediated allergic disease include: provocation–neutralization, hair analysis, Vega analysis, kinesiology, iridology, auriculo-cardiac reflex, and leucocytotoxic testing.

Urinary methyl histamine

Histamine is one of the key mediators of the allergic and pseudo-allergic response, leading to acute urticaria, flushing, tachycardia, and wheeze. It is released from mast cells and basophils and, under normal circumstances, is rapidly destroyed in the plasma; its measurement is therefore technically difficult and is limited to the research setting. Its urinary metabolite, *N*-methyl histamine, is stable and is therefore useful in determining whether mast cell degranulation has taken place in an acute reaction. Few laboratories are capable of measurement of urinary methyl histamine (Protein Reference Units). They suggest urine samples immediately and 24 hours later, to look for changes. Renal function must also be known. Mast cell tryptase may be a better marker.

Venom-specific IgE

Measurement of specific IgE to bee and wasp venom is an essential investigation in suspected insect-sting allergy. Measurement of venom-specific IgG may be helpful in determining the success of desensitization.

14 Cellular investigations

Introduction

The detection of specific cellular products, such as antibodies, cytokines, and shed surface molecules (soluble CD8, etc.) are usually undertaken using EIA or RIA techniques, as already described in Chapter 12. Cytokines may also be detected by bio-assays using cell lines that are dependent for their growth on a given cytokine. Strictly, both types of assays should be used, as EIA techniques may give spurious results due naturally occurring cytokine-binding proteins in serum (soluble receptors, binding factors). However, bioassays are notoriously difficult to standardize and to reproduce and are not suited to routine diagnostic use.

Flow cytometry

Flow cytometry provides the cornerstone of diagnostic cellular immunology and is dependent upon the availability of monoclonal antibody reagents reactive with human surface and intracellular antigens. Because the technique involves the flow of labelled cells past the exciting laser and the subsequent detectors, the method is only applicable to single-cell suspensions. In practice, this means blood-derived cells or cultured cells; however, it is possible to use disaggregated solid tissues, such as tumours. Modern flow cytometers use a single exciting laser (monochromatic light) and can detect up to three different wavelengths of light emitted by the fluorescent dyes. In addition, there are detectors for forward and 90° light scatter, which are related to size and granularity of the cells, respectively. When software for real-time analysis is added, the machine can record six parameters. This gives the potential for extremely detailed analysis.

Mostly conjugated monoclonal antibodies are used against surface antigens, but cell permeabilization techniques are available to permit the entry of antibodies into cells to stain intracellular antigens. Both surface and intracellular stains may be combined. Appropriate controls are required to detect non-specific staining.

The major advantage of flow cytometry for analysis is that it is semi-automated and can analyse very large numbers of cells very rapidly, compared to fluorescence microscopy. It is thus much more accurate. Newer machines can cope with absolute counts, usually through the use of a standardized bead reagent. This obviates the need for a separate haematology blood count.

Tissue culture

In vitro functional studies of cells usually requires that the cells be purified from blood. This is done by density gradient centrifugation, in which the different buoyant densities of blood cells are employed to separate them. Further purification of lymphocyte populations can be undertaken using either older techniques such as rosetting with sheep red cells, or by magnetic separation using monoclonal antibodies coupled to magnetic microspheres. The problem is that the more cells are handled *in vitro*, the more that the cells' characteristics are altered. Cell culture is usually carried out in tissue-culture medium, supplemented with antibiotics to prevent contamination with bacteria, and with fetal calf serum (FCS), human AB serum (no isoagglutinins), or other 'black-box' factors that are required for optimal cell growth. Where proliferation assays are being carried out, it is important to screen the FCS first, as some batches are mitogenic in their own right. Good sterile technique is essential.

Proliferation assays

There are numerous mitogenic stimuli that can be used (see below). However, the gold-standard is still uptake of tritiated thymidine by dividing cells. There is a lot of interest in alternatives, particularly those using the flow cytometer. In my experience, none of the flow cytometric techniques, which either look for DNA doubling or expression of so-called activation markers, are as reliable or as sensitive as tritiated thymidine incorporation.

Immunohistology

Immunoperoxidase and other enzymatic immunostains are used in the diagnosis of lymph-node disease. Multiple monoclonal antibodies are used, which recognize different stages of lymphoid development or particular subsets of cells. Many of the antibodies used will also work on paraffin-embedded sections, but this depends on whether the target antigen is stable under the conditions of fixation. Frozen sections are better at present.

Cytokine assays

These are usually carried out by EIA (see Chapter 11). However, the immunochemical measurement may not reflect the biological activity, as there may be circulating cytokine-binding proteins or antagonists. It may therefore be helpful to use bioassays that measure a biological activity of the cytokine. These are fiddly to set up and are frequently difficult to standardize.

Adhesion markers

Measurement of the surface expression of adhesion molecules is important in the diagnosis of leucocyte adhesion molecule deficiency (LAD). Two types have been identified (see Chapter 2). LAD-1 is associated normally with deficiency of CD18, the common β-chain for the integrins, leading to absence on the surface of CD11a (LFA-1), CD11b (Mac-1, CR3), and CD11c (CR4). The analysis should be carried out using all four markers on both lymphocytes and neutrophils, as the level of expression of the markers differs according to the cell type. However, partial variants may occur in which there is some residual CD18 expression, dependent on the type of mutation. Here it may be necessary to undertake stimulation studies, using PMA or γ-interferon, to see whether the expression of the adhesion molecules can be up-regulated. There have been unpublished reports of LAD due to deficiencies of specific integrin α-chains. LAD-2 is exceptionally rare and is associated with deficiency of the hapten-X receptor on neutrophils (CD15). Under certain circumstances it may be appropriate to look at the expression of the other complement receptors, CR1 (expressed on red cells, eosinophils, and B cells) and CR2 (CD21, EBV receptor, expressed on B cells, NK cells, and follicular dendritic cells). Reduction of red cell CR1 has been found in SLE, and some patients with CVID may lack CD21 on some of their B cells.

Bronchoalveolar lavage (BAL) studies

- Normal values:
    - Non-smokers:
      total cells: $130–180 \times 10^3$/ml
      macrophages: 80–95 per cent
      lymphocytes: <15 per cent
      neutrophils: <3 per cent
      eosinophils: <0.5 per cent
    - Smokers:
      total cells: $300–500 \times 10^3$/ml
      macrophages: 85–98 per cent
      lymphocytes: <10 per cent
      neutrophils: <5 per cent
      eosinophils: <3 per cent.

BAL is a helpful adjunct in the diagnosis of interstitial lung disease, particularly sarcoidosis, hypersensitivity pneumonitis, idiopathic pulmonary fibrosis (IPF), eosinophilic granuloma, and connective tissue diseases. The total and differential cell counts are usually performed on neat BAL fluid as this is more accurate. The identification of lymphocyte subpopulations is carried out by flow cytometry. In sarcoidosis, there is a marked increase in lymphocytes (to about 30 per cent of the total cells), predominantly CD4+ T cells, giving a CD4:C8 ratio (which is normally 2:1) of between 4:1 and 10:1. The values improve with treatment, but the levels and the ratio do not predict the severity of the disease. Occasionally there is an increase in neutrophils and mast cells, which is said to indicate a poorer prognosis. In hypersensitivity pneumonitis, the BAL lymphocytosis comprises mainly CD8+ cells, with the highest levels occurring in the acutely exposed. In IPF, a neutrophilia in excess of 10 per cent, particularly if there is an increase in eosinophils, is associated with a poor prognosis. A lymphocytosis (a rare finding) is associated with a better prognosis and indicates a probable response to steroids. In eosinophilic granuloma (histiocytosis X), there is an increase in OKT6-positive (S-100, CD1+) histiocytic cells, up to 20 per cent of total cells, which is diagnostic.

14 Cellular investigations
Bronchoalveolar lavage (BAL) studies
Complement membrane regulatory factors

Complement membrane regulatory factors

Deficiencies of a group of surface proteins, with an unusual glycosyl-phosphatidylinositol membrane binding, are associated with paroxysmal nocturnal haemoglobinuria (PNH), a clonal disorder leading to unusual susceptibility to homologous complement lysis, particularly of red cells. The proteins in question are regulatory proteins to prevent destruction of cells by homologous complement and include decay accelerating factor (DAF, CD55) and homologous restriction factor-20 (HRF20, CD59), C8-binding protein (HRF65), and acetylcholinesterase. Flow cytometry can be used to identify the abnormality, although the standard test involves a functional test of susceptibility to lysis.

Cytokines

The measurement of cytokines is predominantly a research tool at present and there are no absolute indications for routine measurement. IL-6 rises very early in acute-phase responses, before a rise in the CRP can be detected. Exceptionally rare cases of primary failure of cytokine production (IL-2 and γ-interferon) have been documented. As noted above, there may be problems with EIA assays and under some circumstances bioassays may be preferable. The expense of the EIAs and the difficulties of bioassays render these tests unsuitable for clinical use, as the sort of conditions that are likely to lead to changes in cytokines are those where rapid answers would be required.

Flow cytometric tests for intracellular cytokine detection are now available and may be helpful in determining the predominance of Th1 and Th2 responses. The technique works well for IL-2 and γ-IFN but poorly for IL-4. It has the significant advantage that specific T-cell subpopulations can be studied, using three- or four-colour flow cytometry.

Cytotoxic T cells

Cytotoxic T cells can be generated during a one-way mixed lymphocyte reaction (MLR), stimulating the responding cells with irradiated or mitomycin-treated allogeneic target cells and then assessing the ability of the responders to kill Cr^{51}-labelled targets, in a similar assay to the NK-cell assay (see below). This is a complex and fiddly assay, and is of use mainly as part of the cross-matching procedure (Chapter 15).

Leukaemia phenotyping

Leukaemia phenotyping is undertaken to identify the origin of the malignant cell and to identify the presence or absence of markers that are known to be of prognostic significance. This will always be undertaken in conjunction with other studies, including examinations of blood films, bone marrow smears and trephines, stained for enzymatic cytoplasmic and membrane markers. Usually leukaemia phenotyping is carried out by flow cytometry using a screening set of antibodies to identify the lineage of the cells (T or B lymphoid, myeloid, erythroid, or other). Further studies will then be carried out with a more detailed panel aimed at the particular lineage. Leukaemic cells often correspond to particular stages of cellular differentiation which can be matched to normal cell ontogeny. However, they often express aberrant antigens, out of sequence. This may give rise to biphenotypic leukaemias Studies can be carried out on blood or bone marrow, depending on the number of blasts in the peripheral blood. Bone marrow studies are more complex because of the very different light-scatter properties of the cellular constituents; it is also necessary to be familiar with the patterns of antigen expression at each stage of differentiation for each lineage. The re-examination of bone marrow, after treatment, is important to detect the presence of minimal residual disease. This can be done either by flow cytometry, which can detect one leukaemic cell in 10 000 cells, or by polymerase chain reaction (PCR) techniques where the leukaemic cells carry an abnormal genetic marker (oncogene) or have a specific rearrangement of either the immunoglobulin (B lineage) or T-cell receptor (T lineage) genes. These techniques are even more sensitive. Flow cytometric karyotyping is now possible as an alternative to molecular techniques.

A usual primary panel for acute leukaemias will include the following:
• B lineage: CD10 (CALLA), CD19, CD24, HLA-DR, cytoplasmic Ig (μ heavy chains) and surface Ig;
• T lineage: CD2, cytoplasmic CD3, CD7;
• lymphoblast: TdT;
• AML lineage: CD13, CD14, CD33;
• erythroid: glycophorin A;
• megakaryocyte: CD41.

A secondary panel may be used in difficult cases and may include:
• B lineage: cytoplasmic CD22;
• T lineage: CD1, CD3, CD4, CD8;
• AML: CD15, cytoplasmic myeloperoxidase.

For chronic lymphoid disorders the panel will be slightly different, with panels as follows:
• B lineage, primary: CD10, CD20, CD5, surface Ig;
• B lineage, secondary: CD11c, CD25, CD38, and FMC7;
• T lineage, primary: CD3;
• T lineage, secondary: CD4, CD8, CD11b, CD16, CD57.

649

Lymphocyte surface markers and HIV monitoring

- Normal adult ranges:
  - Total T cells (CD3): $1.0–2.2 \times 10^9$/l
  - T4+ T cells (CD4): $0.6–1.6 \times 10^9$/l
  - T8+ T cells (CD8): $0.4–1.1 \times 10^9$/l
  - Total B cells (CD19): $0.1–0.4 \times 10^9$/l
  - Activated T cells: $0.1–0.4 \times 10^9$/l.

Analysis of lymphocyte markers is now carried out by flow cytometry, using monoclonal antibodies directly conjugated to a fluorochrome. There is no longer a place for fluorescence microscopy. The range of markers available to stain the surface of immunologically relevant cells is now large. However, a relatively small panel is sufficient for most purposes related to the diagnosis and monitoring of immune deficiency. Additional markers rarely add anything to routine care, as opposed to those of interest for research purposes. Identification of T cells (CD3), B cells (CD19 or CD20), NK cells (CD16/CD56), activated cells (CD25 or MHC class II), and the major T-cell subpopulations (CD4 and CD8) will suffice. More rarely, measurement of cells bearing Tcr αβ or γδ, or CD45RA versus CD45RO on either all T cells or on CD4 cells may be helpful, for example in the investigation of rare forms of SCID such as Omenn's syndrome, materno-fetal engraftment (MFE), and kinase deficiencies. In a baby with suspected SCID, the presence of mainly activated CD8+ T cells is suspicious of MFE, while the presence of activated CD4+ T cells, in the presence of large numbers of eosinophils, is suggestive of Omenn's syndrome (T-cell receptor gene rearrangements will show an oligoclonal response). Absence of CD8+ T cells is a feature of ZAP-70 kinase deficiency. Suspected neutrophil defects require the assessment of leucocyte adhesion molecules (see above) and there is interest in the levels of expression of Fcγ receptor abnormalities in recurrent infection. Abnormalities of T- and B-cell populations are also seen in CVID, with CD4+ T-cell lymphopenia, affecting particularly CD45RA+ T cells. Regular monitoring of SCID babies after bone marrow transplant is essential: the appearance of high levels of activated cells suggests impending GvHD.

It is often wrongly assumed that very low CD4+ T-cell counts are a diagnostic feature of HIV disease: they are not. Temporary reductions in the CD4+ T-cell count is seen with a number of trivial viral infections, particularly in the acute phase. There is also often an elevation of the CD8+ T cells and NK cells. Persistent CD4+ T-cell lymphopenia has also been reported as a cause of opportunistic infections in the absence of any evidence for infection with either HIV-1 or HIV-2 (idiopathic CD4+ T-cell lymphopenia). Abnormal lymphocyte profiles are also seen in lymphoma, malignancy, chronic fatigue syndromes, and protein-losing enteropathy. Generalized proportionate reductions in lymphocyte counts are seen with long-term immunosuppressive therapy. Cell marker analysis should never be used as a surrogate for proper HIV testing. The monitoring of HIV+ patients is best undertaken by measuring the

absolute CD4+ and CD8 + T-cell counts, together with a marker of
T-cell activation. Although other markers have been suggested as
being valuable (CD8+ CD29+ T cells), they do not add much to
clinical management. The CD4:CD8 ratio is of little value, as it is
the absolute CD4+ T-cell count that defines the risks of the various
opportunist infections. The measurement of either neopterin or
β2-microglobulin is also helpful. Immunoglobulins are usually
raised, often grossly so, and measurement on a regular basis is of no
value. However, in HIV+ patients with recurrent bacterial infections, i.e. those behaving as though they have a B-cell defect, it is
worth a full humoral investigation as for a primary immunodeficiency (immunoglobulins, IgG subclasses, anti-bacterial antibodies, anti-viral antibodies, and immunization responses). Once
the absolute CD4+ T-cell count declines below 0.05×10^9/l for
two or more consecutive values, there is little further point in
monitoring, as the levels are unlikely to recover, unless it is deemed
psychologically important for the patient.

B-lymphocyte function

The best assay of B-cell function is still measurement of *in vivo* antibody production. This should include IgM antibody (iso-haemagglutinins), and responses to bacteria and viruses. The responses to both protein and polysaccharide antigens should be measured. In choosing which antigens to look at, it is necessary to take a good infection and immunization history. Responses to tetanus, *Haemophilus influenzae* type B (Hib) and *Pneumovax* should always be sought, as patients with low levels can be immunized to test the dynamic response. Remember, no live vaccines should be given to any patients suspected of having an immunodeficiency. In the USA, the bacteriophage ΦX174 can be used as an immunogen: this is a neoantigen, and allows the primary and secondary antibody responses to be tested (see Chapter 11).

In vitro B-cell function is usually tested by stimulation of purified mononuclear cells by pokeweed mitogen (PWM), anti-IgM + IL-2, *Staphylococcus* strain A Cowan (SAC), or Epstein–Barr virus (EBV). IgG, IgA, and IgM production can be measured at 7 days by sensitive ELISA. There are few indications for this at present, although the application of the anti-IgM + IL-2 system may identify prognostically important subgroups of common variable immunodeficiency (Chapter 2).

T-lymphocyte function

T-cell function *in vivo* is tested by delayed-type hypersensitivity. Antigens are pricked through the skin (Multitest CMI®, Merieux) or injected intradermally. There may be early reactions but these are due to mechanisms not involving T cells. At 72–96 hours, in a positive reaction, there will be a cellular infiltrate that is palpable, with overlying erythema. The most useful antigens include PPD, *Candida*, mumps, tetanus, and streptokinase/streptodornase, which are available (some with difficulty) as single antigens, or are part of the battery in the Multitest. Reactivity to the panel is low in early childhood and increases with age. Poor responses are seen in primary T-cell defects, combined defects, in some patients with CVID, in leukaemias, lymphomas and other malignant disease, renal failure, and during some chronic infections (late HIV). Testing is of limited value except in the circumstance of chronic muco-cutaneous candidiasis, where there is often specific anergy to *Candida*, with reasonable responses to other antigens.

In vitro T-cell function is carried out by inducing the T cells to proliferate by exposure to either mitogens or antigens. Mononuclear cells are separated from neutrophils by density gradient centrifugation. Proliferation of the T cells is measured by the incorporation into DNA of tritiated thymidine in replicating cells. The results will be reported as counts per minute (cpm) for the unstimulated and stimulated cells and as a stimulation index: for PHA-stimulated cells the uptake should be >5000 cpm and the increment over the unstimulated cells should be >4000 cpm; the stimulation index should be >10. For antigens such as *Candida*, the response is smaller and an increment of 2000 cpm and a stimulation index of 3.0 are satisfactory. The requesting clinician must also arrange a control sample from a healthy volunteer, where possible of the same age/sex as the patient. This is necessary, as there are wide variations of individual responses, even in healthy individuals and there are variations with age.

The most useful stimuli are:

- Phytohaemagglutinin (PHA), a lectin (sugar-binding molecule) derived from kidney beans. This binds to sugar residues on a number of surface molecules, thus activating cells by several pathways simultaneously, including via the CD3–Tcr complex.
- Concanavalin A (ConA), a lectin derived from jack beans. Its effect is similar to that of PHA except that it is dependent on normal monocyte accessory function.
- Mitogenic anti-CD3 monoclonal antibodies. Soluble and immobilized anti-CD3 cause specific stimulation of T cells via the CD3–Tcr complex, mimicking antigen.
- Phorbol esters (phorbol myristate acetate, PMA). This molecule activates protein kinase C directly in cells, bypassing the need for membrane events. The addition of a calcium ionophore, which raises the intracellular calcium by inserting unregulated calcium channels in the membrane, increases the effect of PMA as it is a calcium-dependent enzyme.
- Interleukin-2. This has very little effect on its own but is synergistic with anti-CD3. Restoration of proliferative responses to

other stimuli by the addition of IL-2 suggests a downstream defect leading to reduced/absent IL-2 production.

- Antigens. Many antigens can be used but the most useful are *Candida*, tetanus, PPD, and viral antigens (CMV, HSV, rubella), as patients are likely to have been exposed or immunized. Responses are lower, as the frequency of T cells with the correct Tcr will be small.
- Anti-CD43 antibodies. It has been reported that proliferation to this antibody is defective in Wiskott–Aldrich syndrome.
- Periodate. Response to this agent (which acts via *O*-linked sugars) is absent in WAS, while responses to neuraminidiase and galactose oxidase, which act via *N*-linked sugars, are normal. This test does not appear reliable.

Other methods used to study T-cell function *in vitro* include a number of flow cytometric tests to measure calcium flux, DNA replication (a non-isotopic alternative to the standard proliferation assay), changes in surface antigen expression in response to activation (IL-2 receptor, CD25, transferrin receptor, CD71, CD69, and the nuclear antigen Ki-67), as well as intracellular cytokines. Cytokine production in culture can be measured, but this is not done routinely, and the flow cytometric determination of intracellular cytokine is likely to be of more value. There is little value in the MLR as a test of T-cell function, although it forms an essential part of cross-matching bone marrow.

In vitro assays of T-cell function are used exclusively to diagnose immunodeficiency states. Monitoring of the proliferative response after bone marrow transplantation in SCID provides a useful marker of returning function that allows the baby to be released from laminar flow isolation.

Lymphoma diagnosis

The diagnosis of lymphoma follows similar principles as leukaemia typing, except that the cells are in a solid organ. While it is possible to work on single-cell suspensions produced by disaggregating the tissue, much more information is gained from looking at tissue sections. The staining is usually done with monoclonal antibodies followed by anti-mouse antibody conjugated to a reagent for developing a colour reaction (peroxidase, alkaline phosphatase-anti-alkaline phosphatase, etc.). Early studies were always carried out on frozen sections but new antibodies have been derived that will react with paraffin sections. Not all antibodies will work on paraffin sections as the antigenic structures may be damaged during the processing and therefore no longer be available to react with the antibody. As with leukaemia diagnosis, the panels of antibodies used are designed to cover the pathways of differentiation of the key elements of the lymphoid system. A first set of antibodies will be used to provide an idea of the type of cell involved; this will be followed by supplementary antibodies to confirm the working diagnosis. The immunophenotyping will always be undertaken in parallel with normal histology, to examine the architecture of the tissue. In the differential diagnosis of an abnormal lymph node the question must be answered 'is this a malignant process or a reactive process?'. This may be quite difficult. However, lymphomas often express aberrant patterns of surface and cellular antigens: $\kappa : \lambda$ ratios >10 : 1; sIg negative, B-lineage antigen positive; co-expression of B-lineage antigens and CD5, CD10, CD43, or CD6; loss of an expected T-lineage antigen; dual expression of CD4 and CD8 (outside the thymus); expression of terminal deoxytransferase (TdT) or CD1a (outside thymus). Lymphoid tumours need to be distinguished from other (metastatic malignancy: cells of lymphoid origin usually express CD45, while other markers are available to distinguish cells from other sources (carcinoembryonic antigen, cytokeratin, chromogranin, desmin, or S-100)). Hodgkin's disease is distinguished by the presence of characteristic Reed–Sternberg cells. These are usually detectable by standard histology, although they may be sparse. They can be identified by their reaction with CD30 and CD15, without reactivity with CD45 or T/B lineage antigens. Evidence of clonality can now be obtained by studies of Ig and Tcr gene rearrangements by molecular techniques. This can be carried out even on DNA extracted from paraffin sections and, because of the use of PCR techniques to amplify DNA of interest, very small samples can be analysed. Considerable interest has also been expressed in the role of EBV genes and oncogenes (particularly *bcl-2*) in the generation of lymphoma, and it is possible to probe for these also. The classification of lymphomas is constantly being revised in the light of new findings: readers are advised to consult an up-to-date detailed text to understand the process.

As for leukaemia diagnosis, an initial screening panel is used, followed by a secondary panel depending on the histology and the results of the primary panel. The primary panel usually includes: CD45 (leucocyte common antigen), CD45RA (minority of T cells and B cells), CD3 (T cells), CD4 (T-helper cells plus macrophages and dendritic cells), CD8, C3bR (follicular dendritic cells, B cells, macrophages), HLA-DR (B cells, activated T cells), and surface immunoglobulins (heavy and light chains). Other T-lineage antigens for the secondary panel would include CD2, CD5, CD7, and CD1, although the latter is also expressed on dendritic cells and macrophages; B-lineage antigens include CD10, CD21, CD22, CD23, CD24, and CD5 (also expressed on T cells). Confirmation of the presence of Reed–Sternberg cells can be obtained by using CD30 and CD15.

657

Neutrophil and monocyte function testing

The function of neutrophils is to ingest and destroy bacteria. This is a complex multistage process, and equally the testing involves several different approaches. Exclusion of chronic granulomatous disease involves the demonstration of normal neutrophil oxidative metabolism. This is usually undertaken using the nitroblue tetrazolium reduction test, in which a colourless intracellular dye is reduced to an insoluble blue compound, formazan, when the neutrophil's oxidative machinery is activated. This test can be done as a simple slide test or as a quantitative assay. Slide NBT tests may miss some cases of chronic granulomatous disease and it is essential, if there is a high degree of suspicion, to perform a more sensitive flow cytometric assay, as dyes are now available that perform the same function on the flow cytometer. Other tests of the oxidative machinery include chemiluminescence (amplified by luminol), and the iodination test, which relates to hydrogen peroxide production. With sensitive assays, heterozygotes for CGD mutations may have half normal activity. Phagocytosis can be measured by simply counting the number of latex beads or yeasts ingested by neutrophils, or more accurately by flow cytometry using labelled bacteria. Bacterial killing assays allow the whole process to be tested, including opsonization, phagocytosis, and oxidative metabolism: a test organism is incubated with patient's serum or control serum and then each is incubated with either normal or patient's neutrophils. At a fixed time thereafter, the cells are lysed and the lysate plated out to allow residual live bacteria to grow. Normally all bacteria will be killed within 30 minutes. This assay may be abnormal in healthy children under the age of two. Chemotaxis is an important part of the process and rare defects due to the lack of anaphylotoxin receptors have been reported. The assays are usually carried out by measuring migration under agarose or by the Boyden chamber method, in which cells migrate into a microporous filter. Both these methods give wide ranges even for normal individuals, so determining what is abnormal is often difficult. Neutrophil function testing should always include testing for adhesion molecule deficiency (see above) and for neutrophil enzymes, especially myeloperoxidase (a common deficiency of doubtful significance) and alkaline phosphatase (reduced in specific granule deficiency).

In many assays, particularly those on the flow cytometer, monocyte function can be studied at the same time as neutrophil function, although defects specific to monocytes are exceptionally rare, having been reported in the context of familial susceptibility to recurrent infection with *Mycobacterium tuberculosis* (due to IL-12 or IL-12R deficiency).

NK cell function

The activity of MHC non-restricted killer cells (natural killer) cells can be assessed *in vitro*. The erythroleukaemia cell line K562 is known to be susceptible to lysis by NK cells. The assay is carried out by incubating mononuclear cells with labelled K562 cells at varying effector target cell ratios and then identifying the death of the targets. The conventional way is to surface label the targets with Cr^{51}, and then measure the release of the isotope into the medium on cell death. Appropriate controls are required to identify spontaneous release of the isotope and target cell death unrelated to effector cell activity; the latter should be less than 5 per cent. An alternative non-radioisotopic assay uses a green fluorescent, membrane-bound dye which is used to label the targets. Cell death is identified by the uptake of propidium iodide, which gives a red fluorescence. Live and dead targets can thus be separated by their staining from the unlabelled effector cells. The flow cytometric assays is more sensitive to minor target-cell damage, permeabilizing the cell to the red dye. The chromium-release assay depends on the complete disintegration of the cell. The assays can be modified using different targets to look at antibody-dependent cell-mediated cytotoxicity (ADCC) and lymphokine-activated killer (LAK) activity.

The clinical diagnostic value of the NK assay remains to be fully evaluated; routine evaluation of ADCC and LAK activity is not undertaken. Excessive NK cell activity has been associated with an increased risk of graft loss in mismatched bone marrow transplants (particularly host NK cell activity). Low/absent NK activity has been reported in rare patients with recurrent infections with herpes family viruses. Very high activity may be found in NK cell leukaemias. The number of NK cells identified by flow cytometry does not necessarily correlate with the activity.

15 Tissue typing

Introduction

The key element to successful transplantation is the ability to correctly identify the tissue types of recipients and donors, and to try and predict whether a graft is likely to be rejected (host-versus-graft disease) or, in the case of a bone marrow transplant, whether the graft will attack the recipient (graft-versus-host disease, GvHD). The antigens of the MHC system are defined and reviewed by WHO which convenes regular workshops to ensure that there is a common approach to nomenclature and typing. The best match of all is an identical twin. However, few individuals requiring transplantation have such a donor and most transplants are from matched unrelated donors (MUDs) or from parents/siblings with a close but not identical match. In the case of a parental donor, this will usually only be a haplo-identical match (half identical) unless there is consanguinity in the family, in which case the match may be better. It is quite clear that for renal and bone marrow transplantation, the better the match, the better the graft will do and the fewer the complications. If a poorly matched sold organ is transplanted, the recipient will require considerable amounts of immunosuppressive therapy to prevent the graft being rejected. This leads to risks of secondary malignancies and of opportunist infections.

The realization of the importance of the best possible cross-match has lead to the generation of highly specific techniques capable of identifying very minor changes in histocompatibility antigens. Tissue typing used to be undertaken by two techniques: MHC class I antigens were identified (and in many cases defined) by serology, using sera derived from multiparous women who spontaneously develop anti-class I antibodies. This technique could not be used directly to identify class II antigens, and cytotoxicity tests had to be used. These had the major disadvantage of the time taken to generate effector cells (up to 6 days), and was therefore of little value in the time scale normally applicable to transplantation of solid organs, which usually has to be teed up within hours of a suitable donor becoming available (if cadaver transplants are undertaken). Molecular biological techniques have rapidly taken over. This has led to problems with the nomenclature, particularly where antigens have previously been defined serologically, as it is now clear from molecular genotyping that some antigens classed as completely distinct by serology are more closely related to each other than some specificities thought, on serological grounds, to be part of a closely related family ('splits' of an antigen). This is important in deciding whether a donor is a good match for a given recipient, as two different B antigens, defined serologically, may differ by only one amino acid, and therefore represent a good match, whereas two splits of the same antigen may differ by five or more amino acids. It is now clear that under the right circumstances even a one-amino-acid change is enough to generate a detectable specific cytotoxic T-cell response, while a five-amino-acid difference may lead to irretrievable graft rejection or GvHD.

In all transplantation there are two steps: first the tissue types must be established and then there is a cross-match stage, in which the suitability of the proposed match is tested. For renal transplantation, the donor will be tissue typed and blood grouped (ABO and rhesus) and screened at regular intervals for the presence of antibodies recognizing allo-MHC. If there are potential living related donors, then these will be tissue typed and blood grouped and then the recipient's sera will be tested against donor cells for anti-donor antibodies, followed by a mixed lymphocyte reaction (MLR), in which the ability of the donor cells to stimulate the recipient's T cells is tested. A good donor will be ABO compatible, with the best match of MHC antigens, a low stimulatory capacity in the MLR, and the recipient will lack anti-donor antibodies (preformed antibodies are a cause of hyperacute rejection). If there is no suitable living related donor, then the patients will be listed to receive a cadaver organ, with their clinical and immunological details stored on a central register. This allows best use of cadaver organs across the country, as cadaver organs can be sent to the best-matched recipients, who are likely to derive most benefit. The cadaver organ will have been ABO/Rh and MHC typed and recipients will be chosen on the best match, with no preformed antibodies against the identified MHC antigens. Immediately before transplant takes place, a fresh sample of patient's serum will be cross-matched against donor lymphocytes, to check that no new antibodies have developed. Normally to ensure that there are sufficient donor lymphocytes to cross-match (as this may have to be done several times against different potential recipients), the spleen is removed to provide a source of cells. Patients who have had previous failed grafts are often highly sensitized, and have high levels of antibodies that make them difficult to cross-match. Interestingly, for liver transplants there is no evidence that MHC matching makes any significant difference, and may even be detrimental: only ABO matching is undertaken. In the case of heart, lung, and heart–lung transplants, the supply of potential donors is so small that MHC matching is impractical, so ABO matching alone is used. In bone marrow transplantation, both the recipient and the donated cells are capable of reactivity, so it is essential that the MLR is done in both directions.

Anti-mouse antibodies

Detection of anti-mouse antibodies is helpful when repeated courses of the therapeutic mouse monoclonal antibody, OKT3, are required. The development of a patient response against the mouse proteins may lead to loss of therapeutic efficacy.

Cross-matching

The purpose of the cross-match is to detect the presence of antibodies in the recipient that would affect the viability of the graft. This is mainly used in the case of solid organs, where the patient's serum is tested against donor cells. The antibodies of interest are mainly IgG anti-class I and anti-class II antibodies. IgM antibodies are often (but not always) considered to be autoantibodies that may cause false-positive responses that are not deemed significant to the outcome of the transplant.

Flow cytometry

The flow cytometer can be used to identify, in a sensitive manner, the presence of antibodies to both T and B cells, if dual-colour fluorescence is used. It does not indicate whether the antibodies are complement fixing and therefore likely to have a major deleterious effect. It can, however, distinguish IgG and IgM antibodies. Because of its increased sensitivity, it picks up weaker antibodies and this makes the positive results harder to interpret in the context of the acceptability of a given match.

Microlymphocytotoxicity

The standard method is to use microlymphocytotoxicity, as used for typing (see below) in which the donor cells are incubated with the serum in the presence of complement and the wells scored for cell death. However, in order to distinguish between anti-class I and anti-class II antibodies, separated T cells and B cells are required. As a control for autoantibodies, the patient's cells will also be put up. If an IgG anti-T-cell antibody is found, this is generally regarded as a contraindication to transplantation. Because B cells express higher levels of class I than T cells, there may be B-cell reactivity with weak antibodies in the absence of a positive T-cell cross-match, and the B-cell reactivities are often titrated to give an idea of their strength: low-titre anti-B-cell antibodies being regarded as only a relative contraindication to transplantation. In these assays, the IgM autoantibodies can be detected by carrying out the assay in the presence of dithiothreitol or dithioerythritol, which disrupt pentameric IgM. If a positive cross-match becomes negative in the presence of these agents, then an IgM antibody can be suspected. Carrying out the reactions at 37 °C also helps to eliminate cold-reactive antibodies that are often of a non-specific nature.

Monitoring

Patients on waiting lists for renal transplants will be screened at intervals by microcytotoxicity against panels of pre-typed cells to identify the presence of any anti-MHC antibodies. This speeds up the process, as cadaver grafts can be selected which lack the antigens recognized.

Genotyping

Determination of the MHC type by genotyping has revolutionized tissue typing and also revealed that the designation of specificities on the basis of serology has been misleading. A variety of methods are in use: which to choose depends on the speed with which an answer is required.

RFLP

This technique uses the ability of certain endonucleases to cut DNA at sites of fixed sequences. By using several endonucleases specific for different sequences, DNA will be reduced to fragments of different lengths. Differences in the lengths will be determined by the underlying genetic structure. This technique, which is very slow (2–3 weeks), also requires significant amounts of DNA and is not sensitive enough to identify all the alleles of class II antigens identified now by other techniques. It is therefore of very limited value.

PCR

The development of the polymerase chain reaction, based on a cyclical synthetic reaction catalysed by the *Taq* polymerase, has been to molecular biology what the monoclonal antibody has been to immunology. Upstream and downstream primers are used to start off the reaction by binding to the denatured single-stranded DNA, which is then re-annealed and allowed to complete synthesis. The new chains then act as the templates for further cycles. Very rapidly, in about 25–30 cycles, many millions of copies of the desired piece of DNA can be produced. Probes can be directed at generic sequences, for example the flanking regions of a gene, or more specific probes can be derived.

Sequence-based typing

This uses probes specific for allelic variants of MHC genes, where the probes are specific for the allelic variant sequence and therefore only amplify that sequence. This is known as sequence-specific primer PCR or SSP-PCR. It is a rapid technique (3 hours) but is of relatively low resolution. It requires minimal amounts of DNA to start with.

Sequence-specific oligonucleotide probes

Here short DNA probes, 18–24 nucleotides long, specific for individual alleles, are used to bind to (hybridize) the patient's DNA under conditions of high stringency (i.e. an exact match is required). The patient's DNA in the region of interest is first amplified by PCR and this is then applied to multiple slots or dots on a filter. The oligonucleotide probes, which carry a radioactive tracer, are then reacted with the filter and the pattern of binding with the panel of probes identifies the sequences present and hence the genotype. This technique is relatively slow and also requires a large number of probes to cover all the possible allelic variants (e.g. 22 probes are required for the DR52 family (DR3, DR5, and DR6) alone). If it is a previously unrecognized allele, there will be no reaction, as no probe will be available.

Sequence-based typing

Here, the sequence of the MHC gene DNA is identified directly. RNA is used as the original template, to avoid amplifying pseudogenes, and DNA is made initially by reverse transcription. This technique is fast (16–24 hours) and very accurate. It will identify previously unknown alleles and has revealed a degree of heterogeneity within the MHC genes that had not previously been recognized.

Genetic identity

Where it is particularly important to know that there is a genetic match between a donor and recipient, as in bone marrow transplantation with matched unrelated donors, two techniques are available to match the DNA directly: heteroduplex analysis, and VNTR typing. Heteroduplex analysis involves mixing the denatured DNA of donor and recipient and then electrophoresing it after allowing it to re-anneal. Where there is a mismatch between recipient and donor, there will be loops of incorrect binding which can be detected as distortions of the banding pattern. Variable N-terminal repeat analysis (VNTR) looks for polymorphisms in the non-coding repeated DNA. It is valuable in identifying engraftment after bone marrow transplantation between MHC identical individuals.

HLA testing as a disease marker

Many diseases are associated with HLA antigens, the best known being ankylosing spondylitis with HLA-B27. Requests are often submitted for tissue typing to identify this particular antigen. However, this is not a diagnostic test, as B27 is a relatively common antigen (8 per cent of Caucasians) and not every positive patient develops the disease. Ninety per cent of patients with AS will be B27+, but 10 per cent will have other antigens. The relative risk of developing AS is 100 times greater in B27+ individuals compared to B27- individuals. It is useful as a confirmatory test. In rheumatoid arthritis, the presence of DR4 is associated with a greater risk of developing erosions and extra-articular disease and a worse prognosis. Typing may therefore provide useful prognostic information which will alter the approach to using disease-modifying drugs. In the absence of full tissue typing facilities, HLA-B27 can be detected by a more economical, simple flow cytometric test.

HTLP and CTLP frequency

These relatively new assays are variants on the mixed lymphocyte reaction, but with a limiting dilution step to identify the frequency of helper (HTLP) and cytotoxic cell (CTLP) precursors. HTLP assays are better established. The higher the frequency of precursors, the more likely that there will be *in vivo* reactivity. These assays are particularly useful in mismatched bone marrow transplants, when they will be done in the graft-versus-host and host-versus-graft directions. They are more sensitive than the ordinary MLR, as the quantitation is more accurate. This allows different recipient–donor combinations to be compared. In the CTLP assay, a primary stimulatory one-way MLR is run to generate effector cells, which are then used to lyse Cr^{51}-labelled targets identical to the stimulating cells.

15 Tissue typing
HLA testing as a disease marker
HTLP and CTLP frequency

Mixed lymphocyte reaction

This test originally defined the class II specificities. It relies on allo-geneic cells stimulating proliferation of specific responder T cells. If the stimulating cells are also lymphocytes, both sets of cells will proliferate (two-way MLR). It is more usual to prevent the stimu-lators from proliferating by exposing them to mitomycin C or irradiating them (one-way MLR). The proliferation assay takes 5–6 days to reach peak proliferation. Proliferation is usually identi-fied by tritiated thymidine incorporation, as for other T-cell pro-liferative assays (see Chapter 14). In the plate set-up, it is usual to do the one-way MLR in both directions, with each person's cells acting as stimulators and responders, and to include the autologous combinations as a background control. This is essential for bone marrow transplantation where the graft will be immunologically active. For solid organ grafts, a one-way assay is all that is required, with the donor cells as the stimulators. Results are reported as a stimulation index or relative response. In detecting differences in class II antigens, the MLR is much more sensitive than serology: T cells may respond to allelic variants differing in a single amino acid.

Tissue typing

The purpose of tissue typing is to identify the expression of MHC on cells. More than one method may be required to give a complete picture.

Class I antigens

For class I antigens (HLA-A, B, C), the standard technique is the microcytotoxicity assay carried out in 20 μl Terasaki plates. In this assay, the patient's mononuclear cells are plated out and typing sera, derived from multiparous women, with known reactivity are added in the presence of a source of fresh complement (normally rabbit). A panel of sera, up to 200, may be used to cover all the specificities. Each serum usually has more than one specificity and some of the antibodies will be against more than one antigen (cross-reacting antigen group) while others will be against a single monospecific private antigen. A dye such as propidium iodide that enters only dead cells is added and the plate is then viewed under fluorescence, so that dead cells show up as red. Other dye systems exist for visualizing the cells (eosin Y). Each well is then scored for the amount of cell death. The pattern of killing is then correlated with the known specificities of the sera to identify the probable pattern: this can usually be done by computer.

Class II antigens

Typing for class II antigens serologically has been difficult, as the antigens are only expressed on a minority of the mononuclear cell fraction (B cells, monocytes, and activated T cells). In order to carry out the tests, purified B cells are required, which can either be obtained by nylon wool adherence (B cells adhere but T cells do not) or by using a monoclonal antibody against a B-cell antigen coupled to a magnetic bead, allowing the B cells to be purified with a magnet. Obtaining adequate anti-class II typing sera is also difficult, as these antibodies tend to be weaker than the anti-class I antibodies. The latter can be removed by absorption with pooled human platelets, which express class I antigens only. As B cells express more class I than class II antigens, the need for reagents free of anti-class I antibodies is obvious if false-positive reactions are to be avoided. These handicaps have meant that serological techniques have been of limited value in defining class II polymorphisms.

The class II antigens have been much better defined by cellular techniques, in which cellular proliferation is induced by the allo-class II in a mixed lymphocyte reaction. However, although these techniques were used originally to define the class II specificities, the techniques are too time consuming to be used routinely for typing, taking 5–7 days. Now, molecular techniques have replaced both serological and cellular techniques for class II typing and are also being used for more accurate class I typing (see Genotyping, above).

16 Quality and managerial issues

Introduction

Clinical and laboratory services do not operate in isolation but are integrated into the clinical and managerial framework of a hospital, and in the UK into a nationwide network (the NHS). This provides a constraint in both managerial and financial terms and also provides a legal framework in which services are delivered. It is essential that no matter where the patient is treated the right diagnosis is reached and the appropriate treatment is given. In this setting, laboratories are at present more tightly regulated than the clinical services but this is likely to change. Quality is a key issue.

Concepts of quality control (QC) in the laboratory

The purpose of quality control is to ensure that the right test is carried out to a high standard of technical competence on the right sample and that the correct result is delivered, with appropriate interpretation, to the requesting clinician. There are many links in this particular chain, not all of which are the direct responsibility of the laboratory. For example, if a sample needs to be transported to the laboratory within 4 hours of venesection for the test result to be valid, it is useless if it sits all day in the back of the delivery van doing the GP rounds, before it is eventually delivered to the laboratory. Once in the laboratory the sample should have an auditable trail, so that at any time in the future, its movement through the process of testing can be charted, with dates and individuals identifiable from the time it enters until the time the report is despatched.

Quality is not only about processing the sample well, but it is also about getting the 'right' answer. A laboratory may be technically excellent, but if staff are using an inappropriate or inaccurate method, then the answer will still be wrong, even though they have carried out their test competently. It is here that problems arise in immunology, particularly when immunological tests are carried out in non-specialist laboratories, without input from immunologists, either clinical or scientific. Furthermore, many immunological tests rely on a high degree of interpretative skill from the technical staff, who will read the immunofluorescence tests that form the backbone of autoantibody testing. If this skill is lacking, then inappropriate reports will be issued.

Unlike biochemistry or haematology, where the result is usually a numerical value which is either normal or not normal, with a quoted range, immunological tests may mean different things under different circumstances and expert interpretation is required before the results are despatched to clinicians, who may not understand the results and interpret them incorrectly (although this book is aimed to help!) . This is the prime role of the clinical immunologist. To offer a results-only immunology service is a waste of time and money, as it frequently leads to inappropriate clinical treatment.

It was to address some of these issues that pathologists in the UK set up an accreditation scheme for laboratories. Once this is fully established, it is unlikely that non-accredited laboratories will be permitted to provide services, at least within the NHS, and probably within the private sector also.

Concepts of quality control (QC) in the laboratory

Clinical pathology accreditation (CPA)

CPA has been set up by the professional bodies and is independent. The key components are the Specialist Advisory Committees (SACs) in each laboratory discipline. An extensive set of standards has been laid down, which is amenable to external review. These standards are tough and all laboratories have had to work very hard, even good ones, to achieve these targets. Once the targets have been achieved, the laboratory applies for accreditation by submitting an application form which gives details of the managerial structure and the repertoires of tests carried out, together with other information. This is then passed to the relevant Specialist Advisory Committee who will then appoint inspectors to visit the centre. Normally all disciplines within a laboratory will submit application forms simultaneously and will be inspected at the same time, but this need not be the case. CPA will decide which disciplines need to send inspectors and there will usually be two inspectors, one clinician or scientist and one senior MLSO. In the case where immunological testing is being carried out by another discipline, that relevant Specialist Advisory Committee will forward the application to the Immunology Specialist Advisory Committee for review and a decision on whether immunologists should be sent on the inspection team; however, this does not always happen, which means that immunological testing is frequently not inspected with the degree of rigour that is required to ensure a high-quality service.

On the visit, the inspectors will gather the night before and review all the documentation relating to the laboratories to be visited. This will, if standards are to be met, fill a large box! The inspection will take all day, and the inspectors will inspect every aspect of the laboratory's work, questioning staff at all levels about technical and managerial matters as well as safety. Facilities will be subject to detailed review with regard to suitability. Over lunch they will meet with senior managers of the hospital plus representatives of the users (hospital and GP representatives) who they will question closely concerning the service that the laboratory provides and its relationships with management and users. This is viewed as a particularly important part of the review.

At the end of the day, the inspection team will usually provide some general views about the visit, but will not indicate whether the laboratory has passed or failed. Their report will be submitted for review by the Specialist Advisory Committees of CPA who will issue the final report to the laboratory some 6–8 weeks later. This may be an unconditional full accreditation, conditional accreditation for a fixed period of time (usually a year) subject to specified conditions that must be met within the period, or failure. Conditional accreditation may be subject to early re-inspection if the unsatisfactory standards are deemed to be of a serious nature. Re-inspection takes place every 4 years.

Other organizations, such as the British Standards Institute, offer quality inspection services leading to certificates. These are not specifically designed for hospital services, although some services have undertaken these as well. The disadvantage of the BSI inspections is that they concentrate only on process, not on the product:

you can make a completely useless article perfectly and still get BSI approval—this is not really very helpful in laboratory medicine where the end product is critical to the whole process!

European legislation regarding laboratory accreditation appears to be taking a rather different line, with the emphasis on the precision of assays and therefore laying down regulations about which tests can and cannot be used, while ignoring the importance of obtaining the 'right' rather than just a precise answer. This represents the lack of involvement of medically qualified specialists in laboratory testing in Europe. How this will affect accreditation in the UK remains to be seen.

Quality control—internal

One of the major features of the CPA standards is the requirement to have written documentation of all procedures within the laboratory, which are reviewed at regular intervals. This includes not only the standard operating procedures (SOPs), which are the detailed recipe by which tests are carried out, but all other departmental policies, such as safety, training, induction of staff, in fact everything that the laboratory does. Producing these is a mammoth but essential task that frequently reveals major deficiencies in process. It is essential that SOPs are used, rather than left to gather dust, and it is important to monitor regularly, through good laboratory practice (GLP) reviews, that these are being followed.

The SOP needs to identify the name and purpose of the test, all the reagents used, and then a detailed method, which someone with normal laboratory competence should be able to follow successfully. The SOP should include all the details of the hazards of the reagents, as required by COSSH regulations, and any special precautions. The SOP will indicate how and by whom the test results will be reported and must specify what internal control samples will be run. Run failure criteria will be documented. When carrying out the tests, it is advisable to have a printed worksheet or a workbook which will include the date of the assay, the operator, batch numbers of reagents, the patients' names and laboratory identifiers and results. There should also be a validation step by a senior MLSO or scientist if the operator is a junior MLSO or MLA.

To ensure that the test is carried out correctly it is essential practice that internal QC samples are included in each run or, if this is not possible (e.g. flow cytometry), that run rejection criteria are established. The internal QC will be a sample whose value has been defined by repeated analysis, at least 20 times, followed by calculation of the mean and standard deviation. Thereafter, all values for the internal QC sample will be recorded, which will allow running plots to be produced which give warning of deterioration in assay performance or running bias. There are a number of ways in which these can be plotted. The Shewart chart plots the value of the internal control in absolute values against time, with one and two standard deviations and the mean marked out. The values should be arrayed equally either side of the mean. Usually, action will be taken if more than four points are on the same side of the mean or if two sequential points are beyond 2SD (although this should also result in run rejection). A more complex plot is the Youden chart, where a high and a low standard are used and the plot is the same as for the Shewart plot but in two dimensions. Here one value is plotted with its mean horizontal and the other with its means vertical. Each point represents the value for the high sample plotted against the value for the low sample. The points should be randomly arrayed around the intersection of the means. The third useful plot is the Cusum chart, which plots the difference of the day's result from the calculated mean value (with sign included). This plot will reveal whether the mean has been set correctly and will also reveal changes in accuracy.

In order to ensure that all laboratories are measuring the same thing, it is necessary to have widely agreed reference preparations which have agreed values for a given analyte. For many analytes there are now WHO approved standards. These have defined values in either mass units or internationally agreed units. Most countries have their own collaborating reference laboratories which will produce secondary standards calibrated against the WHO standard, which can be distributed to working laboratories. Manufacturers of analysers and kits will also use these standards to produce calibration reagents or kit controls. Such primary and secondary standards should not be run in routine assays, but used to calibrate internal control samples. Obviously if there is a major problem with an assay, then the original standards should be used to help with troubleshooting. A recent exercise has led to the establishment of a much improved reference preparation for protein chemistry, including immunoglobulins, although this has led to wholesale changes in normal ranges. The provision of standards for autoantibody detection has been much harder, mainly because of the multiplicity of antigens. There are, however, standards for several ANA patterns, for rheumatoid factors, and anti-thyroid antibodies. Where standards are distributed, it is standard practice that they should test negative for hepatitis B and HIV.

Another important facet of internal quality control is the evaluation of reagents. This applies particularly to any fluorescence reagents. The conjugated anti-human immunoglobulin reagents used in direct and indirect immunofluorescence need to be titrated to determine the optimum (and most economical) working dilution. This is done by a chequerboard titration, where serial dilutions of the conjugate are titrated against serial dilutions of a serum of known specificity and titre. Similarly, reagents for use of the flow cytometer should also be titrated against increasing cell numbers. Ideally, this process should be carried out each time a new batch is purchased, particularly with polyclonal antisera.

Immunological tests require a significant amount of interpretation. The major role of the clinicians in the department is to ensure that appropriate interpretation is provided to users, together with guidance to users on test selection. This should involve telephone calls to users when abnormal results are detected that may influence management. This process should be assisted by the production of a laboratory handbook, giving essential information to users. Compliance with the standards in both of these areas is viewed as essential by CPA.

Quality control—external

External quality control is an essential tool for the laboratory manager in ensuring that his laboratory is indeed performing satisfactorily and getting the same answers as other laboratories. Satisfactory participation in external QC is a mandatory standard of CPA accreditation. There are a number of schemes, both within the NHS (UK National External Quality Assurance Scheme, UK NEQAS) and provided by manufacturers. Participating laboratories are assigned a number by which they are identified, so that only they and the scheme organizers know who is who.

An essential element is the distribution of unknown samples at regular intervals. These are run by the standard process for the designated analyte. It is important that the samples are treated in the same way as normal patient samples for the results to be meaningful. Once the returned results have been analysed, participants are sent a summary showing their performance and how it compares with other laboratories. This will often be broken down by method used, which allows laboratories to see whether a method is performing particularly well or badly.

For each sample there will be a designated value (DV). For quantitative analytes (i.e. protein chemistries) this is usually the trimmed mean (i.e. the mean recalculated with outliers excluded), while for qualitative analytes (e.g. ENAs) the designated value is determined by the consensus of a small group of specialist reference laboratories. Performance is assessed by calculating the variance index (VI) from the difference of the obtained value from the designated value corrected by the chosen coefficient of variance (CCV), a scaling factor dependent on the type of assay being used, according to the formula:

$$VI = (xDV)/DV \times 1000/CCV.$$

For the variance index, the sign is ignored, but for the bias index the sign is kept. The variance (VIS) and bias index (BIS) scores are calculated as VIS (or BIS) = VI where VI < 400. If VI > 400 then the maximum score of 400 is applied. For many analytes, these are plotted graphically as running performance scores by using the mean running VIS (MRVIS) or mean running BIS (MRBIS), which are calculated by taking the mean of the last 10 VISs or BISs.

For qualitative reporting, overall performance is judged by scoring 1 point for each misclassification compared to the designated value (misclassification score, MIS). The running performance is looked at by adding the scores of the preceding 10 circulations to give the overall misclassification score (OMIS), which will have a maximum dependent on the maximum number of answers that can be given wrongly. Perfect performance gives a score of zero.

The problem about this type of EQA scheme is in the determination of the 'right' answer. If in a quantitative scheme 90 per cent of the laboratories use a method that gives the 'wrong' answer and 10 per cent use a method that gives a different but correct answer, then the apparent performance of the 10 per cent will appear poor as the mean and SD will be determined largely by the majority. This is difficult to address, although the Department of Health does sponsor methodological evaluations which are published as 'blue book' reports.

There are obvious difficulties in obtaining sufficient material for large distributions and there is reliance on plasmapheresis samples. These samples may behave very differently from serum samples in some assays. An alternative is to pool donations from multiple donors, but this is most undesirable in immunological assays, particularly for autoantibodies, and has mostly been dropped in favour of single-donor pools. Unfortunately scheme organizers do not usually have the resources to troubleshoot problems, and it is left to individual laboratories and manufacturers to chase up unexpected results.

Another difficulty with the NEQAS schemes is the lack of feedback about why the answer was wrong; this is being addressed through regular workshops. Feedback is particularly important in interpretative tests such as immunofluorescence, and here regional QA schemes have a role, as it allows participants to meet regularly and discuss the results and problems. The scheme organizers will only intervene if performance is persistently poor over a long period, and according to pre-determined standards will report failing laboratories to the chairman of the relevant National Quality Assurance Panel (NAQAP). The chairman will then write to the head of the laboratory pointing out the problem and asking what steps are being taken to remedy the problem, as well as offering help (usually a visit from a panel member). Lack of a response or an inappropriate response to this letter will lead to fiercer letters and, if necessary, a report direct to CPA so that the laboratory's accreditation status can be reviewed.

CPA inspectors will also inspect the results from EQA schemes and are keen to see that poor performances are treated seriously and lead to an investigation and rectification of faults in a way that is documented and disseminated to all staff.

Clinical standards and audit

Clinical work has been less amenable to such detailed quality assessment. Clinical audit should, if carried out correctly, assist in improving standards. The audit cycle starts from the definition of a 'standard', which may be set on the basis of existing evidence or empirically. The audit process then reviews clinical care against the standard. The outcome of the audit may lead to changes in practice to achieve the standard or to a revision of the standard, or both. Up until now practitioners have been free to treat in any way they see fit, with the fallback being litigation to keep them on the straight and narrow. The Bolam principle in law has held that a practitioner shall not be held negligent if his practice is that which would be endorsed by a body of his peers. The transfer of indemnity insurance for doctors within the NHS from the Defence Unions to the NHS Trusts has meant that the hospitals are suddenly very interested in clinical standards. Equally, there is pressure from purchasers, via contracting, that clinical practice should be limited to treatments where the benefits are proven (evidence-based medicine). This has led to pressure to develop guidelines or protocols, which are evidence based, which will form the backbone of clinical practice. How this will affect the courts' view of practitioners who deviate for whatever reason from the established guidelines remains to be tested. None the less, guidelines are here to stay and, provided that they are developed by the involved clinicians and regularly updated, they can only serve to improve the quality of clinical practice. The problem for purchasers of healthcare is that 'best practice' may be significantly more expensive, and this will lead to more pressure for rationing.

Audit should also take place in the laboratory, both internal, looking at compliance with CPA standards and internal standards, and external, where the usage of tests is evaluated in collaboration with clinical users. This provides a valuable way of improving users' knowledge of the services that the laboratory can provide.

The government's review of the NHS (1997–98) has placed an even greater emphasis on standards through the proposed formation of a National Institute for Clinical Excellence (NICE) and the Committee for Health Improvement (CHIMP). In the wake of the Bristol affair, clinical governance is now the watchword, with tighter controls on consultant practice and a higher level of accountability. Regular hospital inspections (like CPA, but worse!) and more aggressive approaches to CME and re-accreditation for specialists will follow. There will be a greater emphasis on the use of best-practice guidelines and, as a result, far less freedom of action in terms of managing patients. Whether any of these steps will lead to better medicine, rather than salving the collective consciousness of ministers and civil servants, who are seen 'to be doing something about the bad doctors', remains to be seen.

Health and safety

Hospitals, and particularly laboratories, are subject in most countries to a significant legal framework. In practice this means that the employers are responsible in law for ensuring that this legal framework is implemented. In the UK, a number of organizations have the right to make unannounced inspections to ensure compliance. The Health and Safety Executive has wide powers regarding the workplace, including, as a last resort, the power to close an installation down and to bring prosecutions. Heads of departments can be held accountable directly for breaches. Particularly important are the regulations regarding all chemical and biological materials (COSSH regulations), which require a full safety assessment to be carried out on any substance in use or held in the laboratory, which must be held in a written form and read by all employees using the substances. This information must contain information on dealing with spills. There are commercially available directories from which this information can be obtained and most manufacturers include such information in the packaging.

Strict regulations apply to the use and handling of radioisotopes, in particular the route of disposal and the amount of permitted discharges. Every hospital will have a radiation protection officer, usually a member of the medical physics team, who will provide guidance and monitor local compliance. Breaches of the legislation are viewed seriously and both hospitals and individuals have been prosecuted by HM Inspectorate of Pollution.

The handling of biological high-risk samples is governed by the guidance produced by the Advisory Committee on Dangerous Pathogens. In the guidance, pathogens are graded according to the potential risk to workers, and handling facilities and other precautions are laid down. Those working in laboratories should treat all samples as being potentially high risk and take sensible precautions, i.e. wearing gloves, appropriate laboratory coats (Howie coats, properly buttoned up!), and disposing of samples safely via an autoclave. All staff should be fully immunized, particularly against hepatitis B.

All staff (including doctors), as part of their induction, should read the necessary statutory documentation and also local policies, which need to be fully documented as one of the CPA accreditation standards. The induction should also include regular Fire Safety training (an obligatory requirement). This training should be documented for all staff and is included in the logbooks for trainee clinicians and scientists.

Laboratory and clinical organization

In the UK, recognized and accredited immunology laboratories will usually have a clinician or top-grade scientist as head of department, assisted by a laboratory manager (senior MLSO or scientist). These two will be responsible for the management of the department. The laboratory will usually be part of a Directorate of Laboratory Medicine, with a clinical director (either a clinician or top-grade scientist) who has overall responsibility for the directorate and will usually be a part of the Trust Hospital's higher management structure. Heads of department will usually be responsible for a devolved budget and should be involved in the negotiation of contracts, budget setting, and personnel matters, with appropriate support from Finance and Personnel. CPA expects to see a clear chain of command in the hospital, with evidence of regular meetings and consultation. Within the department, they also expect to see documented evidence of regular staff meetings to discuss operational matters and review QC performance.

Management of staff is a major role and heads of department need to be aware of the employment legislation, particularly in regard to equal opportunities and discrimination. Staff development is important and CPA expects to see some form of performance appraisal for all grades in place. At present, there is no formal scheme of appraisal for consultants, except those in managerial posts (clinical directors), nor is staff appraisal yet related to performance-related pay, although both will come. It is wise to ensure that all staff involved in appraisal receive formal training.

Clinical heads of department will now also be responsible for all types of staff, although usually assisted by a senior nurse. All junior clinical staff will have nominated consultants who are responsible for the supervision of their training. Regular appraisal meetings for junior medical staff are now expected, with reports going to the Regional Postgraduate Dean.

Budget and price setting is a major function of departmental managers. This is usually done as a 'top-down' exercise, which is usually used for clinical services. However, for laboratory work each test needs to be costed accurately ('bottom-up'). This exercise requires accurate information on departmental overheads (space, light, heat, laundry, phones, etc.) which can then be applied to the costs of actually doing the test (consumables, labour, and equipment). The costing of tests is complex. The time and effort taken in doing tests must be calculated; this may be reported in Welcan units, although most laboratories require a modification to this, depending on assay types, and as this system has not been updated it does not accurately reflect current practice. Weightings may be given, depending on the seniority of staff required to perform a test. Where equipment is used, an element of depreciation of the capital cost needs to be included, apportioned across all tests using the machine, together with the costs of maintenance. Many laboratories now prefer not to buy equipment, but to rent it in reagent rental schemes. This has the major advantage that when the equipment is upgraded the laboratory will get the new equipment immediately without the need to argue the case for another capital purchase. Every pricing exercise requires good information on the volume of tests carried out, and when prices have been set, then the recovery needs to be checked. This exercise tests that, on the set prices, all the costs (staff, equipment, overheads and consumables, less any other income from service increment for teaching – SIFT) will be covered on the workload projected. If the workload exceeds the minimum required to cover the fixed costs, then the tests can be marketed at marginal costs (the variable costs associated with the test, i.e. the consumables only). There are ground rules covering what may be included in test prices. NHS laboratories are not permitted to make a profit from services to other NHS units, nor are they permitted to subsidise services to one section, at the expense of another. Thus differential pricing to different NHS users is not permitted, although this is sometimes flouted. However, in dealing with external contract work, laboratories may charge whatever they feel appropriate (i.e. what the market will bear), and a significant profit element may be built in. For testing carried out to support bona fide NHS or academic research, as fixed costs will have been recovered, it is usual to charge at marginal rates.

Contracts can be of three types:

- Block contract, where a fixed sum is agreed for the provision of the service regardless of the volume of work actually done. These contracts may have a review mechanism if the workload deviates wildly from that used to project the initial cost. The monitoring is crude.

- Cost-volume. Such contracts set a baseline price based on a given workload, with agreed additional costs depending on the deviation from the projected total. Additional work is often charged at a reduced rate or marginal cost.

- Cost-per-item. Here the charge is the full cost for each item of service. This is the most desirable for the provider but less desirable for the purchaser, who may get a very large bill if the workload increases substantially, as they have an open-ended commitment. This method also has the heaviest requirement for accurate monitoring.

Research and teaching

Considerable amounts of research and teaching are undertaken in hospitals in the UK. The majority of this is undertaken in the hospitals associated with the medical schools and various specialist postgraduate institutes. The additional costs that these activities incur was recognized many years ago and the hospitals received an enhanced budget, the enhancement being the service increment for teaching and research (SIFTR). There was also a complicated knock-for-knock arrangement whereby NHS staff would teach and university staff would carry out NHS duties. The whole system is now being dismantled at huge effort. The medical schools are now contracting for specific teaching of their undergraduates, not always with the teaching hospitals, and the knock-for-knock arrangements are being unpicked. Subsequent to the Culyer Report on research in the NHS, the 'R' element of SIFTR is being analysed and hospitals are required to contract with the NHS R&D directorate to reclaim the money. These activities have had a seriously destabilizing effect on teaching hospital budgets as the SIFTR components have long been built into baseline budgets. The non-teaching hospitals getting SIFT for the first time are, of course, getting cash windfalls!

Training

Training in immunology in the UK takes place at three levels: clinical, technical (Medical Laboratory Scientific Officers, MLSOs sometimes also known as biomedical scientists, BMSs), and clinical scientists. For doctors wishing to embark on a career in immunology, the training will take 8 years from first qualification. After pre-registration, 2 years of general medicine are required, culminating in the MRCP (UK) or equivalent. The next stage is to obtain a higher specialist training post (specialist registrar). Two years of core training follow, including basic science, clinical practice related to immunology, and laboratory practice, culminating in the Part I examination of the MRCPath, which includes both written papers, practical examination, and an oral examination. Training then divides into two arms: either allergy, usually taken with another medical speciality such as respiratory medicine, or immunology, both of 3 years' duration. For those wishing to take the allergy arm, the MRCPath Part I examination is optional, although the core training will otherwise be similar. After a further 2 years, trainees in immunology will take the MRCPath Part II, which may be in the form of a thesis (this may have been submitted for a Ph.D. or MD), a case book, or submission of a collection of published papers. The trainees will be expected to broaden their clinical and laboratory experience during this period. Up to 1 countable year may be spent in research.

MLSO training can be undertaken in many ways, dependent on previous qualification. For those entering a trainee post with an approved degree in biological sciences, the training is 1 year. However, many obtain their degrees through part-time day release over a longer period (3–4 years). The regulations are laid down by the Council for Professions Supplementary to Medicine (CPSM). At the end of the training period, the trainee undergoes an oral examination by external assessors. If performance is satisfactory, state registration is awarded. Progress up the career scale for MLSOs is dependent on acquisition of further qualifications, either fellowship of the Institute of Biomedical Scientists, or an M.Sc. Appointment above MLSO-2 is unlikely without one of these. In addition some MLSOs obtain specific diplomas in laboratory management.

The training for non-clinical scientists has been defined. Trainees will usually start as Grade A scientists having undertaken a primary degree in a relevant subject at university. However, scientists are often employed directly into higher scales (B and C) who have undertaken their training in academic departments and obtained Ph.D.s. The fact that many MLSOs are graduates has blurred the role of the Grade A scientists, and direct recruitment of Ph.D.s into the higher grades has meant that the career path is insecure. With the improvement of the quality of recruits into the MLSO structure, it is debatable whether two parallel tracks are now desirable.

Private finance and private practice

All NHS consultants are entitled to carry out private practice, the amount being dependent on their contractual commitment to the NHS. Some NHS hospitals are getting more particular about where and for whom such private work is carried out, particularly if there may be a conflict of interest. This is important in the light of government policy, enunciated in their 'Strategic Review of Pathology Services' to 'market test' pathology services, i.e. offer them to private laboratories to run, as working as a consultant to a private laboratory which then tenders for NHS work might well be construed as a significant conflict of interest. There has been significant concern over market testing (back-door privatization of NHS services), particularly with regard to the role of the clinical head of the department, as it has been made clear that consultants will remain hospital employees. They will therefore be responsible for reporting and interpreting results produced by a laboratory owned and run by a private company and over which they have no control in terms of assessing quality standards, appropriate test selection, etc. This back-door privatization will be more widely applied through the requirement that all capital schemes in the NHS above a certain cash limit are required to be put out for private finance. The return on investment that private companies will require makes it highly unlikely that this will result in cheaper NHS services and it may be that the sources of private finance will take over other support services, or even clinical services, so that they can market them directly outside the NHS and increase their profit.

Index

The user is reminded of the list of Abbreviations at the front of this volume.

epidermal antibodies 260–6, 272, 554
epidermolysis bullosa acquisita 266
Epstein–Barr virus infection 106, 118, 122, 229
lymphomatoid granulomatosis 340
rheumatoid-associated nuclear antibodies (RANA) 596
X-linked lymphoproliferative syndrome 34
erythema elevatum diutinum 348
erythema nodosum 348, 362
erythrocyte antibodies 556
exercise, and infections 377
extrinsic allergic alveolitis 186–7
eye disease
autoimmune 268–74
ocular cicatricial pemphigoid 272
retinopathy 274
sympathetic ophthalmitis 272
uveitis 270, 272

factor VIII antibodies (acquired haemophilia) 256
familial hypercatabolism 91
familial Mediterranean fever 366
Fanconi anaemia 84, 130, 298
Felty syndrome *see* rheumatoid arthritis
fetal alcohol syndrome 62
fibromyalgia 368
fibrosing alveolitis 228, 244, 246
finance, and private practice 698
flow cytometry 642
cross-matching 668
fludarabine 435
fluorescein isothiocyanate (FITC) 528
fluorescence reagents, evaluation 685
follicle-stimulating hormone (FSH) 208
food allergy 178–81, 242, 368
food challenge tests 624
food intolerance 179–80
fungal infections 116
fungal precipitins 498

galactosaemia 142
ganglioside antibodies 221, 556

gastric parietal cell antibodies 206, 558
gastrointestinal tract 238–42
gut antibodies 564
post-gastrectomy syndrome (fistulae) 140
see also inflammatory bowel disease
Gaucher disease 132
Gell & Coombs sensitivity reactions 182
genetic studies 13–14
genotyping 670–1
genetic identity 671
PCR 670
RFLP 670
sequence-based typing 670, 671
sequence-specific oligonucleotide probes 670–1
giant-cell arteritis 342
gliadin antibodies (IgG and IgA) 242, 560
glomerular basement membrane antibodies 232, 236, 562
Goodpasture's syndrome 236
glomerulonephritis 232–5, 246, 356
necrotizing crescentic 232
post-streptococcal 234
glucose-6-phosphate dehydrogenase, deficiency 78
glutamate receptor antibodies 218
glutamic acid decarboxylase antibodies 198–9, 202, 217, 564
glycogen storage disease type Ib 90
glycoprotein antibodies, myelin-associated (MAG) 578
goitre, sporadic 196–7
gold 440
gonadal autoimmunity, and infertility 208
Goodpasture (anti-GBM) syndrome 236–7, 562
mimicked 326
graft-versus-host disease (GvHD) 396, 664
graft-versus-leukaemia effect (GvL) 396
granulomatous disease (CGD) 24, 74, 292
granulomatous thyroiditis 195–6
Graves' disease 194–5, 202